U.S.News
& WORLD REPORT

BEST
Hospitals

EXCLUSIVE RANKINGS

The 2017 Edition

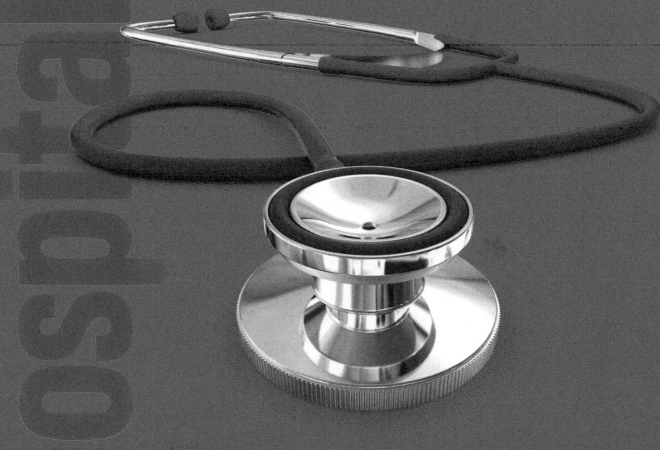

▶ Get Expert Care in Cancer, Cardiology, Neurology, Orthopedics and More

▶ The Best Children's Hospitals

▶ The Top Hospitals in

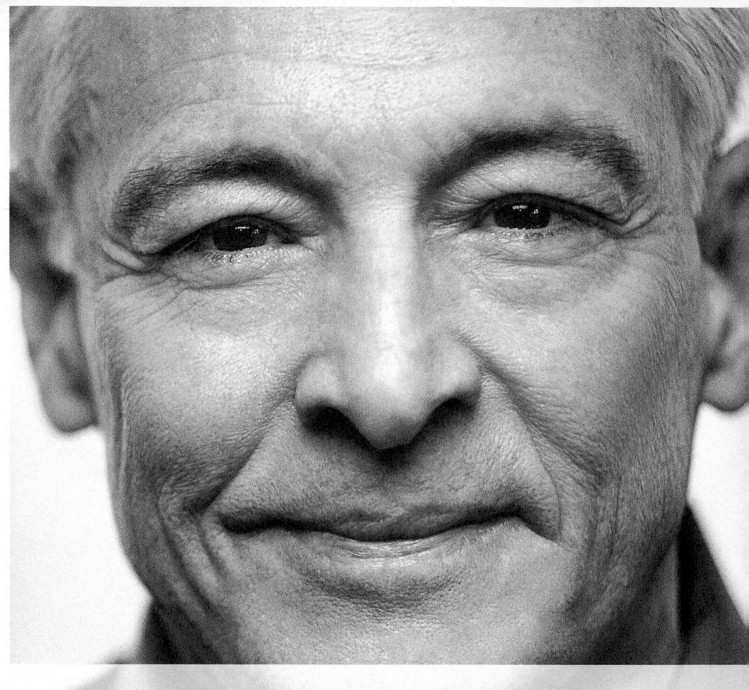

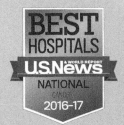

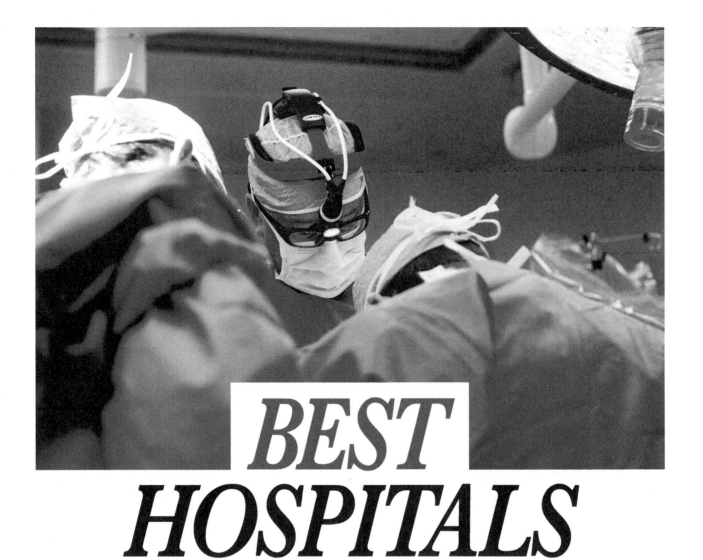

U.S.News & WORLD REPORT

BEST HOSPITALS

2017 EDITION

HOSPITAL FOR SPECIAL SURGERY

BRETT ZIEGLER FOR USN&WR

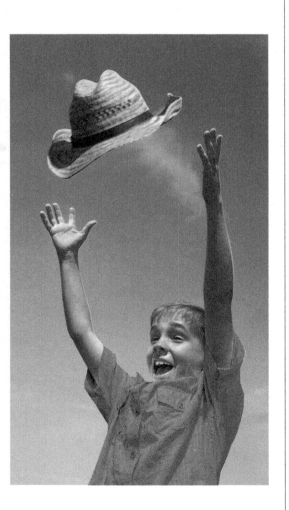

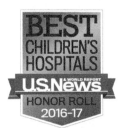

CONTENTS

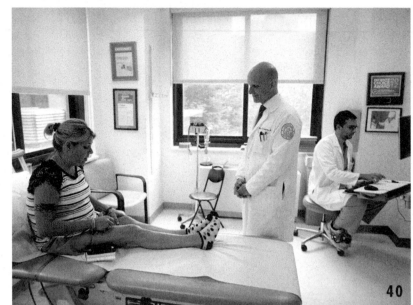

40

CONTENTS CONTINUED ON PAGE 4 ▶

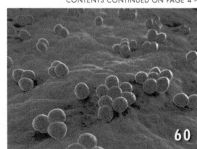

60

FROM TOP: BRETT ZIEGLER FOR USN&WR; GETTY IMAGES
COVERS: GETTY IMAGES (2)

The Lone Star State is known for its independent spirit and pioneering culture. So is Texas Children's Hospital. As one of the top four hospitals in the nation for children's care, we've spent six decades conducting and providing the most innovative research and treatments in pediatric medicine, pushing boundaries and exploring new territory.

Best in Texas.
4th in the U.S.

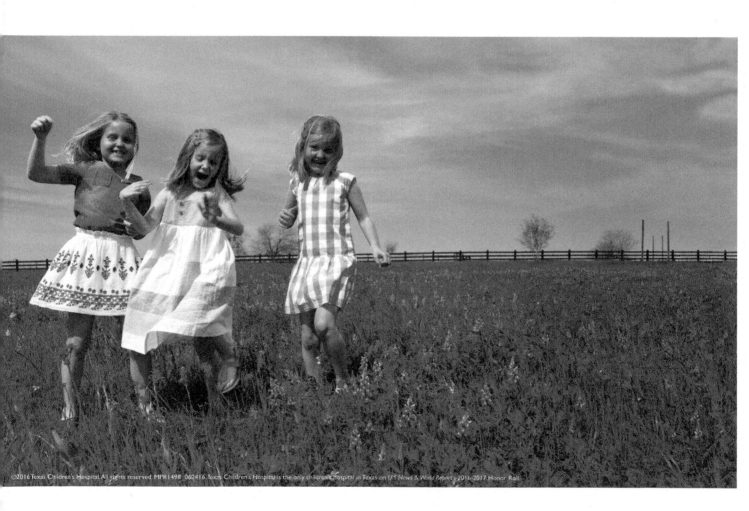

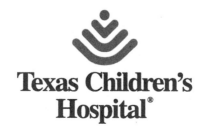

Texas Children's Hospital®

CONTENTS

THE U.S. NEWS RANKINGS

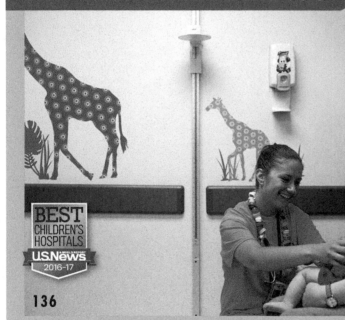

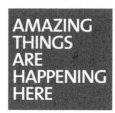

AMAZING
THINGS
ARE
HAPPENING
HERE

NEW YORK'S #1 HOSPITAL.
16 YEARS IN A ROW.

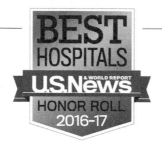

BEST
HOSPITALS
U.S.News & WORLD REPORT
HONOR ROLL
2016-17

Our commitment to patients every day is recognized every year.

Once again, NewYork-Presbyterian has been ranked the #1 hospital in New York and the highest ranked New York hospital in the nation. Thank you to all the doctors, nurses, staff, and volunteers for their expertise and commitment. And, of course, a special thanks to all the patients who put their trust in us each and every day.

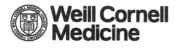
Weill Cornell Medicine

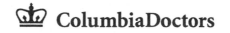
ColumbiaDoctors

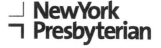
NewYork Presbyterian

@ USNEWS.COM

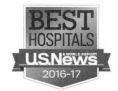

NUTRITION & LIFESTYLE

BEST DIETS

A look at some of the most popular and most researched diets, with reviews by a panel of health experts. Discover the top diets for weight loss, diabetes management and heart health, as well as the best plant-based and commercial diets.
usnews.com/bestdiets

EAT + RUN

Doing what it takes to stay in shape can be tough to manage. Eat + Run serves up expert advice daily.
usnews.com/eat-run

INSURANCE

BEST MEDICARE ADVANTAGE PLANS

State-by-state ratings of Medicare Advantage and Medicare Part D plans, plus tips on choosing one of these plans vs. original Medicare.
usnews.com/medicare

HEALTH INSURANCE GUIDE

We help you select the right coverage for you or your family.
usnews.com/healthinsurance

MEDICAL CARE

HEALTHCARE OF TOMORROW

Health reform, technological innovation and big data are transforming hospitals and care delivery. U.S. News explores how the industry is adapting.
usnews.com/
healthcareoftomorrow

BEST HOSPITALS HONOR ROLL

A VISUAL TOUR OF THE TOP 20

See the best of the Best Hospitals – 20 medical centers that lead the pack in a host of specialties, procedures and conditions, excelling in both breadth and depth of care.
usnews.com/hospitalphototour

BEST HOSPITALS

IN SPECIALTIES, PROCEDURES & CONDITIONS

We've evaluated more than 4,000 hospitals in up to 16 medical specialties, from cancer to urology, and in nine procedures and conditions, including hip replacement, knee replacement, heart bypass surgery, congestive heart failure and COPD.
usnews.com/best-hospitals

SENIOR CARE

BEST NURSING HOMES

We've analyzed government data and published ratings of nearly 16,000 facilities.
usnews.com/nursinghomes

PHARMACIST PICKS

TOP RECOMMENDED HEALTH PRODUCTS

Which over-the-counter products do pharmacists prefer? Check out Top Recommended Health Products.
usnews.com/tophealthproducts

PHYSICIAN SEARCH TOOL

DOCTOR FINDER

A searchable directory of more than 800,000 doctors, created with Doximity, a professional network for physicians. Patients can find and research doctors who have the training, expertise and hospital affiliation they need. With free registration, physicians can expand or update the profile patients see.
usnews.com/doctors

Morristown Medical Center. Top Rated.
Again. Again. Again. Again. Again.

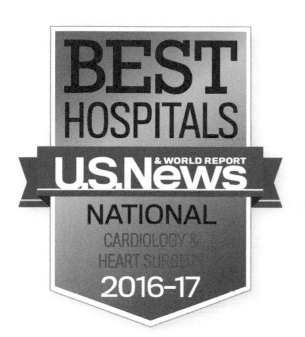

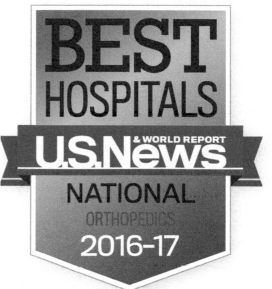

U.S. News & World Report has named Morristown Medical Center a top hospital in the entire country for Cardiology & Heart Surgery FIVE YEARS in a row.

We've also been ranked a top hospital for orthopedics THREE YEARS in a row.

We give our best. You get the best.

Morristown Medical Center, part of Atlantic Health System.

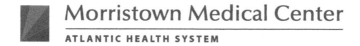

Morristown Medical Center
ATLANTIC HEALTH SYSTEM

AtlanticHealth.org | 888-4AH-DOCS

WE'RE COMING AT CANCER

IN WAYS CANCER

DOESN'T SEE COMING

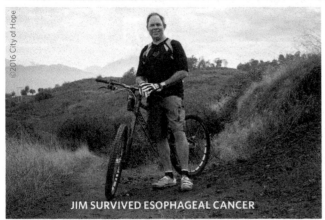

JIM SURVIVED ESOPHAGEAL CANCER

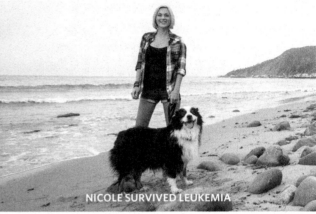

NICOLE SURVIVED LEUKEMIA

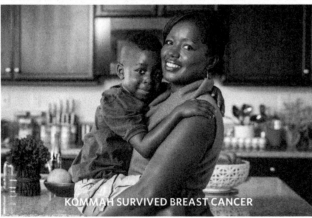

KOMMAH SURVIVED BREAST CANCER

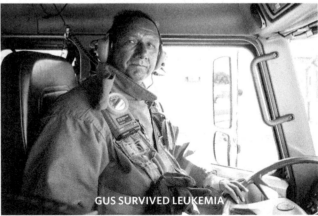

GUS SURVIVED LEUKEMIA

Every day, just northeast of Los Angeles, City of Hope's cancer researchers are pioneering some of the most innovative cancer breakthroughs of our time: from developing the technology behind four of the most widely used cancer medicines to advancing immunotherapy to teach the body's T cells to destroy cancer. Each of our patients is treated as an individual by world-renowned doctors working together as a team. At City of Hope, we combine science with soul to create medical miracles. For more about how we're saving lives as never before, go to **CityofHope.org** or call **800-826-HOPE.**

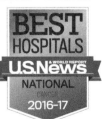

BEST HOSPITALS
U.S.News & WORLD REPORT
NATIONAL
CANCER
2016–17

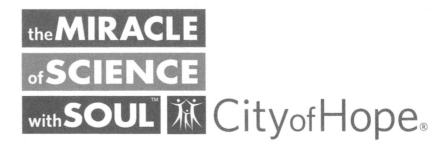

the **MIRACLE** of **SCIENCE** with **SOUL**™ City of Hope®

ON MEDICINE'S FRONT LINES

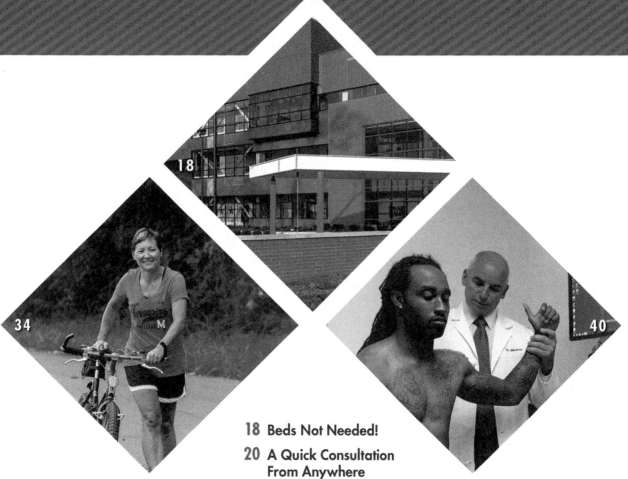

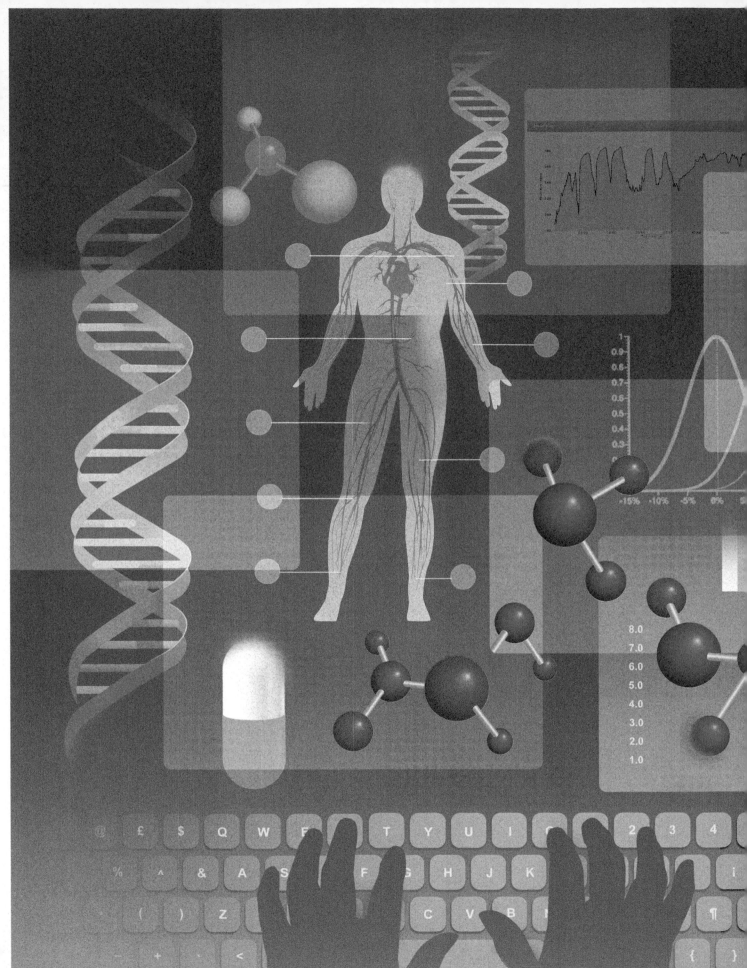

HEALTH CARE
of the
FUTURE

Virtual doctor visits, bedless hospitals, wireless patient oversight from afar. Technology is revolutionizing how, where and when you can receive care, from consulting with a doctor on your iPad for an ear infection to having your vital signs monitored remotely as you're "hospitalized" at home. And the day is coming when a computer crunching billions of pieces of data from patient records, medical literature and your DNA will pinpoint the cancer treatment most apt to save your life. Read on for how these changes will affect you.

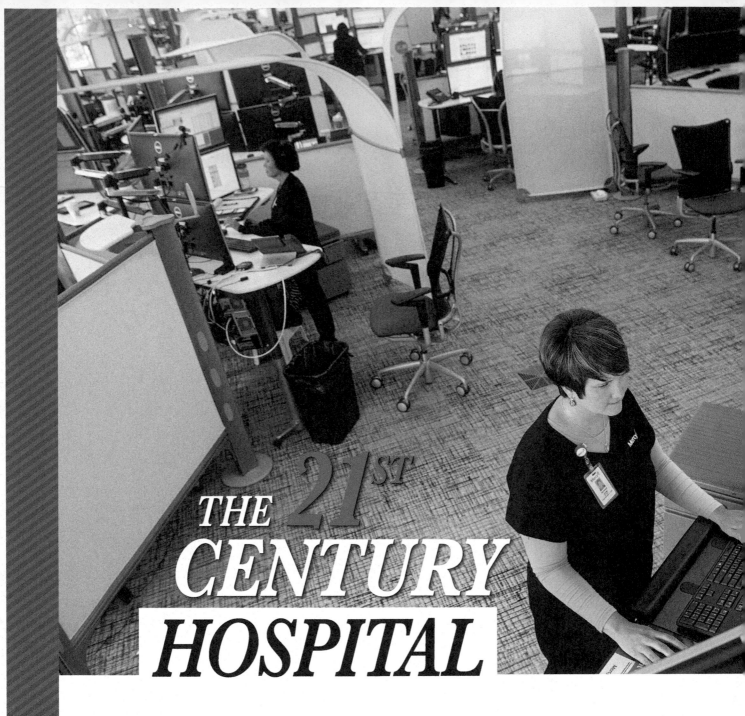

THE 21ST CENTURY HOSPITAL

Are virtual care clinics the wave of the future?

BY BETH HOWARD

James Hoevelmann of Sullivan, Missouri, used to work in hospital construction. But these days, even though he suffers from severe chronic obstructive pulmonary disease, the retired carpenter, 74, doesn't want to go anywhere near a medical facility. And he doesn't need to, even though his COPD has been bad enough in the past to regularly land him in the emergency room and the intensive care unit. The reason: Hoevelmann now gets his care from Mercy Virtual Care Center some 50 miles away in Chesterfield.

Equipped with an iPad and devices such as a blood pressure mon-

itor and scale that stream his vital signs and other data from his home to the Mercy Virtual "command center," he and his providers have been able to detect subtle health shifts in time to avert the cascade of deterioration that put him in the ICU. "We can trend the data on a daily basis and intervene in many cases even before patients experience symptoms," says Gavin Helton, Mercy's medical director. Says Hoevelmann: "I feel safer knowing I have those people behind me."

Hoevelmann and his Mercy team are pioneers in the next big thing in telemedicine, the virtual care clinic, whose physicians,

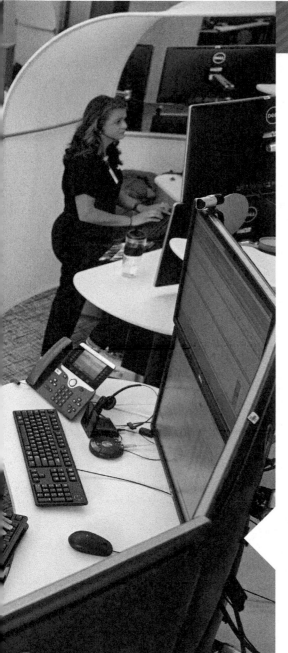

front of monitors and computer displays, watching over the care of patients at 38 hospitals in seven states. In addition to intensivists who observe patients and direct care at distant ICUs, neurologists provide guidance on stroke treatment to community hospitals. A team of virtual hospitalists orders and reads tests, and nurses field questions about everything from nosebleeds to sinus infections. Other clinicians, like Hoevelmann's doctors, stay in near continuous touch with chronically ill patients at home – though these patients may venture to town occasionally for checkups at their doctor's office nearby.

THE CONCEPT IS WORKING. Mortality in the ICU "is trending 40 percent less than predicted," says Randall Moore, Mercy Virtual's president. "By virtually monitoring ICUs 24/7, we're getting to problems earlier." The result, he says, is that Mercy in the past year sent home 1,000 ICU patients who otherwise would have been expected to die and saved $40 million.

While no other institution is demonstrating the promise of this type of care on a similar scale, patients in a growing number of health systems are getting a taste of the virtual clinic experience. Many hospitals, including CHI Health, which runs 14 hospitals serving Nebraska, southwest Iowa and northern Kansas, and

MERCY VIRTUAL'S 300 PROVIDERS GUIDE AND MONITOR THE CARE OF PATIENTS IN 38 HOSPITALS ACROSS SEVEN STATES.

Virginia Mason in Seattle, have partnered with the telehealth company Carena to create what the firm calls 24/7 private-label virtual clinics. Web portals carrying the health system's brand connect patients to primary care doctors in the system or to one of the board-certified family practice doctors or nurse practitioners ("virtualists") on Carena's payroll, who work at a patientless clinic near Seattle. When patients access the portal, they request a visit and can expect to interact with a physician in 30 minutes or less, day or night.

"The next thing you know, you're in a virtual exam room on the screen. The doctor is there and the visit starts," says Carena President and CEO Ralph C. Derrickson. Treatment recommendations rely on evidence-based guidelines, and because care is provided within the health system, the results are integrated into the patient's electronic health record. "It's on demand, like streaming a movie," says Frank Twiehaus, head of strategic business development for virtual care at CHI Health. "We are now bringing care to patients wherever they are."

Thomas Jefferson University in Philadelphia has a similar arrangement with different companies, using only Jefferson physicians to deliver care. Besides primary care, the virtual clinic, called JeffConnect, allows consults in 18 different medical specialties from urology to psychiatry.

"People should be cared for in any way they want," says Judd Hollander, associate dean for strategic health initiatives at Jefferson's Sidney Kimmel Medical College and a professor in the department of emergency medicine. The virtual clinic enabled more than 3,000 doctor-patient interactions in the last year and now averages 20 to 30 a day. Jefferson is able to resolve the health

nurses and therapists provide the bulk of the care from miles away. Virtual care itself isn't new: For a number of years, hospitals have contracted with remote critical care specialists to monitor their ICU patients and have relied on teleconsults with specialists at major academic centers to provide guidance or second opinions. But Mercy Virtual, which opened last fall, takes the concept to a whole other level.

The $54 million, 125,000-square-foot facility has no waiting rooms, hospital beds or patients on site. Instead it houses more than 300 medical professionals who sit in problems for over 85 percent of the patients who connect; others are sent to their own doctors or to the ER.

Jefferson also offers "virtual rounds" to inpatients' family members who can't get to the hospital. Using an iPad equipped with video camera and telehealth software, patients and doctors connect from the hospital room to family members across town or the country.

A first-of-its-kind app being developed at the University of Southern California will add one more level of remoteness: Patients will meet with a lifelike avatar of their doctor. Using virtual reality technology and artificial intelligence, computer scientists at the university are working with Keck Medicine of USC to capture doctors' faces and create avatars that can interact with people and guide them through complex medical decisions. These "virtual doctors," which will have the ability to recognize emotion and show empathy, will have the knowledge base to diagnose problems and provide

MERCY *SENT HOME* **1,000 ICU** PATIENTS *WHO OTHERWISE* WOULD LIKELY HAVE DIED.

information personalized to the patient: the best treatment path for someone diagnosed with prostate cancer, say, based on age, tumor characteristics, and levels of prostate specific antigen, or PSA. Eventually, sensors worn by the patient will also feed data back to the virtual (and actual) doctor to provide a fuller picture of the patient's health.

The app will make it possible to access world-class medical expertise over a smartphone. And while it may sound like an impersonal way to serve patients, an avatar has advantages in that department, too. "Often people will disclose more to a virtual human than a doctor," says Leslie Saxon, a professor of medicine at Keck and executive director of the USC Center for Body Computing. "They don't feel judged." ●

YOUR DIGITAL DATA FILE

In an ideal world, your electronic health record would be a complete trove of your medical data, accessible with a click by all of your doctors and other providers. The risk of treatment errors and of duplicate tests would plunge, and any emergency room physician nationwide could instantly call up your history. All EHR systems would "talk" to each other, so vast numbers of patient records could be tapped to quickly identify which treatments are proving most effective for certain conditions.

Six years after health reform mandated EHRs, the dream has yet to materialize. Some 94 percent of U.S. hospitals do have at least rudimentary EHRs, up from just 9 percent in 2008. But they generally

don't communicate with each other – at least not yet.

Still, there are encouraging signs of change. EHR tech companies are working with the medical community to do a better job of connecting systems. "It's mind-bogglingly complicated," says Margo Edmunds, vice president for evidence generation and translation at AcademyHealth, a national health research organization. It hasn't helped that "the IT industry doesn't know much about health care and vice versa."

Many patients now log into portals where they "can look at X-rays, refill prescriptions, make appointments and email the doctor," says Robert Wachter, author of "The Digital Doctor." Patients at Weill

Cornell Medicine in New York, for example, can track their blood test results, cholesterol and blood sugar levels. Orthopedic patients at the University of Rochester Medical Center get iPads at check-in to answer questions about their pain, activity levels, sleep and mood. The data is transferred to their EHR, where it can be compared to their previous scores and to how other people are faring on the same treatment.

Indeed, the EHR dreams are getting even loftier. Wachter foresees that doctors will be able to verbally record information and that the data will suggest diagnoses, tests and treatments. Future EHRs might also constantly comb the patient's database to assess his or her risk of infections or falls before they happen. –B.H.

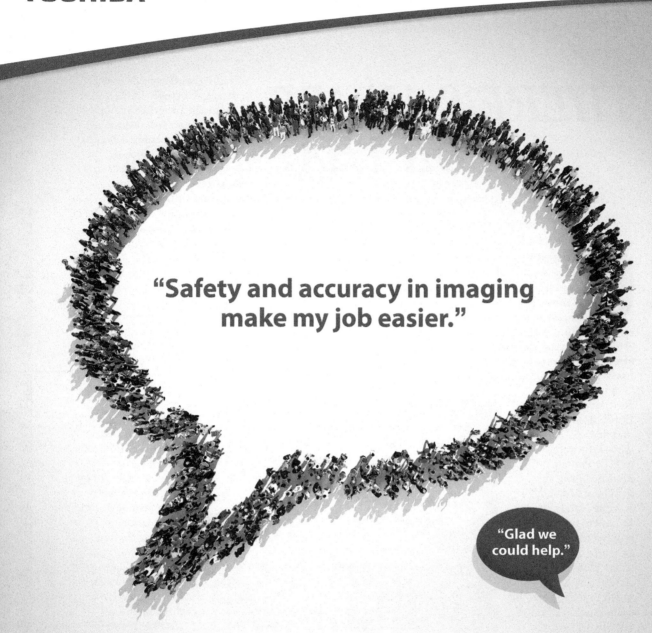

TOSHIBA

"Safety and accuracy in imaging make my job easier."

"Glad we could help."

When your imaging partner is all talk, talk to one who listens. At Toshiba we hear you out first, then create solutions working closely with you.

We build richly featured, worry-free solutions for hospitals across America. Our systems let clinicians focus on what matters most: providing the best imaging experience.

When you're ready for a solution that fits, Toshiba is here to listen. Share #YourVoice.

Toshiba gives you a voice. What's yours?

COMPUTED TOMOGRAPHY

MAGNETIC RESONANCE

PET/CT

ULTRASOUND

VASCULAR X-RAY

X-RAY

medical.toshiba.com

THERE'S AN APP
FOR THAT

Patients will increasingly manage their ills themselves

Cardiologist Eric Topol, a professor at the Scripps Research Institute in San Diego, knew that medicine had reached a turning point when a patient sent him a screen shot of the electrocardiogram he'd run on himself with a smartphone app. "I'm in afib," his text read, referring to atrial fibrillation. "Now what do I do?" As Topol, who is the author of "The Patient Will See You Now: The Future of Medicine is in Your Hands," sees it, patients are rapidly gaining the power to generate and interpret many kinds of medical data and will become much more engaged in managing their health. Ideally, he says, the shift "will lead to much better outcomes."

INDEED, THE MORE THAN 165,000 health-related apps now available for download go well beyond counting steps, guiding meditations and otherwise promoting wellness. There are now apps that, alone or paired with another device or sensors, take blood pressure readings and monitor blood glucose levels, for example. With the Dexcom G5 app, patients place a sensor

just under the skin to take continuous glucose readings that are transmitted to and graphed on a phone, all without drawing blood. And using AliveCor's Kardia app, patients can touch sensors attached to their smartphones to make sure their heart is in rhythm. Data can often be

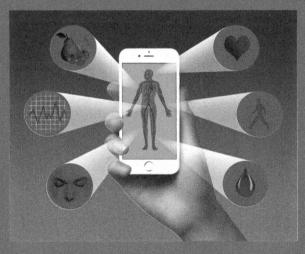

sent to a provider or uploaded into the patient's electronic health record for review.

And that's just the beginning, according to Iltifat Husain, assistant professor of emergency medicine at Wake Forest School of Medicine in North Carolina and founder of iMedicalApps, which reviews new entries for doctors and patients. Now being tested are apps that allow people with Parkinson's disease to

measure their finger dexterity and record changes in their gait to gauge the progression of their disease or their response to a drug. Others are being designed to diagnose sleep apnea by interpreting breathing patterns and to detect postpartum depression by tracking how often new mothers text or talk with friends and how far they travel each day, measures of social isolation.

This revolution couldn't come at a better time, experts say, given a growing shortage of primary care providers and health reform's emphasis on prevention and improved outcomes. Not only does shifting responsibility to the patient reduce the burden on providers, but also it helps patients stay on top of their symptoms. "Hundreds of people have avoided an ER visit by being able to record and get an algorithmic interpretation of their heart rhythm," Topol says.

Doctors will get help prescribing disease management technology from firms like iPrescribeApps, a service that iMedicalApps is rolling out later this year. The program curates apps aimed at conditions from asthma to diabetes to obesity that have been shown in trials to be effective; doctors can quickly choose and prescribe one to a patient, who then receives instructions. "We need to give ownership of health back to patients," Husain argues. Technology is showing the way. –B.H.

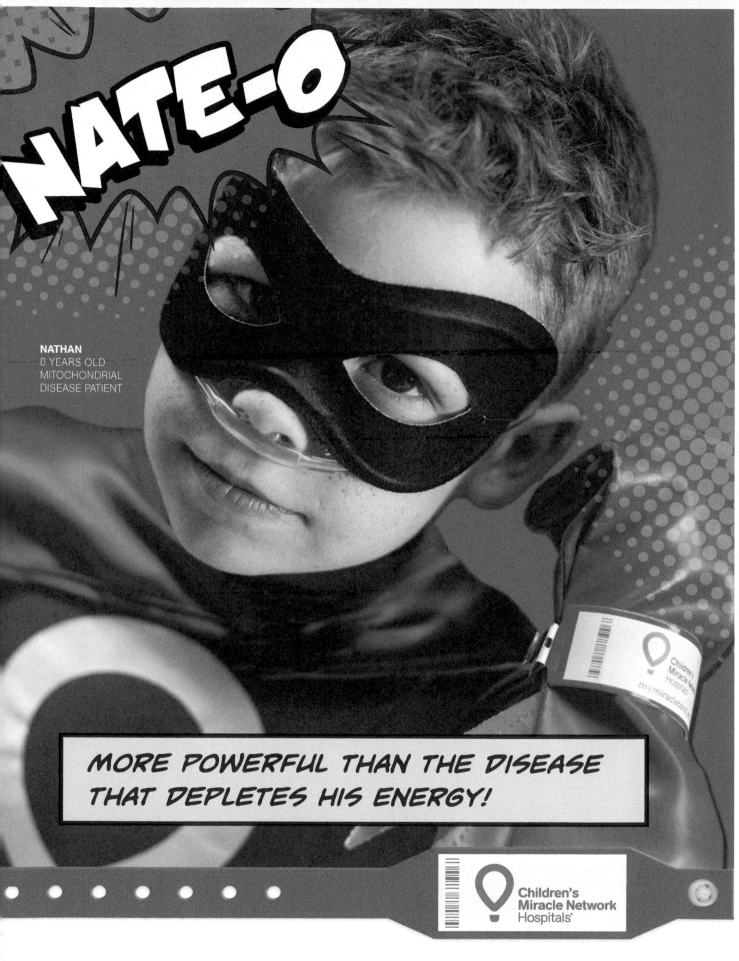

NO BEDS NEEDED

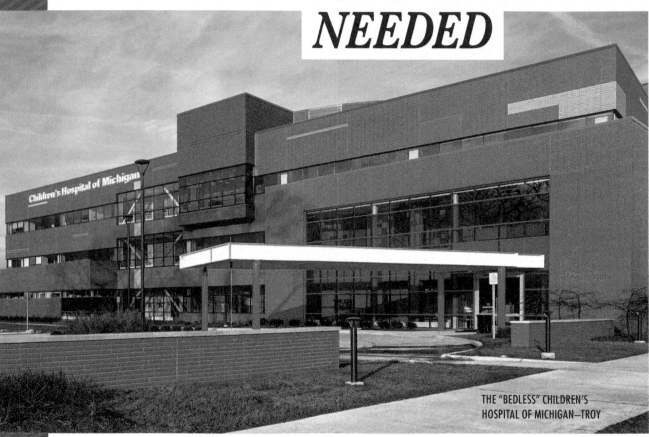

THE "BEDLESS" CHILDREN'S HOSPITAL OF MICHIGAN—TROY

New ambulatory care centers aim to improve the patient experience

People needing surgery at Memorial Sloan Kettering Cancer Center may no longer have to submit to the whole hospital routine. Those coming in for a mastectomy or breast reconstruction, a prostatectomy or a cervical biopsy, for example, may now head instead to the gleaming new Josie Robertson Surgery Center nearby for a same-day release or at most a one-night stay. Rather than wait to check in, they'll wear a radio frequency badge to track their movements, allowing staffers to come to them as they wander to a sitting area or snack bar. During surgery, family members can check status boards to see when a procedure is

underway and when the patient moves to a private recovery room. Often, patients meet with their surgeon via videoconferencing before discharge. "The whole place is focused on not being sick, but on getting better," says Brett Simon, an anesthesiologist and the center's director.

Josie Robertson is one of a slew of state-of-the-art ambulatory centers being opened by health systems to reduce costs and hospitalizations while also drumming up business. The aim is "a high-end patient experience," says Rudolph P. Valentini, chief medical officer at Children's Hospital of Michigan, of the striking new pediatric center in Troy that opened in February. These centers are all equipped to handle an emergency, and patients can quickly be moved to the inpatient hospital if necessary.

Instead of cooling their heels in the waiting room, families arriving at the bright primary-colored center

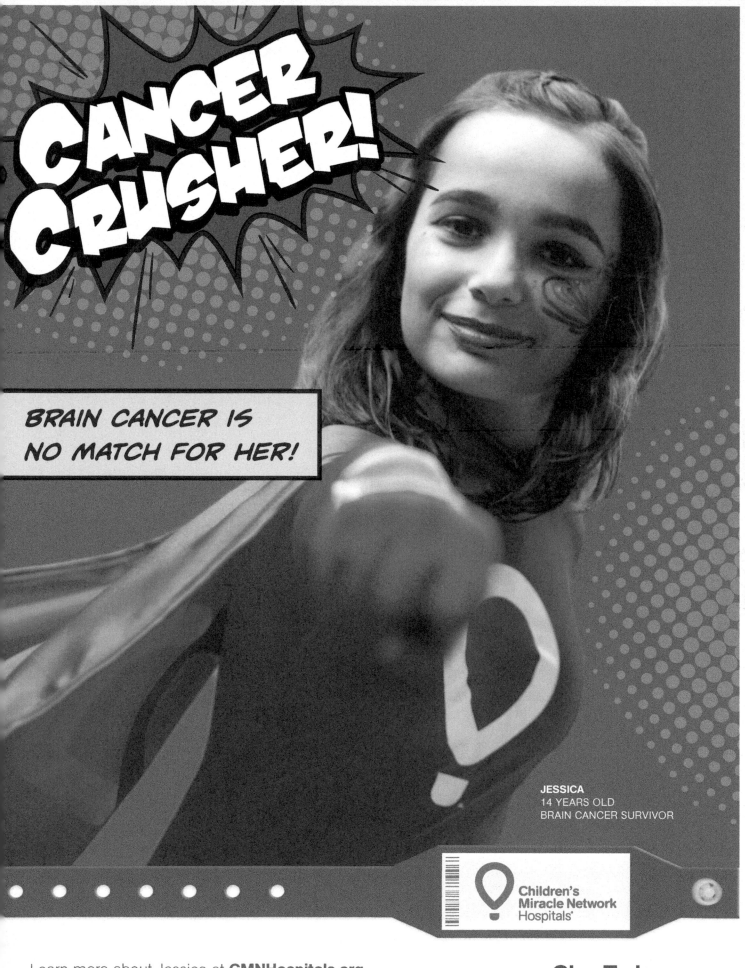

in Troy move directly to an exam room, where the provider meets them. The cheery hospital has just about everything you'd expect – a pediatric emergency room, rehabilitation facilities, a laboratory, imaging capabilities and a pharmacy. The only thing missing: inpatient beds. Radiology services are next to the trauma rooms, so injured kids don't have to travel to get an X-ray. Kids needing to lie still for an MRI can put on movie goggles and watch a show.

PATIENT COMFORT AND CONVENIENCE are also a major focus at the 500,000-square-foot Naval Hospital Camp Pendleton in California, which opened in 2013. Featuring green roofs, gardens, and a private meditation space with ocean views, the facility "bears very little resemblance to military medical facilities of the past," says Lieutenant Commander Stephen Padhi of the U.S. Navy's Civil Engineer Corps. The hospital has 96 procedure rooms as well as labor and delivery and exam rooms, allowing everything from immunizations to colonoscopies. The facility does have some beds just in case, but patients who need true inpatient care rely on the nearby Naval Medical Center San Diego.

Montefiore Health System's new ambulatory center in the Bronx, Montefiore Hutchinson Campus, performs 15,000 outpatient operations each month while also offering laboratory and imaging services, a pharmacy and doctors' offices. By focusing on relatively simple, routine surgeries, the 11-story facility doesn't have to worry about "long complex cases where anything can happen and throw a monkey wrench into the schedule," says Susan Solometo, vice president of clinical services. That allows the center to accommodate more patients. "Pulling ambulatory services out of the acute care facility is allowing us to grow the practice," she says.

Like the amenities at other new ambulatory centers, the center's valet parking, hotel-like ambience and breathtaking views of Long Island Sound play an undeniable marketing role. But they also serve another purpose: to convey that "patients aren't really sick," Solometo says. "They just need a procedure," and then they're headed home. –*B.H.*

DOCTORING
AT A DISTANCE

Get your checkup by phone or video

When 11-month-old Jack Causa's eyes became red and developed a yellow discharge last winter, his mother Izzy immediately recognized the problem: pinkeye. Because the pediatrician's office was closed, she used a service called Teladoc, provided through her health benefits, to reach a physician on her smartphone. A moment of consulting by video allowed the doctor to look at the baby's eyes and confirm

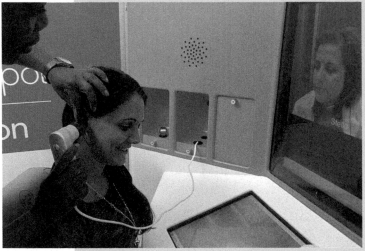

GETTING A REMOTE EAR CHECK IN A PALM BEACH COUNTY SCHOOL DISTRICT KIOSK

the diagnosis. "In less than 20 minutes, I had a consult with a doctor and an eyedrop prescription was sent to our pharmacy," says the 31-year-old Reston, Virginia, mom.

Teladoc is one of several services, including MDLIVE, American Well, and Doctor on Demand, offering secure access to a doctor anytime, anywhere to anyone with a smartphone or tablet. This year Americans are expected to rack up about 1.25 million phone and video interactions, primarily to address nonurgent matters such as sore throat, rashes, sinusitis,

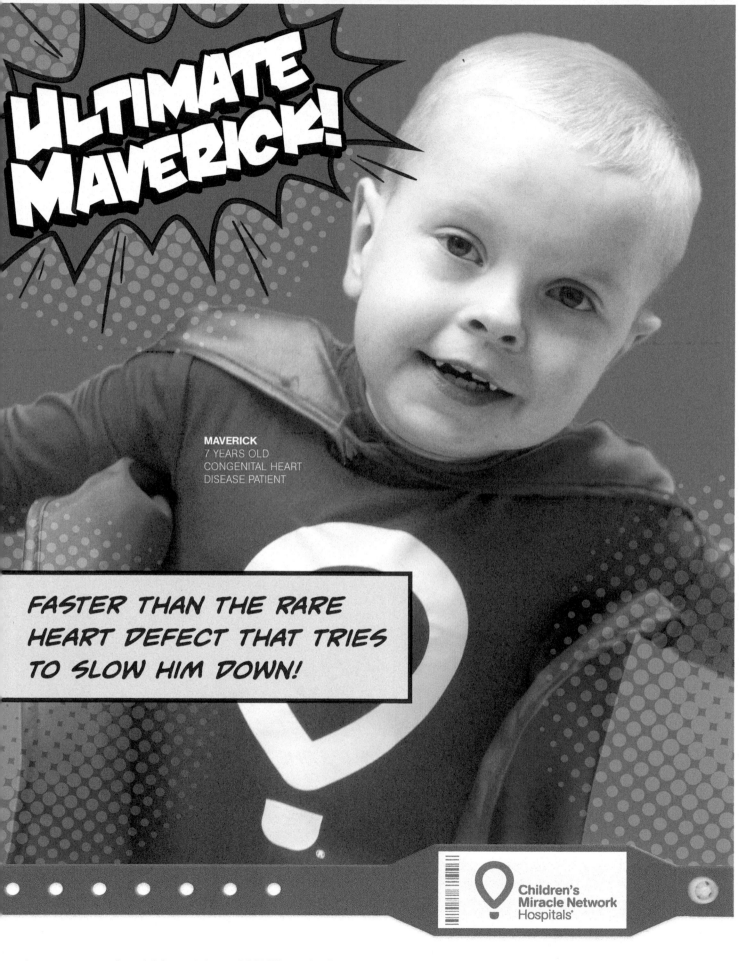

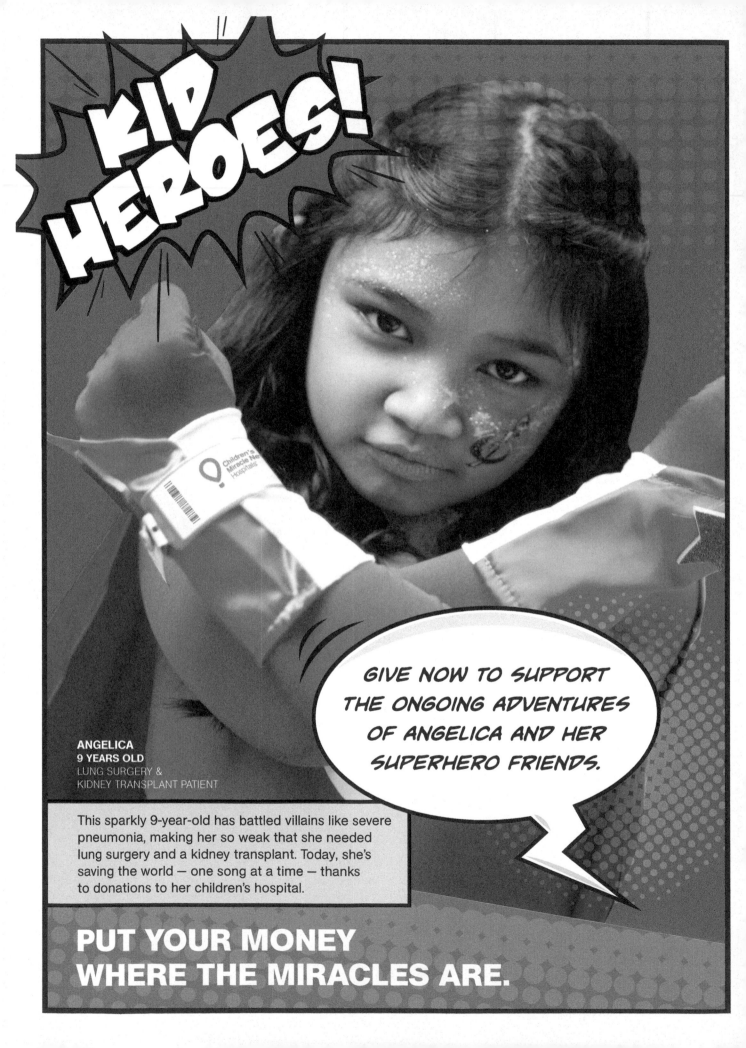

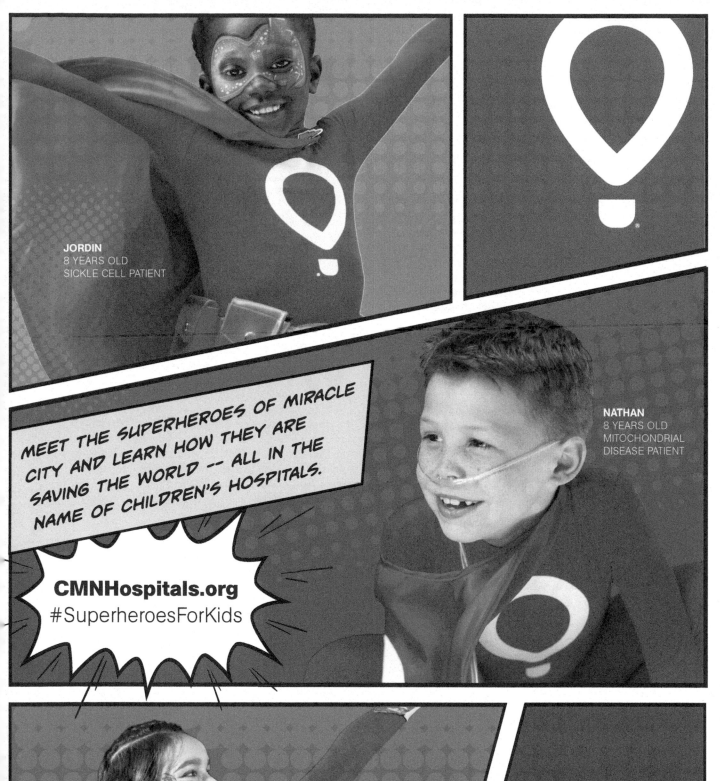
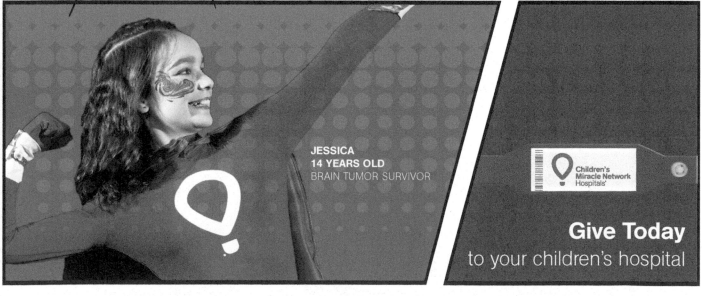

YOUR HOME, THE HOSPITAL

Get set for the modern house call

bronchitis and ear infections. Other patients will consult with a provider remotely from a kiosk in a pharmacy or at their job site, for example, outfitted with blood pressure cuffs and other devices to measure body functions.

THE DRIVING FORCE BEHIND these e-health encounters: "Convenience, convenience, convenience," says Ateev Mehrotra, an associate professor of health care policy and medicine at Harvard Medical School and a hospitalist at Beth Israel Deaconess Medical Center in Boston. Patients also like the price: Most phone consults cost $40 to $50, paid with a credit card. (Employers providing the service may pay a monthly per-member fee.) "The fact that they know ahead of time the actual cost is a big plus," he says. "You can't get that information from your own doctor." And "think how many emergency room visits can be avoided," notes Ranya Habash, chief medical officer for Everbridge, a company that makes technology that enables doctor-patient communications compliant with privacy regulations. Moreover, these services show promise for reaching underserved groups. "If you're on Medicaid, try getting a dermatologist to see you," Mehrotra says.

But there are concerns. Research suggests that doctors delivering telemedicine are more likely to prescribe broad-spectrum antibiotics rather than one targeting a specific bug. That is worrisome, since it could contribute to the growing problem of antibiotic resistance. Other data reveal a related trend of undertesting for conditions like urinary tract infections and strep throat, which could result in using antibiotics needlessly. And as any doctor will say, some information about a patient can only be gleaned through a hands-on physical.

Whether the option saves the patient and the system money, an oft-touted perk, is also up for debate, since it's not yet clear that such visits replace in-person appointments. "They may just increase utilization of health services," Mehrotra says. In either case, the trend seems bound to grow. "People are voting with their feet," he says. "This sector of medicine is only going to get bigger." –B.H.

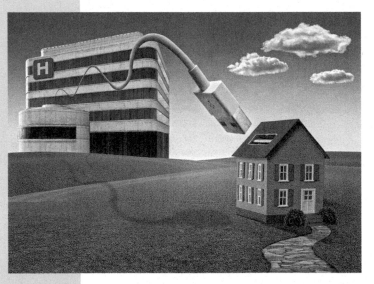

When Tiana Thomas went to the Mount Sinai emergency room last winter with an infection in her transplanted right kidney, she expected to be admitted to the Manhattan hospital for a round of high-potency intravenous antibiotics. But she was worried. "The guy next to me in the ER was hacking like he had the flu," says Thomas, 30, a resident and community services manager for the Workforce Housing Group in New York. And she feared being exposed to far more menacing threats on the hospital ward. The immunosuppressant medication she takes to keep her body from rejecting the organ makes her vulnerable to infection.

To her relief, Thomas was sent back to her apartment. Over the next 10 days, while she prepared her own meals and worked from home, nurses dropped by to administer the antibiotic infusion

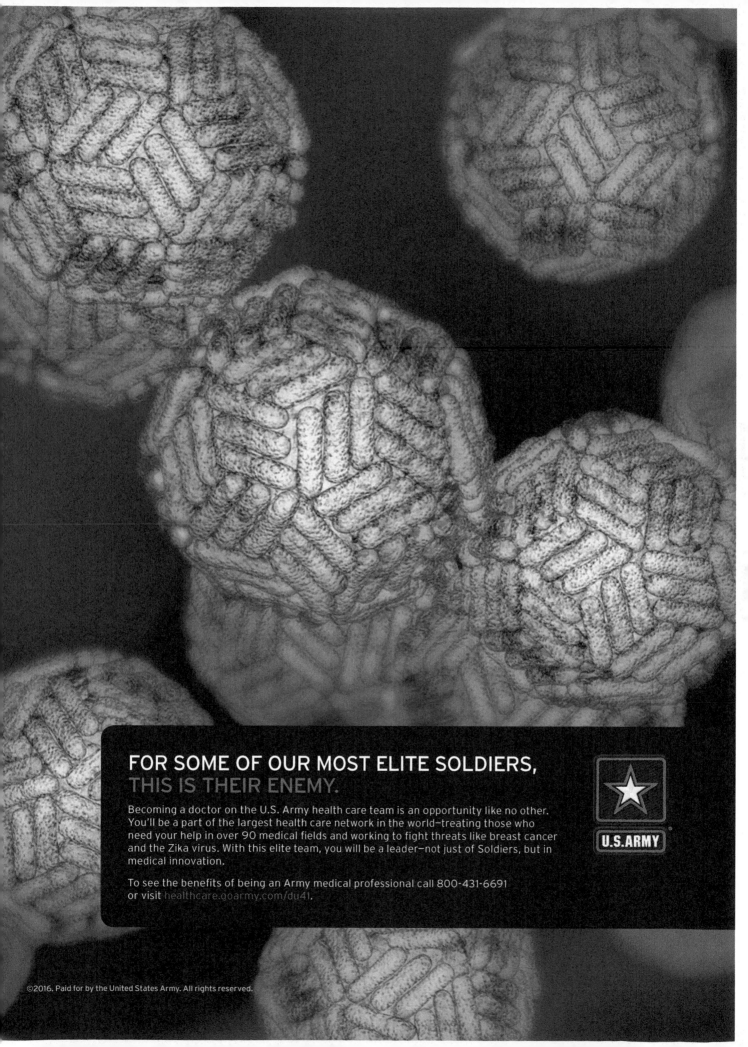

FOR SOME OF OUR MOST ELITE SOLDIERS,
THIS IS THEIR ENEMY.

Becoming a doctor on the U.S. Army health care team is an opportunity like no other. You'll be a part of the largest health care network in the world—treating those who need your help in over 90 medical fields and working to fight threats like breast cancer and the Zika virus. With this elite team, you will be a leader—not just of Soldiers, but in medical innovation.

To see the benefits of being an Army medical professional call 800-431-6691 or visit healthcare.goarmy.com/du41.

U.S.ARMY

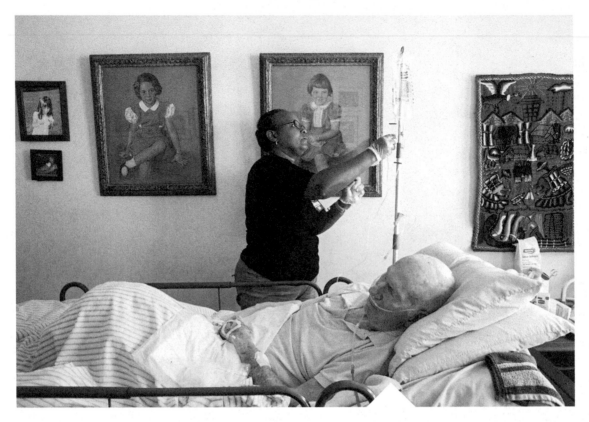

and check her vital signs, and a doctor visited via video. She was "discharged" having never left home. "No one should be in the hospital who doesn't have to be," she says.

That's the underlying philosophy of Hospital at Home, a novel health delivery model that is being tested at Mount Sinai and hospitals around the country. Conceived by Bruce Leff, director of the Center for Transformative Geriatric Research at Johns Hopkins University School of Medicine, the program aims to reduce costs while avoiding the discomforts, falls, infections, deconditioning and delirium that often accompany a hospital stay, particularly among older adults. "The hospital can be a very difficult and dangerous environment for old and frail people," Leff says. "One

of the most challenging decisions we make is whether to send a patient to the hospital when there's a significant likelihood that they will suffer" from being there.

A multitude of enabling technologies – such as videoconferencing and sensors that feed data on blood oxygen levels, blood pressure and other vitals back to providers – will over time make these modern-day house calls even more attractive. New penalties for hospital readmissions will help, too. The setup benefits both older patients needing care for chronic conditions and younger ones getting post-surgery rehab.

A SIMILAR PILOT PROGRAM called Independence at Home allows Medicare patients to get their primary care in house calls; partic-

MOUNT SINAI NURSE LINDA CHENET TAKES CARE OF JULES TEWLOW IN HIS OWN HOME.

ipants include Boston Medical Center, Virginia Commonwealth University Medical Center in Richmond, and the University of Pennsylvania Health System. Bringing the doctor or nurse practitioner to the patient allows better management of complex issues, experts say, and can head off hospital care or a move to the nursing home. A plus of both programs is that providers get a window into patients' lives and factors like housing, family situation and socio-economic status, all of which affect well-being.

Although some patients need the monitoring that only a hospital can provide, research shows that patients with certain conditions – heart failure, some types of pneumonia, flare-ups of chronic obstructive pulmo-

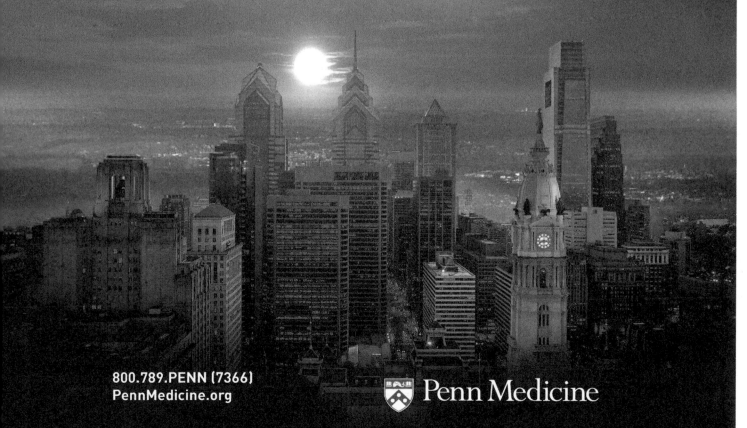
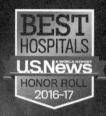

nary disease, and stubborn bacterial skin infections known as cellulitis – do as well or even better outside the hospital than patients inside. Hospital at Home patients cost less to treat and recover more quickly. Moreover, in the familiar environs of home, they are less likely to experience disorientation and delirium, Leff says.

And patients are sold. "Ninety-five percent of eligible patients pick the option," says Karrie Decker, administrator of Presbyterian Healthcare at Home, a program of Presbyterian Healthcare Service in Albuquerque, New Mexico, that launched 11 years ago. Over the past 10 years, Presbyterian has avoided 2,000 admissions and saved over $4 million thanks to the hospital at home program. A recent Centers for Medicare and Medicaid Services study found that the Independence at Home service saved over $25 million at the 17 sites where it was being tried in 2015.

THE VETERANS HEALTH ADMINISTRATION has seen similarly positive outcomes with its 15-year-old Hospital at Home Program, says David J. Shulkin, the VA's undersecretary for health. And other perks have emerged. Hospital at Home proved particularly useful in New Orleans after Hurricane Katrina closed the VA hospital, says Kenneth Shay, director of the Veterans Health Administration's geriatrics programs, who helped implement the program at a handful of VA hospitals. And home-based care lends itself to patients with spinal cord injuries, the focus of the program in Tampa, since wound care and complications like urinary tract infections and pneumonia can often be easily treated at home.

In integrated provider/payer systems like the VA and Presbyterian, care at home is covered; CMS is funding it in the pilot programs. But a way is needed for hospitals to bill for the unconventional delivery in a fee-for-service system. Still, it seems just a matter of time before a solution is found. "When an individual with multiple medical issues is confined to a hospital bed, it takes very little time to slide down in function," Decker says. "It's a slippery slope. Being able to get up to get a glass of water or prepare a simple meal at home can make all the difference." –B.H.

THE POWER OF
BIG DATA

How computer analytics is offering medicine better answers

BY ARLENE WEINTRAUB

In an era of genomics and big data, medicine is getting to be as much about computer analytics as it is about listening to patients' complaints and asking them to say "ah." Imagine a day when your oncologist can sequence your genes and pinpoint the treatment most likely to save your life based on your genetic makeup – in minutes, with just a few clicks. That's the goal of Watson for Genomics, a technology launched by IBM in 2014 to capitalize on the data processing power of Watson, the computer that famously won "Jeopardy!" in 2011 (and whose $77,147 in prize winnings went to charity).

More than 20 cancer centers are now collaborating with IBM to collect DNA data from patients and then use a new cloud-based software program based on Watson's wisdom to personalize treatment plans for patients battling lymphoma, melanoma, ovarian cancer and many other tumor types. The computer processes all sorts of data from patient records to doctor's notes and millions of pages of medical literature – at a rate of 800 million pages per second – and learns the material as it goes. It then produces information about potential treatments based on individual patients' DNA profiles.

at simplifying what has been a cumbersome and time-consuming process. In cancer, for example, it's now possible to analyze and test up to 500 genes for inherited cancer risks and other mutations that may guide treatment choices, says Jennifer Klemp, director of cancer survivorship at the University of Kansas Medical Center, one

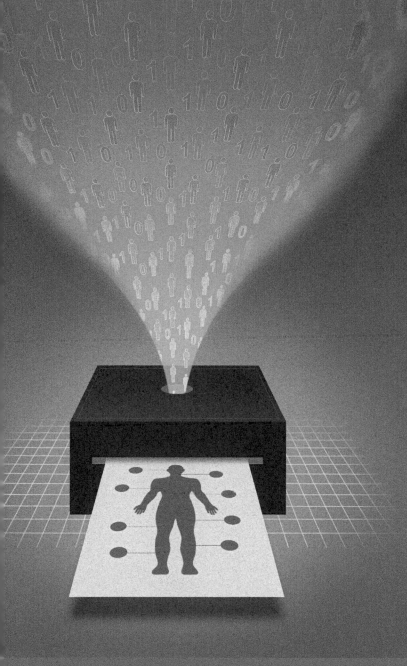

into for insights on the molecular makeup of many cancer types.

IBM has been expanding Watson's role in oncology. In 2012, the company teamed up with Memorial Sloan Kettering Cancer Center in New York to develop software that suggests treatment regimens based on scientific evidence and the prior experiences of other MSK patients. That product is now being rolled out to other cancer centers. And in April, the American Cancer Society teamed up with IBM to work on deploying Watson as a navigator for individual patients, providing tips on how best to manage their care given their particular diagnosis and the information they feed back to Watson about their race, income, location and other factors.
                                    in low-income areas tend not to adhere to their drug regimens, for example, says Richard Wender, chief cancer control officer at the American Cancer Society. With Watson's help, "we'll be able to identify features that put people at high risk," he says, and from the moment of diagnosis offer them guidance that has been useful to similar patients in the past. IBM has also formed a partnership with the U.S. Department of Veterans Affairs, which will tap Watson to provide personalized care to 10,000 veterans with cancer.

It's not just oncologists and cancer patients who stand to benefit from big data. Watson is also being tapped to create apps to assist people recovering from joint surgery and tools that patients can use to control their diabetes, for example. In January, IBM and medical device-maker Medtronic debuted a smartphone app prototype that can flag impending trouble for people with diabetes up to three hours before the patients themselves would realize that something is wrong. By analyzing data from 10,000 people who use Medtronic's insulin pumps and glucose monitors, Watson figured out how to predict a dangerously low blood glucose level in plenty of time to help prevent it. The app will roll out later this year. ●

of IBM's partners. "The problem is, what do we do with the information? Figuring out how to apply it can be overwhelming for providers," she says. Several companies are developing tools that can come to physicians' aid in improving the prognosis for each patient. Besides IBM, the players include Craig Venter, one of the first scientists to sequence the human genome, whose San Diego-based firm Human Longevity is partnering with pharmaceutical companies to look for links between genes and several diseases.

And in June, Vice President Joe Biden, who is heading up President Barack Obama's cancer "moonshot" initiative, announced that the National Cancer Institute would launch an open-access database containing anonymous genomic and clinical data from 12,000 patients that any scientist or doctor can tap

A NEW WEAPON AGAINST CANCER

Researchers are arming patients' immune cells to fight their disease

BY ARLENE WEINTRAUB

When Karen Koehler was diagnosed with chronic lymphocytic leukemia in 2011, she was told not to worry. She had a mild case that could simply be monitored, her doctor said. But two years later, the cancer took a turn for the worse when a genetic mutation made it aggressive and difficult to treat with chemotherapy. "I was told I had 10 months to live," says Koehler, 59, a retired teacher who lives in Park Ridge, New Jersey. At best, she was told, chemo might stretch that to two years.

Then Koehler was accepted into a clinical trial at Memorial Sloan Kettering Cancer Center in New York that aimed to turn her own immune cells into cancer killers. Within a month of treatment, her leukemia had vanished. "There were no cancer cells whatsoever," says Koehler, who remains cancer-free today.

The MSK oncologists whose research has helped Koehler are working on the latest entry in the booming arena of cancer immunotherapy. The potential of boosting the immune system's natural ability to fight off cancer was first realized with so-called checkpoint inhibitors, promising new drugs like Keytruda and Yervoy whose job is to block proteins that normally suppress immune function. These medicines are now being used to turn melanoma and lung cancer, once almost certainly terminal prognoses, into diseases that some patients can manage over the long term.

The newer therapy, dubbed CAR T for "chimeric antigen receptor T cell," is the next generation of immunotherapy: personalized one-time infusions of cells that destroy cancer and theoretically work in perpetuity to prevent it from coming back. In addition to the trials in blood cancers, these T cells "are being explored in ovarian, pancreatic, lung and brain cancer trials," says Jae Park, Koehler's oncologist at MSK. "There is definitely great potential here."

Working with biotechnology companies, doctors are creating the individually tailored treatments by removing T cells from patients' immune systems, engineering them to recognize and attack the patient's own particular cancer, expanding the population of the cells in a lab, then infusing them back into the body. The technology was designed to solve a fundamental problem: Because cancer involves a collection of normal cells growing out of control, the immune system doesn't recognize it as a foreign invader.

AFTER KOEHLER'S DOCTORS harvested T cells from her blood in late 2014, the cells were altered to recognize a protein called CD19 that resides on the surface of blood cells that malfunction in chronic lymphocytic leukemia. These CAR Ts would thus be equipped to home in on the blood cells, known as B cells, and eliminate them. Koehler returned to Sloan Kettering in early 2015 to have the cells infused back into her body. Her doctors had

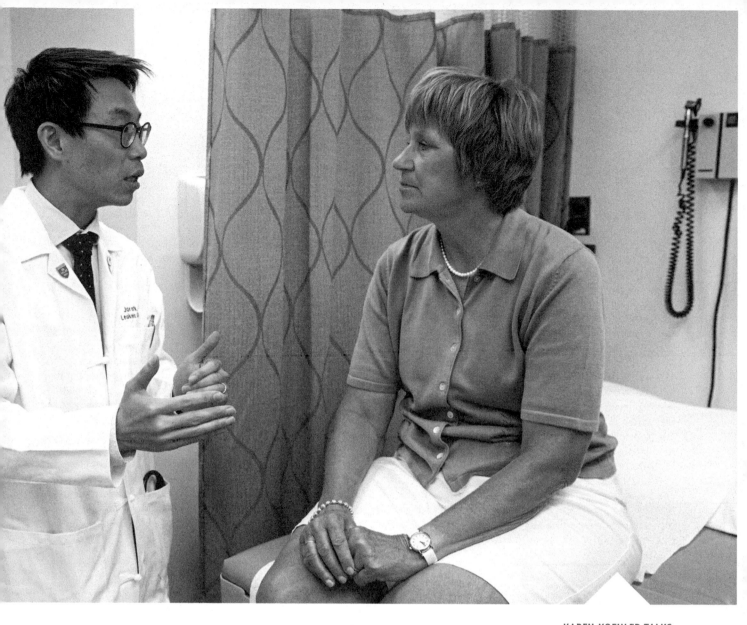

KAREN KOEHLER TALKS WITH JAE PARK, HER ONCOLOGIST, DURING A RECENT CHECKUP AT MEMORIAL SLOAN KETTERING.

warned that tests might show cancer for several months longer, though that didn't happen.

The first suggestion of the power of CAR Ts came from the University of Pennsylvania's Abramson Cancer Center, which is developing another CD19-targeted technology with the backing of the drug company Novartis. In early 2014, Novartis announced that 27 out of 30 patients with acute lymphoblastic leukemia who had not responded to traditional chemotherapy, most of them children, were in complete remission after having been treated. Novartis, Juno Therapeutics (the company working with MSK), and a third developer, Kite Pharma, predict that the Food and Drug Administration could approve their CAR Ts next year.

"THE IDEA OF REPROGRAMMING immune cells made sense to me," says Douglas Olson, 69, a retired medical device company executive from Bucks County, Pennsylvania, who received CAR Ts in a Penn trial in 2010 after his leukemia returned. He gets regular check-

ups and blood tests several times a year, all of which have been clean since three weeks after his treatment. Olson has even taken up running since his cancer battle and has finished five half marathons. Eight of the 14 patients in the trial Olson participated in responded to the engineered cells. One of the questions researchers at Penn, MSK and other cancer centers hope to answer is why the engineered cells work for some patients but are ineffective in others.

Since the treatment affects some normal immune cells as well as the cancer cells, Olson, Koehler and other recipients may need infusions periodically to restore normal immune cells to their bloodstreams. That's a manageable effect of treatment. For some patients, the one potentially serious effect is what's called "cytokine release syndrome," a dangerous overwhelming immune response that occurs shortly after the treatment when CAR T cells encounter cancer cells and begin working.

The disorder can cause high fevers and dangerous drops in blood pressure and kidney function, putting some patients in intensive care.

Neurological symptoms like confusion and seizures are also a risk. Steroids can be helpful in managing some of the symptoms, and an immune-suppressing drug called tocilizumab, usually used to treat rheumatoid arthritis, has been shown to be effective in controlling these short-term problems.

"WE'RE WORKING ON trying to prevent" side effects, says William Wierda, a professor in the department of leukemia at Houston's MD Anderson Cancer Center, which is participating in several CAR T clinical trials. "In some cases, we can identify patients who are at higher risk of cytokine release syndrome. And now we're discussing whether tocilizumab could be used to prevent it."

Researchers are also developing CAR Ts that will work against other cancers, including tough-to-conquer solid tumors like ovarian and pancreatic cancers and glioblastoma, the aggressive brain cancer. The biggest challenge in fighting solid tumors is finding targets like the CD19 pro-

THESE ARE *ONE-TIME* INFUSIONS OF *CELLS* THAT DESTROY CANCER.

tein. "Solid tumors have unique ways of avoiding the immune system that blood cancers do not," says David Porter, a physician and director of blood and bone marrow transplantation at Penn's Abramson Cancer Center. "One issue is that solid tumors are all wrapped up in a mass, making it difficult for T cells to be able to get in and kill the cancer cells." Penn scientists are examining one potential target on glioblastoma tumors called EGFRvIII. About 30 percent of patients have tumors that produce this protein, and trials are now starting of CAR Ts that have been engineered to attack those tumors.

The process of using CAR Ts to treat cancer will not only extend to many more tumor types, it will also become more streamlined and easier for patients, predicts Sloan Kettering's Park. He believes the T-cell collection process will eventually "be like getting a blood draw from your doctor's office." The engineering time will be shortened and perhaps even automated, he says. "It only gets better from here." ●

AIMING AT OTHER TARGETS

assuming that engineered T cells can trick the immune system into recognizing and destroying cancer, it stands to reason that a similar approach might help conquer autoimmune disorders, chronic viruses and other diseases that logically would be vulnerable to an enhanced immune response. That's the thinking behind several early-stage research programs aimed at manipulating T cells:

HIV. In 2013, scientists at the University of Texas and Stanford University showed they could insert genes that are resistant to HIV, the virus that causes AIDS, into T cells that would

normally be attacked by the virus. Similar research at the University of Pennsylvania has yielded engineered T cells that could potentially replace drugs for the long-term control of HIV. Penn's Perelman School of Medicine has launched human trials of the cells, which are ongoing.

Diabetes. Type 1 diabetes occurs when the immune system mistakenly destroys insulin-producing cells in the pancreas. This process is often exaggerated by a lack of so-called regulatory T cells – the good guys that normally keep the immune system in check. An international study in 2012 that included the University of Chicago showed that infusing

regulatory T cells into children who were coping with Type 1 diabetes prompted them to enter prolonged remissions.

Multiple sclerosis. MS occurs when an abnormal immune response causes some T cells to attack a key component of the central nervous system – the myelin, or fatty sheath that surrounds and protects nerve fibers. That knowledge has led to the development of drugs that can inhibit those T cells. But what's emerged more recently is an understanding that the B cells that are the target of CAR Ts in chronic lymphocytic leukemia (story) might also contribute to the neurological decline that is seen in MS patients. Therapies that deplete B cells may prove useful in battling this disease, as well. –A.W.

NEVER UNDERESTIMATE THE POWER OF 7,000 PEOPLE FOCUSED ON ONE GOAL.

As pioneers of "disease management teams," we understand the importance of collaboration. Each week, our cancer specialists gather to discuss not just individual patients' treatment options, but also their personal challenges and goals during and beyond treatment. We believe there's nothing more powerful than a group of dedicated people ensuring the best care for you — a belief that has helped make us a top-ranked hospital for the 27th year in a row. **Learn more at MSKCC.ORG/MORESCIENCE**

**MORE
SCIENCE.
LESS
FEAR.**

Memorial Sloan Kettering
Cancer Center

MANHATTAN · BROOKLYN · LONG ISLAND · WESTCHESTER COUNTY · BASKING RIDGE, NJ
In-network with most health plans. Ask about financial assistance.

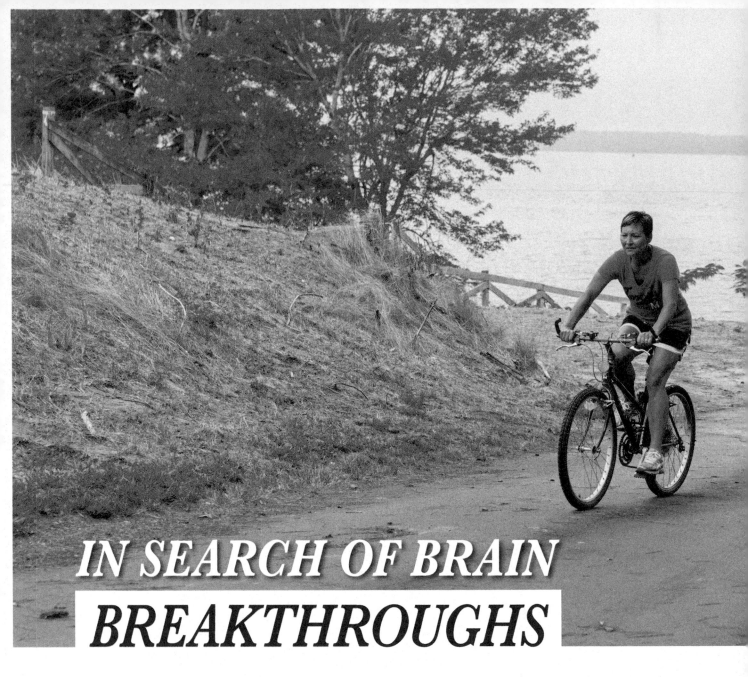

IN SEARCH OF BRAIN
BREAKTHROUGHS

A look at where research stands on some of the most devastating brain diseases

BY LINDA CHILDERS

Several years ago, when Kim Spletter began experiencing stiff muscles and difficulty walking, she chalked it up to her exercise regimen. Yet even after she'd scaled her workouts back, the symptoms continued to worsen. Soon Spletter, who lives in Frederick, Maryland, was experiencing tremors in her left leg and muscle rigidity. When doctors ultimately diagnosed the retired Montgomery County sheriff, who was then 45, with Parkinson's

disease, she was devastated.

Then last year, her physician encouraged Spletter to participate in a new clinical trial at the University of Maryland Medical Center that would target and heat the brain cells interfering with her motor skills. Over the course of four hours, Spletter received a series of focused ultrasound waves applied through her skull. After the 11th wave, she'd regained 70 percent of her strength on the side of her body affected by her condition.

"The results were instantaneous," says Spletter nearly a year after the treatment. "I feel like I've been given a second chance. I'm biking, running and even teaching an indoor cycling class specifically designed for people with Parkinson's."

As aging Baby Boomers usher in what is expected to be a "silver tsunami" of neurodegenerative disease, researchers are working urgently to speed up the search for more effective treatments, if not cures. At the moment, 1 million Americans have Parkinson's, and by 2030 that number is expected to jump by 80 percent. The Alzheimer's Association predicts that the number of Americans 65 and older suffering from the devastating brain disorder will almost triple to 13.8 million by 2050. A national effort known as the BRAIN Initiative (for Brain Research through Advancing Innovative Neurotechnologies) was launched by the White House in 2013 to unlock the mysteries of the brain by developing tools to examine how

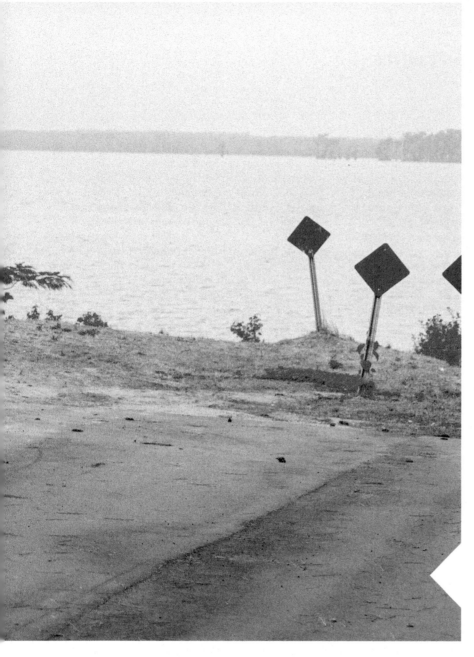

"I'M BIKING, RUNNING AND EVEN TEACHING *AN INDOOR* CYCLING CLASS."

KIM SPLETTER, WHO HAS
PARKINSON'S, REGAINED
70 PERCENT OF HER STRENGTH
AFTER A PROCEDURE CALLED
FOCUSED ULTRASOUND.

"individual brain cells and complex neural circuits interact at the speed of thought." Scientists hope that this sort of brain "mapping" could lead to better answers not only for people with Alzheimer's and Parkinson's but also with brain tumors, depression, multiple sclerosis and other neurological conditions. Meantime, here are a few promising updates from the brain research front lines:

Progress against Parkinson's disease

The best that medicine can do at the moment to fight Parkinson's, a disorder in which the motor cells stop communicating properly due to a lack of the neurotransmitter dopamine,

is to control the symptoms: tremors, stiffness, difficulty with walking and balance, depression and dementia. Current treatments generally rely on drugs that replace or act like dopamine. When drugs don't suffice or side effects interfere, a surgical procedure known as deep brain stimulation can sometimes be helpful. DBS therapy involves drilling a hole in the skull and inserting a thin electrode to target motor circuits that an MRI can identify as not functioning properly. Electrical pulses from a device similar to a cardiac pacemaker, implanted under the skin of the abdomen or near the collarbone, stimulate the brain region and block nerve signals that cause symptoms.

The focus of research lately has been

on less invasive ways to improve quality of life, as well as on the continued quest for medications that slow the rate at which Parkinson's progresses. (Some drugs that look promising are currently in clinical trials, as is gene therapy.) The procedure performed on Spletter, focused ultrasound guided by MRI, creates a heat lesion at a targeted neural circuit that essentially resets the damaged circuit. The patient is awake and monitored in real time so that doctors can precisely aim the beam and conduct physical tests to see if symptoms are fading.

It's known that focused ultrasound can make Parkinson's symptoms less debilitating, says Howard Eisenberg, principal investigator and a neurosurgeon at the University of Maryland

Medical Center. "What we don't know yet is how long the results will last. Kim was our first patient," he says, and she is "doing great." It's still too early in testing to know if the treatment could be repeated.

Spletter, who arrived for the procedure in a wheelchair and walked out without assistance, says she's been given a new lease on life. "I am hoping the focused ultrasound treatment will last long enough for researchers to find a cure or improve the current medications," she says.

New approaches to tackling deadly brain tumors

Treating brain cancer is a notoriously difficult matter. Drugs are often blocked by the blood-brain barrier; surgery carries the risk of damaging tissue responsible for vital functions.

ONE TACK *DOCTORS* ARE TAKING IS APPLYING HEAT TO KILL *CANCER CELLS.*

For inoperable tumors, radiation is often the answer, but it, too, can damage healthy tissue. And at a certain point a maximum dose may be reached.

One tack doctors are taking when tumors recur or can't be safely accessed through standard surgery is applying heat – in this case generated by a laser – to kill rogue cells. Although laser treatment for cancer isn't new, the technology has advanced, allowing greater precision. And in contrast to radiation, repeating the procedure is sometimes an option. Guided by MRI, doctors thread a laser catheter about the size of a pencil lead through a small opening in the skull and into the center of a tumor.

"Traditionally, brain surgery has been a very intensive procedure, requiring multiple night stays, hours of surgery and postoperative recovery time," says Julian Bailes, chair of the department of neurosurgery and co-director of the Northshore Neurological Institute at Northshore University Health System in Chicago. The laser procedure "only requires an incision the size of a coffee stirrer, one stitch, and an overnight hospital stay." He and his colleagues are among the first in the country to use the MRI-guided laser system Visualase to treat inoperable tumors including glioblastoma and high-grade gliomas and metastases to the brain from elsewhere. A similar device, NeuroBlate, is being used at the Cleveland Clinic and other hospitals.

While the data on how patients fare is still extremely limited, Bailes says the outcomes he is seeing are very encouraging; early results are showing the procedure can extend lives, even if only by weeks or months.

Will the promise of immunotherapy, which is now being used to treat lung cancer, melanoma and leukemia, extend to brain cancer? A number of approaches enlisting the immune system are being tried, including one against glioblastoma that removes the patient's T cells, engineers them to attack the tumor, and reinfuses them (story, Page 30).

And a treatment developed by researchers at Duke University was recently designated a "breakthrough therapy" by the Food and Drug Administration for its success attacking glioblastoma through the injection of a modified poliovirus directly into the tumor. The virus infects the tumor, signaling the immune system that it is an enemy. A phase one clinical trial showed a 22 percent three-year survival rate, compared to the normal 4 percent rate. The first two patients, who were treated in 2012, are still cancer-free. The breakthrough designation means the FDA will expedite getting the treatment developed and approved.

Attacking Alzheimer's before symptoms arise

It's long been thought that a buildup of amyloid beta protein, which accumulates outside nerve cells and begins to block communication between neurons, is largely responsible for the ravages of this disease. All people naturally produce the protein, and a May study from Massachusetts General Hospital adds evidence that it may even play a role in the immune system, protecting the brain against pathogens. But certain genetic and environmental factors may contribute to some people's handling the protein poorly.

This theory of the disease has focused efforts on finding effective anti-amyloid agents. Those that have reached the testing stage so far have

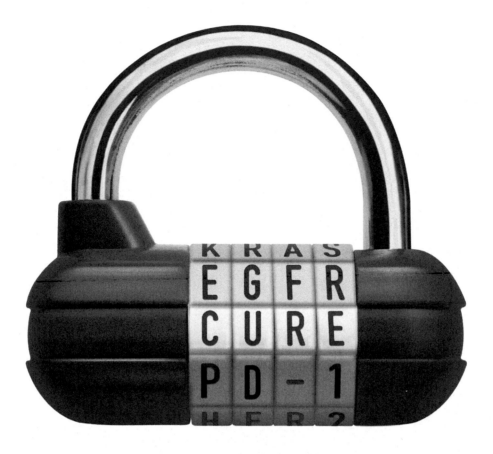

Who will crack the cancer code?

It's the question that millions of people are asking. Pushing us to explore every idea, continually refining our approach, and collaborating with innovators across the globe to explore cancer genomes as never before. Leading us to identify cancer mutations and mechanisms, like PD-1 interactions and EGFR, discoveries that help all of us develop more targeted therapies. Together, we can find solutions to the toughest problems, because the more answers we find, the more lives we save.

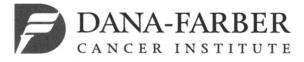

DANA-FARBER
CANCER INSTITUTE

Discover. Care. Believe.

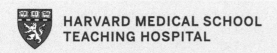

**HARVARD MEDICAL SCHOOL
TEACHING HOSPITAL**

Videos, whitepapers and more at
DiscoverCareBelieve.org/code

worked only modestly and not well enough to impress the FDA. Researchers now think that's because amyloid beta begins to do its harm, damaging brain cells' synapses, long before the characteristic plaques form and symptoms are distinguishable. And drugs to date have only been tested in people who already have symptoms. Current medications for Alzheimer's may ease symptoms for a time by supporting neurotransmitters involved in cell communi-

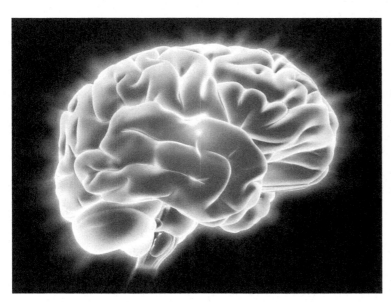

THE NUMBER OF **AMERICANS** WITH **ALZHEIMER'S** WILL ALMOST *TRIPLE BY 2050.*

cation, but they do not treat the underlying disease or delay its progression.

A number of avenues are now being investigated to intervene much earlier, says Lawrence Honig, director of the Clinical Core of the Alzheimer's Disease Research Center at Columbia University. Rather than focus on amyloid, Frank Longo, a professor of neurology and neurological sciences at Stanford University, is working on a way to keep brain cells from degenerating. He's testing a molecule called LM11A-31 that binds to receptors on the cells and triggers the receptors "in a way

that counteracts that degenerative signaling inside the cell," he says. The drug is moving to phase two trials now.

Another clinical trial just getting underway, organized by researchers at Brigham and Women's Hospital in Boston, will focus on an anti-amyloid antibody called solanezumab. The trial will rely on advanced brain scan technology to spot early amyloid buildup in people who have no signs of Alzheimer's and will test whether the drug could have an effect at this stage.

"We hope that starting treatment much earlier in the disease, before symptoms are present, as well as treating for a longer period of time, will slow cognitive decline and ultimately prevent Alzheimer's disease dementia," says Dennis Selkoe, a Harvard Medical School neurologist and co-director of Brigham's new Ann Romney Center for Neurological Diseases. A thousand participants across more than 60 sites in the U.S., Canada and Australia will be monitored for three to five years to determine whether solanezumab can help the brain to clear the amyloid beta and delay or prevent the onset of symptoms.

The Ann Romney Center was designed to accelerate treatments for and prevention of all the major brain diseases by gathering researchers focused on the different disorders in one place to share their work. It grew out of a conversation that Ann Romney, the wife of former Massachusetts Gov. Mitt Romney, had with Howard Weiner, director of the Multiple Sclerosis Program at Brigham and Women's. Romney has MS, and Weiner, who is her neurologist, mentioned how MS research was leading to breakthroughs in Alzheimer's disease; protollin, a drug he had studied for MS, for example, unexpectedly cleared plaques from the brains of mice. Fascinated by that potential for collaboration to speed results, Romney spearheaded a fundraising effort. The center will house up to 300 researchers as well as serve patients with a range of brain disorders.

Weiner and Selkoe have been collaborating to develop vaccines for MS and Alzheimer's. In the case of Alzheimer's, Weiner says, they are now working with several pharmaceutical companies to manufacture a protollin-based nasal vaccine that could be tested as a way to clear plaque in people. Like the solanezumab trial, the nasal vaccine is aimed at slowing the disease or even preventing it. ●

With Peter Rathmell

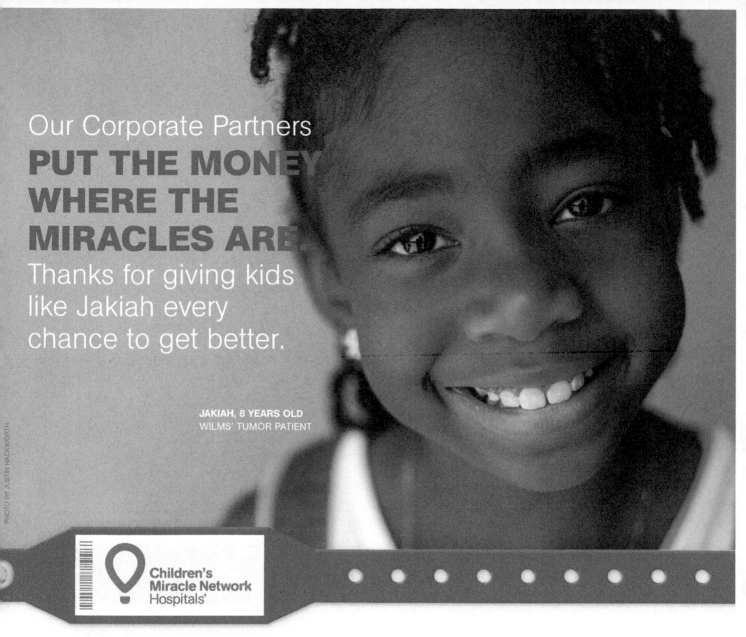

Our Corporate Partners
PUT THE MONEY WHERE THE MIRACLES ARE.

Thanks for giving kids like Jakiah every chance to get better.

JAKIAH, 8 YEARS OLD
WILMS' TUMOR PATIENT

PHOTO BY JUSTIN HACKWORTH

Children's
Miracle Network
Hospitals

Because they give, Children's Miracle Network Hospitals® provide the best care for local kids.

Thank you to our top corporate partners for raising funds that save and improve the lives of local kids. Since becoming a CMN Hospitals partner, each has raised more than $50 million, totalling more than $2 billion, collectively, for member children's hospitals across North America.

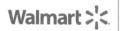   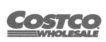

  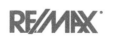 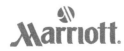

CMNHospitals.org

Give Today
to your children's hospital

SKELETON CREW

The relentless focus of the Hospital for Special Surgery
BY MICHAEL MORELLA

NEW YORK – Lea Marie Medina has been gently turned facedown, arms at her sides. Inside an operating room at the Hospital for Special Surgery, the 16-year-old from Queens is undergoing selective thoracic fusion to correct the scoliosis in her spine. The condition, in which vertebrae in the back curve improperly to the side, is a common one in adolescents that often does not require surgery. But Medina's curve is greater than 50 degrees, so the risk of arthritis and future

LEA MARIE MEDINA, 16, IS PREPPED FOR THORACIC FUSION SURGERY TO CORRECT THE SCOLIOSIS IN HER SPINE.

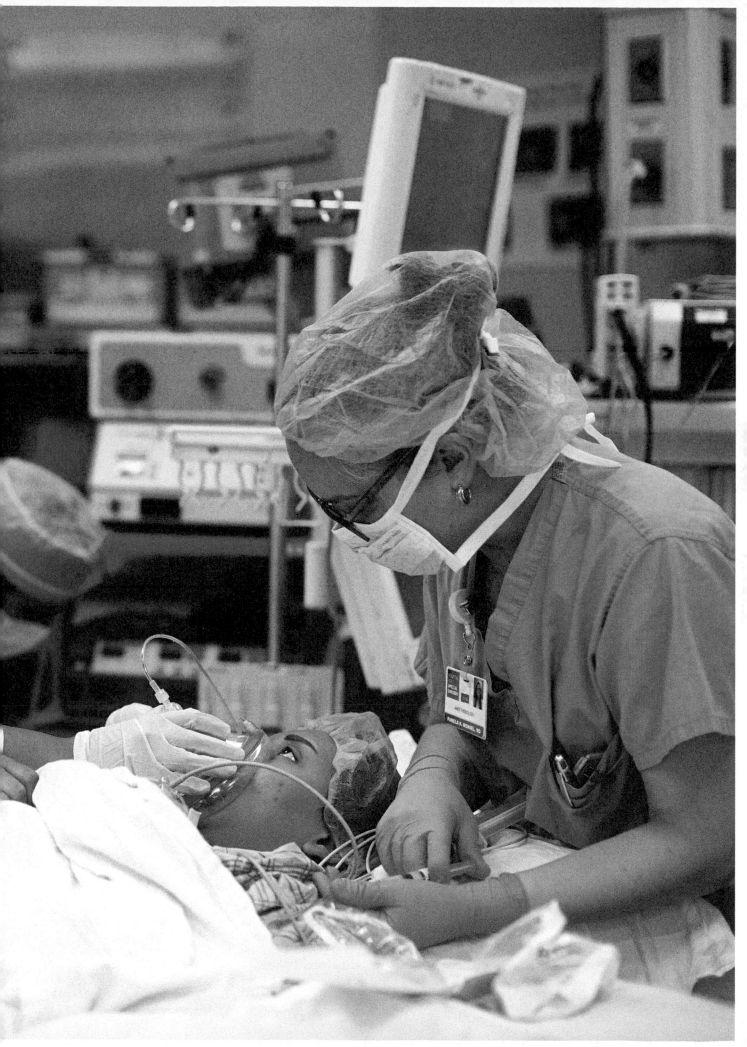

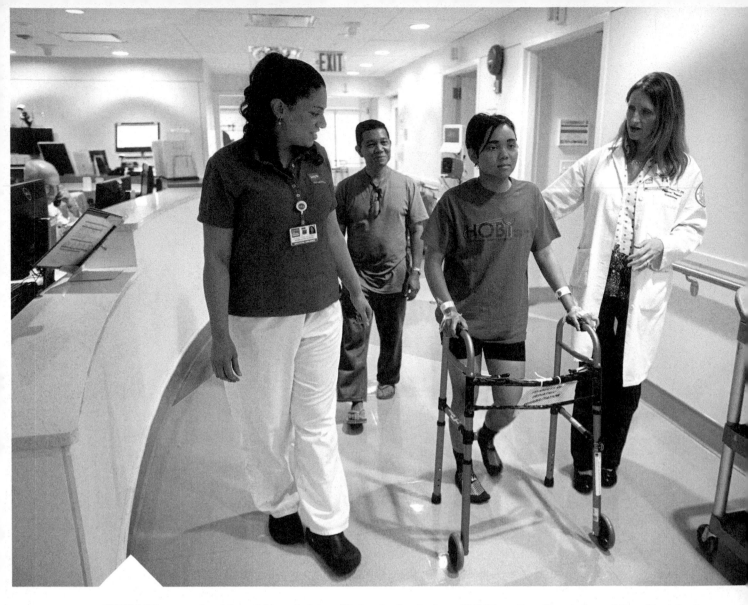

health problems in her still-developing body are a concern. She was also forced to give up swimming competitions because of pain. "Swimming is my life," Medina says shortly before her surgery.

Today, in the OR, surgeons led by Roger F. Widmann, chief of pediatric orthopedic surgery, cut into Medina's back and move away muscle to reveal her spine. They use an osteotome and mallet, resembling a chisel and a hammer, to expose joints between each vertebra from roughly her shoulders to the top of her stomach. Widmann and his team insert screws at most points, install a rod on either side of Medina's spine, and move the vertebrae into the proper alignment. Finally, they graft a combination of bone from Medina and a tissue bank into the spine to make sure the alignment holds. The grafting is "kind of the glue that keeps it all together," Widmann says. After about four hours, the curve is largely corrected.

Both complex surgeries and everyday procedures like hip and knee replacements are commonplace at HSS, the nation's top-ranked hospital for orthopedics, according to the latest U.S. News Best Hospitals rankings (Page 108). Founded during the Civil War, the 215-bed specialty hospital on the Upper East Side of Manhattan performed more than 31,000 surgeries in 2015, up from about 18,000 a decade ago; it handled more than 20 times as many hip and knee replacements in Medicare patients as the average U.S. hospital in 2012-13. People come for care or second opinions from all 50 states and over 100 countries. While many hospitals are expanding their service lines or being swallowed up by large health care chains, HSS has grown and earned its reputation by maintaining a "relentless focus" on conditions affecting the muscles, bones and joints, says Louis Shapiro, the hospital's president and CEO. "It's never taken its eye off the ball." U.S. News spent several days this summer shadowing patients and clinicians to find out what makes HSS so special.

Alex Douglass sits on an exam room table as Joseph Feinberg, HSS physiatrist-in-chief, attaches a small electrode to his right foot. Feinberg, whose focus is nonsurgical physical medicine and rehab, sends a small impulse

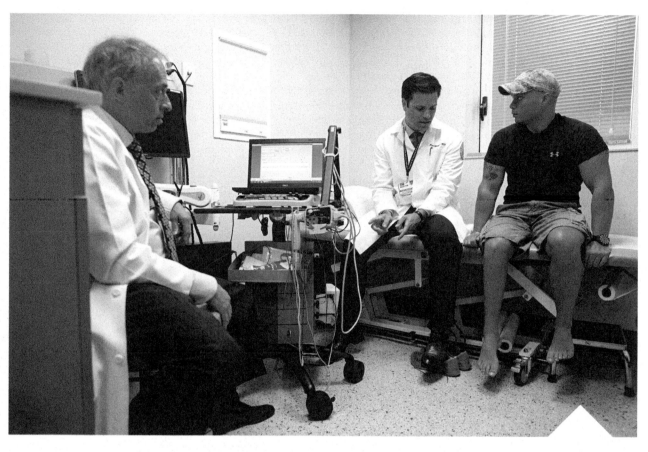

into nerves in Douglass' knee, measuring any response in his foot before moving to a different point on his leg. He prods Douglass' lower leg with a needle at various points to further check if nerves are regenerating below the knee.

Douglass, 33, cannot move his right leg below his shin, but the fact that he has any mobility in his leg at all is a testament to the care he has received at HSS for the last year and a half. Two years ago, Douglass, a Pennsylvania state trooper from near Scranton, was shot in his side with a .308-caliber rifle round by a sniper firing outside the police station barracks. The bullet sent a shock wave through Douglass' body, fracturing his pelvis, part of his thighbone and his sacrum, the bone at the base of the spine near where the nerves emerge; it also punctured his bowels, causing a widespread infection. Doctors at a nearby hospital treated him for the infection and installed metal plates to stabilize his hip. But after a month of rehab and recovery, when Douglass was still troubled by constant fevers and pain, his doctors reached out to HSS.

Orthopedic surgeons David Mayman and David Wellman, who specializes in trauma,

took the case, along with infection experts and Feinberg, who would handle the returning function of Douglass' nerves and muscles.

"When we went in, it was a pretty dreary situation," Wellman says. He and Mayman operated together to treat the breaks in the femur, pelvis and sacrum. They cleared out debris and infection and replaced the metal hardware the other doctors had implanted with a temporary prosthesis that dispersed antibiotics over about six weeks. When the infection had cleared, Mayman removed the antibiotic implant and performed a full hip replacement, using a joint made of titanium, ceramic and polyethylene plastic that should be durable for many years in a young patient like Douglass, Mayman says.

Today, after plenty of rehab closer to home, Douglass walks without crutches and only an occasional lurch. Muscle in his abs and hamstring has returned, and his hip feels strong and pain-free. A brace on his right ankle allows him to move around, drive and exercise; without it, his ankle and foot flop down. "As soon as I came here, it was like progress nonstop," says Douglass, who hopes to eventually return to

DOCTORS JOSEPH FEINBERG (LEFT) AND DAVID WELLMAN MEET WITH STATE TROOPER ALEX DOUGLASS, 33, WHOM THEY TREATED AFTER A SNIPER'S BULLET SEVERELY DAMAGED HIS HIP, PELVIS AND LEG TWO YEARS AGO.

work. "And it still is." He comes in every three months to see Feinberg, who has monitored his nerve function. "Why it hasn't come back further down, I don't know," Feinberg says. Says Mayman: "We just treat it one step at a time."

Such a team approach to treatment is a hallmark of HSS and "really optimizes care," Feinberg says. The wide range of orthopedic conditions treated here range from traumatic injuries like Douglass' and ultracomplex limb and ankle reconstruction surgery, for example, to infusion therapy for rheumatological diseases like arthritis, lupus and other autoimmune conditions affecting the muscles and joints. While it might seem logical that a hospital with surgery in its name would push surgery, only about 31,000 operations were performed on the 120,000-plus patients who visited last year; many came for physical therapy and rehab for

sports-related injuries and noninvasive treatments to manage back pain, for instance. Nearly 2 in 5 patients who come seeking a second opinion receive a different treatment recommendation – and not infrequently, it's to skip surgery in favor of something else.

Jessica Markus, a special education preschool teacher from the Bronx who has lupus, is faring much better since she came to rheumatologist Joseph Markenson and started a new monthly drug infusion regimen. Markus, 39, no longer suffers from the recurring headaches, fatigue and extreme joint pain that the autoimmune disorder causes. "It's a part of me every day," she says, "but it's not the whole me anymore."

Research and treatment are closely integrated, and HSS has several specialized centers focused on cartilage repair and spinal conditions, for instance. Another focus is computer-assist-

ORTHOPEDIC SURGEON FRANK CORDASCO EXAMINES BUFFALO BILLS CORNERBACK STEPHON GILMORE, 25, WHO HAD SHOULDER SURGERY IN DECEMBER AFTER AN INJURY.

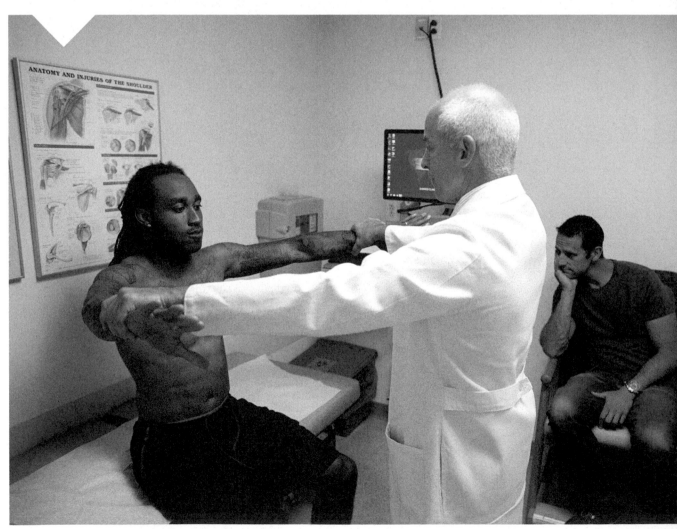

ed surgery, which allows surgeons to incorporate X-rays and other data about a patient to develop a virtual plan of attack before they even make an incision. In 2013, the hospital established a research center to investigate genetic causes and targeted therapies for lupus and other autoimmune diseases. Researchers are also exploring using 3-D printing to create precisely customized replacements for torn meniscus cartilage in the knee, doing the printing with synthetic material infused with a patient's own cells to cause genetically matched new cartilage to grow.

Like Douglass, Susan Perry is taking her recovery step by step. Sitting with orthopedic surgeon Austin Fragomen, the former nurse and nursing professor from Whitesboro, New York, discusses several options for what will be hip surgery No. 30.

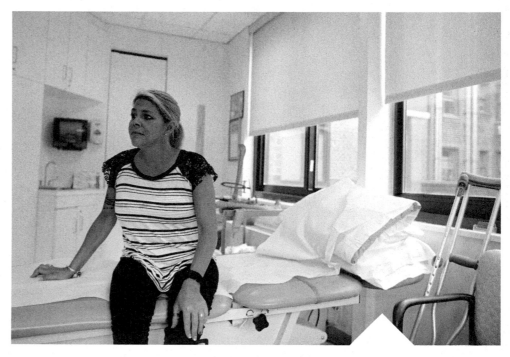

Perry, 45, was born with congenital hip dysplasia, a condition in which the ball and socket of her left hip joint weren't properly developed. She has had multiple reconstructive surgeries and hip replacements since she was young. Now, her left leg is about 4 inches shorter than her right.

Today Fragomen, fellowship director of the hospital's Limb Lengthening and Complex Reconstruction Service, advises Perry on several surgical approaches to even out her legs. He could insert a nail into her femur that could be gradually stretched with an external magnet as new bone fills in around it over time. Alternately, Fragomen could surgically cut her thighbone and attach an external device to each end of it with quarter-inch pins, and Perry could crank the device at home to create room for new bone. A third option is something of a hybrid: using a nail and magnet to internally lengthen Perry's shinbone while attaching the external device to lengthen her femur. Limb lengthening is performed regularly at HSS, Fragomen says, but it's a surgery that most residents elsewhere "never even see."

Perry first came to HSS a year ago, after a bad infection led to removal of her hip and pelvis and two and a half years in bed in a body brace. Her doctors had "just said that's the way it's going to be," she says.

Here, orthopedic surgeon Seth Jerabek worked with the hospital's biomechanics team to design a custom implant that took six months to build and included replacement parts for her pelvis and femur. Perry's pelvis and the muscles around it were so eroded that her leg almost became completely motionless, so a plastic surgeon had to transfer some extra muscle from her buttock to the area around her hip to support her implant. After several months of physical therapy, Perry is walking again with a crutch, a shoe lift and a slight limp. "I'm very happy I'm actually standing up," she says. Jerabek has reviewed today's X-rays and discussed limb lengthening with Fragomen.

"The safest is to split it up" and expand both the tibia and the femur, Fragomen decides. They plan the surgery for later in the summer, after which the expanding and rehab process could take about a year. "Maybe next year at this time I will be totally mobile," Perry says.

The department of radiology and imaging has a key role to play, working closely with physicians to give them the information they need to formulate "a game plan," says Hollis Potter, chairman of the department. Cutting-edge imaging techniques range from highly sensitive X-rays that allow doctors to examine the components of Perry's implant or the precise angles of the curves in a spine like Medina's, for example, to advanced magnetic resonance imaging that offers a three-dimensional look at soft tissue, spinal discs or a meniscus in the

SUSAN PERRY, 45, WAS BORN WITH CONGENITAL HIP DYSPLASIA. AFTER AN EARLIER OPERATION FITTED HER WITH A CUSTOM-BUILT HIP IMPLANT, SHE'S BACK TODAY TO DISCUSS SURGERY TO LENGTHEN HER LEFT LEG, WHICH IS ABOUT 4 INCHES SHORTER THAN HER RIGHT LEG.

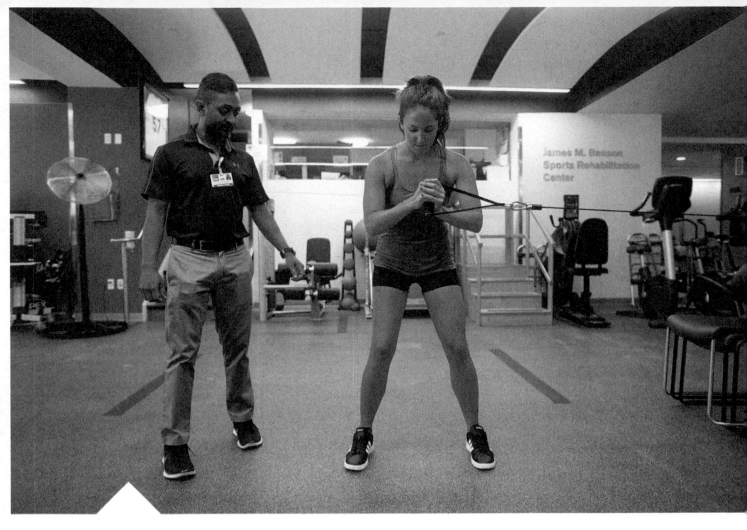

knee, say. In May, the hospital won a grant from the National Basketball Association and GE Healthcare to explore one of the next frontiers of imaging: using noninvasive ultrasound and MRI to forecast what will happen with particular individuals. The goal is to identify players at risk for tendinopathy, a disease of the patellar tendon in the knee, and incorporate motion analysis to predict future performance and recovery. "This technology is going from just taking a picture of something and diagnosis to predicting function," Potter says.

Elsewhere at the hospital, Stephon Gilmore sits in an exam room, while his orthopedic surgeon, Frank Cordasco, examines his left shoulder. Cordasco assesses whether both shoulders look symmetrical and checks for any muscle atrophy or tenderness. He gauges Gilmore's range of motion, which is full and pain-free. "He looks fantastic," Cordasco says. "He's completely ready to play football."

Gilmore, a cornerback for the Buffalo Bills, is one of the many professional athletes whose injuries and aches and pains HSS treats each year; 372 pro players passed through in 2015. HSS is the official hospital of several professional, Olympic and college sports teams, including the Brooklyn Nets; New York Giants, Mets, Knicks, and Liberty; and USA Basketball and

USA Swimming. On Dec. 6, Gilmore took a big hit in a game against the Houston Texans, fracturing parts of his shoulder socket and shoulder blade and dislocating his shoulder.

Out for the rest of the season, Gilmore, 25, came to Cordasco for a surgery to fix the socket fracture by augmenting it with part of the fractured shoulder blade. It was Gilmore's second time on Cordasco's operating table; he had injured the same shoulder late in the 2014 season and needed surgery to repair a torn labrum, the cartilage that connects ligaments to the shoulder socket and holds it in place. Today, after six months of rehab, "everything is going great," says Gilmore. "I'm just ready to roll."

Three days after surgery, Lea Marie Medina walks gingerly around her hospital room. She begins with the aid of a walker and, before long, is taking a lap of the hallway without one. "You have progressed completely according to plan," says Siobhan Clarke, clinical specialist and section manager of pediatric rehabilitation. She works with Medina as she steps up and down several stairs with no issues. "It feels different," Medina says. "I think I'm taller." Widmann checks one more set of X-rays before releasing the teen from the hospital. Medina will continue with a few months of rehab closer to home. And she will be back in the pool by mid-summer. ●

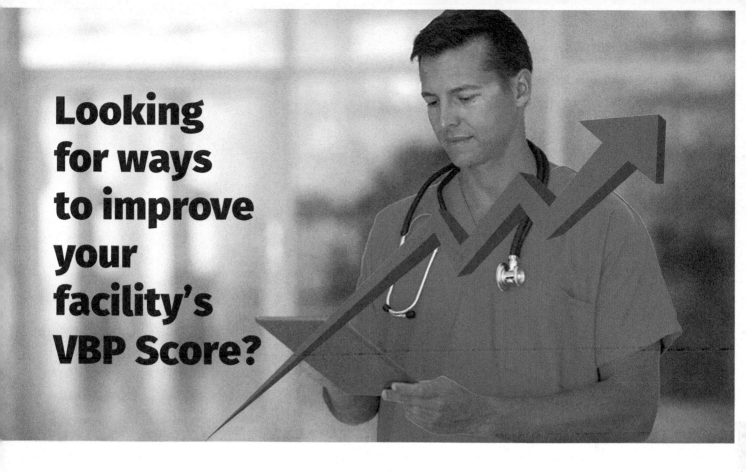

Looking for ways to improve your facility's VBP Score?

A recent independent study shows that U.S. hospitals using **Lippincott Solutions** performed better in the Value-Based Purchasing (VBP) model, than hospitals not using Lippincott Solutions.

Hospitals using **Lippincott Procedures** performed 9% better in Patient Outcomes and 23% better in the Clinical Process of Care, in the CMS VBP Outcomes model, and showing a 12% overall improvement in the VBP Total Performance Score.

Visit **LippincottSolutions.com/VBP** to learn more!

Lippincott
Solutions

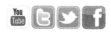

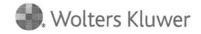 . Wolters Kluwer

6-P153

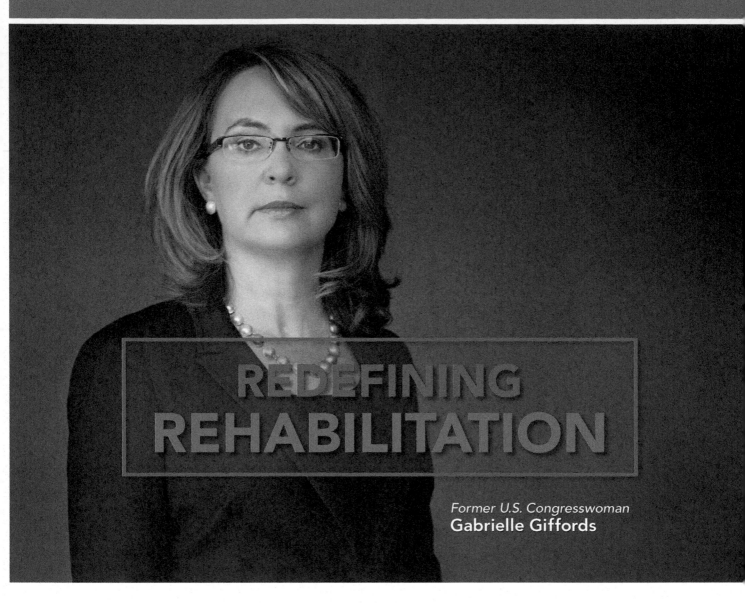
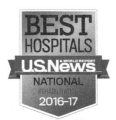
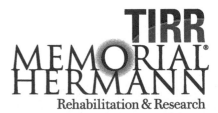

THE SAFETY FACTOR

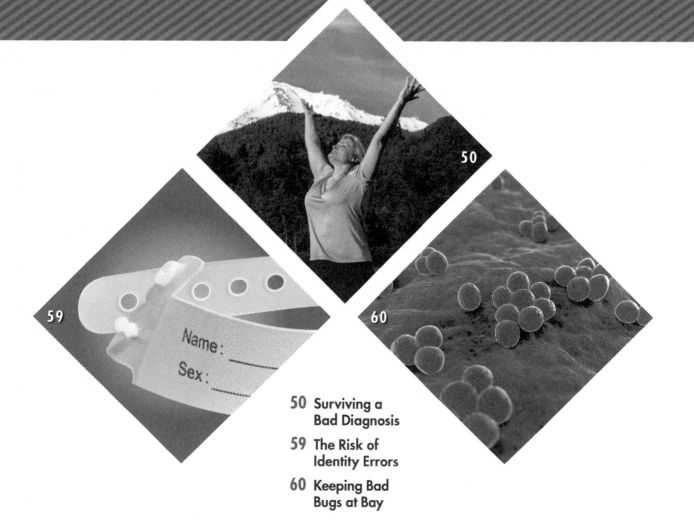

SURVIVING
A BAD CALL

Diagnostic error is one of medicine's most serious failings
BY KATHERINE HOBSON

Peggy Zuckerman was on her way to a concert at the Hollywood Bowl back in 2004 when her doctor called. Blood work she'd had in preparation for minor surgery showed she was dangerously anemic, he said, and she needed to get to the emergency room. Instead of enjoying "Madama Butterfly," Zuckerman spent that night and the next at the hospital, getting three blood transfusions, an endoscopy and a colonoscopy to figure out where the problem might lie. She was told the bleeding was likely due to a tiny, scabbed-over stomach ulcer and sent home. But seven months later, she still wasn't feeling well. "By this time, I was just dragging tail," recalls Zuckerman, 67. Finally, an ultrasound revealed a softball-sized mass on her right kidney. The cancer had also spread to her lungs.

Zuckerman was fortunate. She responded well to surgery and immunotherapy, and has been free of kidney cancer since. (She's now receiving care for a separate early-stage breast cancer.) But as she recovered, she started to look into why she hadn't been diagnosed earlier. "When I was well enough to lift my head up and read," she says, she learned that hemoglobin levels as low as hers would have required significant bleeding, not "a small, theoretically scabbed-over ulcer." She reviewed her records and spotted missed opportunities, including an ER physician's recommendation – never passed on to her – that she see a rheumatologist or a hematologist, and a pathology report showing no ulcer. Misdiagnosis is common with kidney cancer, which often presents with seemingly unrelated symptoms. As Zuckerman, who is now a patient advocate, did more research, though, she realized poor calls are a far broader problem. "It's not just odd cancers or rare diseases," she says.

THAT WORRISOME REALITY was underscored last year by the National Academies of Sciences, Engineering, and Medicine in a report on the urgent need to improve diagnosis. The authors defined diagnostic error as the failure to establish an accurate and timely explanation of the problem or to communicate that information to the patient. And they concluded that most people will experience at least one diagnostic error, "sometimes with devastating consequences." Autopsy reports suggest that these mistakes contribute to about 10 percent of patient deaths, while medical record reviews suggest they cause up to 17 percent of adverse events in hospitals.

One way doctors err is by leaping to conclusions before all the evidence is in. Tamara Patterson, a 35-year-old therapeutic yoga instructor in Mount Shasta, California, recalls telling her physicians over and over again that her lower abdominal pain wasn't alleviated by a hernia repair and that her pain and bleeding varied with her menstrual cycle. "I said, 'I don't think it's the hernia.' And I literally had four clinicians look at me like I was a lunatic." It turns out she had endometriosis. In other cases, key information isn't passed on from one clinician to the next. Or test results fall through the cracks. "This is a safety issue," says Mark L. Graber, a member of the committee that authored the report and president and founder of the Society to Improve Diagnosis in Medicine. "It might be the biggest one."

A report in the journal Diagnosis in October 2014 described one example. A feverish patient had walked into a Dallas emergency department complaining of dizziness, nausea, abdominal pain and headache. He told the nurse that he'd recently traveled to Liberia, which should have raised a red flag. But according to the case report, that information "was not appreciated or acted upon." The patient was prescribed antibiotics, told to take Tylenol, and discharged. He was

> **THIS IS A SAFETY ISSUE. IT *MIGHT BE* THE BIGGEST ONE.**

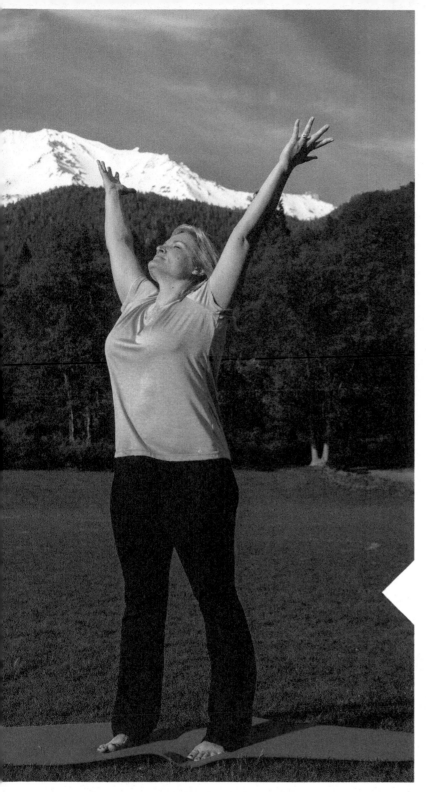

Baylor College of Medicine, who co-authored the Ebola case report.

Singh is one of the researchers trying to get a handle on the problem. A 2013 study in JAMA Internal Medicine that he co-authored found that in primary care, commonly missed conditions included pneumonia, heart failure, cancer and infections. The breakdowns happened most frequently during the patient-clinician encounter – a medical history or physical exam was incomplete, for example. But many cases also went wrong because of factors such as a specialist referral not made or incorrect test interpretation. Experts say much more work needs to be done to characterize and measure misdiagnosis so they know where to focus their efforts.

IN THE MEANTIME, some hospitals and physicians have begun to tackle the problem in multiple ways, from changing the processes that lead to a diagnosis and the health system culture to teaching physicians to think differently about, well, how they think.

One important innovation: encouraging reporting. "Diagnostic errors were having a significant effect on patient safety, but we weren't identifying or responding to them in the way we did to other safety problems," says Robert Trowbridge, a hospitalist and medical educator at the Maine Medical Center in Portland. In 2011, he led a six-month pilot program that educated doctors about misdiagnosis and let them anonymously report diagnostic errors by clicking a computer desktop icon and briefly describing what went wrong.

The findings: 36 mistakes, none of which had been flagged by other monitoring systems. The ability to report diagnostic mistakes is now built into the error reporting system, and while there's no hard evidence, Trowbridge thinks the system is reducing their frequency.

The switch to electronic medical records is often blamed for missed signals because a focus on the computer screen can divert clinicians' attention from the patient. But plenty of experts think health IT has the potential to improve diagnosis. For example, involuntary weight loss is associated with a higher risk of death since it can indicate a serious health problem. But changes in a patient's weight over time may not be noticed by his or her physician, says Gordon Schiff, an internist and associate director of the Center for Patient Safety Research and Practice at Brigham and Wom-

back two days later, severely ill with Ebola, and he infected two nurses who were caring for him before he died.

That misdiagnosis made headlines. Most aren't even identified. It can be extremely difficult to pin down exactly how often the diagnostic process goes wrong or at what step, or even to define exactly when that occurs. A rare disease, for example, may take a while to diagnose correctly, not because physicians missed clear signals but because knowledge of or experience with the condition is lacking, says Hardeep Singh, a patient-safety researcher at the Houston Veterans Affairs Health Services Research Center of Innovation and an associate professor of medicine at

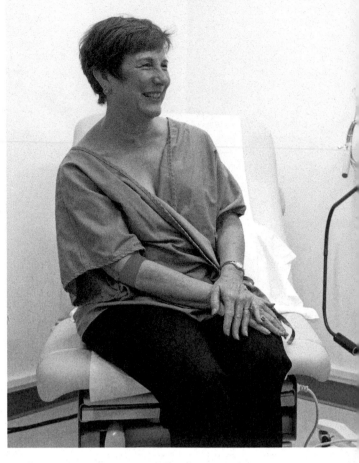

en's Hospital in Boston. When he and colleagues crunched electronic medical record data, they found that 45 percent of patients who unintentionally lost 10 percent or more of their body weight in a year had medical conditions emerge in the next two years that might have been related. What if software automatically searched for that kind of pattern? "We have to make the computer work harder," says Schiff.

KAISER PERMANENTE IS ALREADY using such triggers. The SureNet system is a series of alerts that tips health professionals off to potential lapses in care "before harm comes to the patient," says Michael Kanter, regional medical director of quality and clinical analysis at Kaiser Permanente, Southern California Permanente Medical Group. Take chronic kidney disease, which is diagnosed on the basis of two elevated blood creatinine levels taken three months apart. With SureNet, if there's no second test in the record within 90 days of the first, the system alerts both the physician and patient that another one is needed. A study published last year found that over a four-year period SureNet identified 12,396 people in need of a repeat test, and that 30 percent of them had chronic kidney disease confirmed.

While systems are clearly important, physicians are ultimately the ones making a diagnosis. That process – gathering information, framing a problem, evaluating possible solutions and choosing one – "is no different from the way we solve any other problem in our life," says Gurpreet Dhaliwal, professor of clinical medicine at the University of California–San Francisco. It's similarly subject to the mental shortcuts and biases everyone relies upon to get through the day. Even an experienced doctor who sees a particular infection several times in a week, for example, is going to be more likely to suspect his next patient's

identical symptoms are due to the same problem. Or a doctor might see an initial test result and quickly home in on a diagnosis, then filter out subsequent information that points to something else entirely.

Doing away with those cognitive shortcuts is neither feasible nor desirable, says Dhaliwal, since they often aid correct diagnosis, too. But it's important to teach clinicians to be aware that their thinking is sometimes flawed. He urges physicians to follow up on their diagnoses to see if they made the right call and,

A RAISED BAR FOR TESTS

I t's one of medicine's nightmare scenarios – a missed diagnosis that fails to spot a cancer at its most treatable stage, or an incorrect analysis that leads to an unnecessary surgery. Patients rely on diagnostic and screening tools to provide an accurate picture of their health status and to guide treatment decisions. But there's a growing concern that many of the tests that doctors routinely use may provide misleading or downright false information.

These so-called laboratory-developed tests, or LDTs, are in-house screening and diagnostic tools developed and performed by a single

laboratory. Hospitals often use tests devised in their own labs, for example, and doctors ship tissue samples off to these facilities.

While traditional widely marketed tests or kits have been closely regulated by the Food and Drug Administration since the 1970s and go through careful testing to prove their accuracy, lab-developed tests were excused from the oversight because they were typically simple and their use was so limited. But in the years since, rapid and quantum leaps in medical science – the arrival of genetic testing, for example – have spawned a billion-dollar industry that exploits the regulatory loophole to

quickly create and sell these new diagnostic tools. The FDA is now pushing for more oversight and plans to issue tougher guidelines later this year.

"SOME LDTS HAVE clearly been beneficial," says Elizabeth Mansfield, deputy director for personalized medicine and molecular genetics in the Office of In-Vitro Diagnostics and Radiological Health at the FDA. "But because we haven't been regulating them, we don't know which ones are good and which ones aren't." The agency reported last fall that an analysis of 20 of these tests uncovered several examples of inaccurate results that could lead patients to take the wrong drugs or undergo unnecessary surgeries.

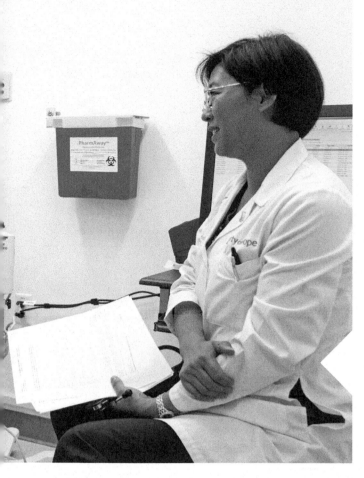

To be sure, it's impossible for every doctor to be deeply familiar with the latest science on every possible illness. So in some cases, fixing misdiagnosis may just be a matter of more widely and quickly disseminating new knowledge, says David Newman-Toker, an associate professor of neurology at Johns Hopkins who will head up a new diagnostic innovation center there. For example, he says, an estimated 4.4 million people show up in the ER with dizziness every year, and 3 to 5 percent of them are having a stroke. Specialists can help identify those people using tests that measure certain eye movements. Hopkins is starting to test a "tele-dizzy" program that would capture those eye movements with video goggles and send the recordings to specialists for evaluation, all within an hour.

CANCER PATIENT PEGGY ZUCKERMAN IS NOW MONITORED BY ONCOLOGIST YUAN YUAN AT CITY OF HOPE.

Patients, too, play a key role in the process. You can improve your odds of getting good answers by providing an accurate description of symptoms, a list of your medications, and your personal and family medical histories.

To help reduce mental shortcut mistakes, patients also have to ask questions. "The universal antidote for patients is, when given a diagnosis, to ask 'What else could this be?'" says Graber. You should also ask how the illness is expected to evolve, and what to do if it doesn't go away or worsens. Ask for a second opinion if you receive a worrisome diagnosis.

You can help to protect yourself by getting copies of all your medical records, checking for obvious errors, and making sure they reflect what you've been told. And, says Dhaliwal, "you can't work under the assumption that no news is good news." Follow-up, he says, "should land on your to-do list as well as ours." ●

if not, to figure out how they can do better next time. At the University of Pittsburgh Medical Center, William Follansbee, the master clinician professor of cardiovascular medicine, is using a checklist to help trainee doctors break the decision-making process into five specific steps, including describing the case briefly and asking themselves whether any available information is discordant with the diagnosis. "We can't turn every physician into a cognitive psychologist, but we can make them more aware of when they might be getting into trouble," says Follansbee.

Industry officials counter that their tests are accurate and even lifesaving, and point out that some FDA-approved tests are already obsolete by the time they get through the lengthy review process. Alan Mertz, president of the American Clinical Laboratory Association, says that "LDTs can be created within a matter of months or even weeks, like the tests for Ebola and SARS, which helps public health laboratories do tests in the middle of these pandemics." Tests developed to recognize HIV infections greatly helped control their spread and guide treatment, he says.

At least 50,000 LDTs are routinely employed to assess saliva, tissue and blood samples. "LDTs are ubiquitous in hospitals and in health care," says Roger D. Klein, medical director of molecular pathology at the Cleveland Clinic. "Where I work, almost everything is an LDT."

USES RANGE FROM screening newborns for a number of illnesses and prenatal testing for Down syndrome to helping women found to have certain mutations make decisions about preventive mastectomy. A few instances of faulty test results have caused women to get mastectomies only to find out later that their mutation had no significance, says Otis Brawley, chief medical officer of the American Cancer Society. "Because

these sorts of things happen, there does need to be some science to justify a test," he argues.

Until the oversight situation changes, patients are wise to discuss the chance of error with their doctors before moving forward. Because the FDA-approved tests can become outdated with technology advancing so swiftly, your best bet may be an LDT. "Talk to your doctor and do some research," advises Klein. "Many LDTs, like ones for oncology applications and heritable diseases, are usually quite accurate." Many insurers insist that tests are proven, so if yours is unwilling to reimburse for one, he says, that might be a red flag. –Linda Marsa

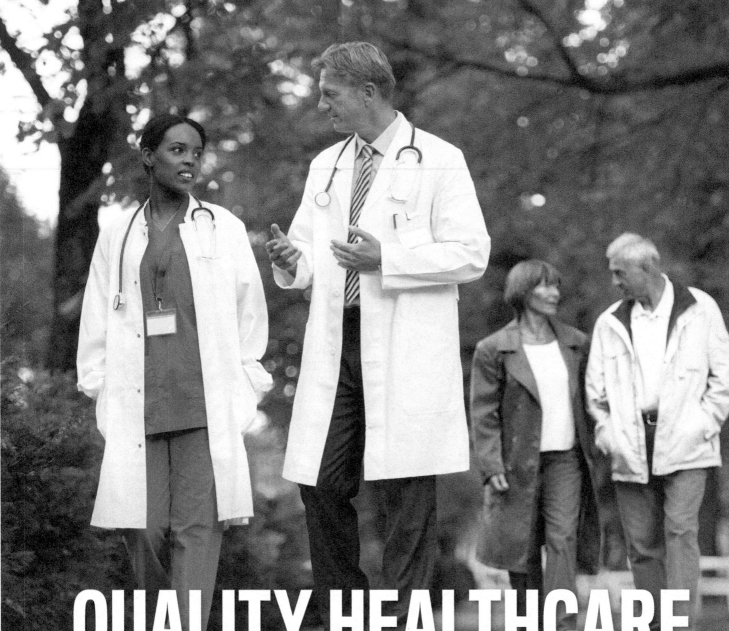

QUALITY HEALTHCARE
Could Be Closer Than You Think.

Too often, we don't consider hospitals until life events make it necessary. But it's never too soon to research where to receive the best care, and fortunately, the best care could be located in your area. Find your best option from this list of recognized hospitals, all of which are dedicated to providing up-to-date, scientific, guidelines-based treatment to the patients in their communities.

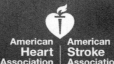

American Heart Association | American Stroke Association

life is why™

U.S. News Brand*Fuse*

THE HEART-SMART PATIENT

The key is to start with modest goals, then stick to them.

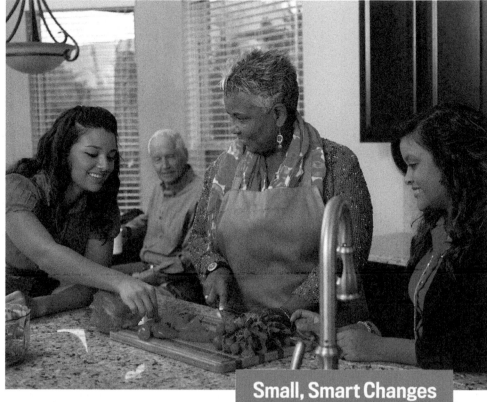

Heart disease strikes someone in the U.S. about once every 42 seconds. It's the No. 1 cause of death in this country, killing more than 370,000 people a year. Fortunately, there are simple, inexpensive lifestyle changes that lead to big improvements in your heart health.

Just starting with these seven changes will have a big impact on many heart-risk factors.

1. Eat healthy. Try fruits, vegetables, whole grains, low-fat dairy, poultry, fish and nuts, and limit red meat and sugary foods and beverages. To get on track, look carefully at nutrition labels. Pick products with the least amount of sodium, added sugars, saturated fat and trans fat.

2. Manage blood pressure. Known as "the silent killer," asymptomatic high blood pressure (higher than 140 systolic or above or 90 diastolic or above) often leads to heart attack, stroke, kidney damage and vision loss.

To make a change, try a different diet. Your doctor may recommend reducing salt consumption, avoiding tobacco smoke, getting regular physical activity and maintaining a healthy weight.

3. Control cholesterol. High levels of low-density lipoprotein (LDL) cholesterol contribute to plaque, the waxy substance that clogs arteries and leads to heart disease and stroke. But low levels of high-density lipoprotein (HDL) cholesterol (which helps remove LDL cholesterol from your arteries) can increase the risk of heart disease.

Healthy eating and increased exercise will help you achieve the right balance. According to the American Heart Association's Chief Medical Officer for Prevention, Dr. Eduardo Sanchez, "What a person eats and portion sizes may contribute to high cholesterol and a higher risk of heart attacks and strokes. Eating more fruits and vegetables, in place of fatty, calorie dense foods, is one approach to improve the heart healthfulness of our diets."

4. Lower blood sugar. Blood sugar acts as fuel for the body. High levels can lead to diabetes, which can cause damage to your heart, kidneys, eyes and nerves. Controlling portions and reading food labels are important, as is limiting simple carbohydrates, such as table sugar, soda and candy.

5. Get moving. "Regular physical activity must also be part of a plan to improve heart health," Dr. Sanchez says. If you haven't been exercising, start with walking just 20 to 30 minutes every day. Physical activity can help lower your blood pressure and cholesterol.

6. Keep the weight off. This will reduce the strain on the heart, lungs and blood vessels. To do so, you'll need to burn more calories than you take in. One pound equals 3,500 calories; most people need to subtract about 500 calories daily from their diet to lose about a pound each week.

7. Quit smoking. This is one of the most important steps to improving heart health. Some people are able to quit on their own, but others need help. An M.D. may recommend smoking cessation classes and support groups. You may also benefit from medical therapy, such as nicotine replacement medicines and non-nicotine prescription medicine, which can reduce the urge.

Small, Smart Changes

Cook fresh foods.
East less red meat and more fruits and vegetables.

Get a stationary bike.
It's easy and safe. Start with five minutes at a time.

Talk to your doctor.
In addition to a healthy lifestyle, you might need a prescription to lower cholesterol or blood pressure.

Want more tips?
Read the full "Heart-Smart Patient article at usnews.com

A KEY TO THE AWARD LEVELS

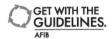
GET WITH THE GUIDELINES. AFIB

SILVER ACHIEVEMENT
These hospitals are recognized for 12 consecutive months of 85% or higher adherence on all achievement measures applicable to atrial fibrillation (AFIB)

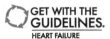
GET WITH THE GUIDELINES. HEART FAILURE

GOLD PLUS ACHIEVEMENT
These hospitals are recognized for two or more consecutive years of 85% or higher adherence on all achievement measures applicable and 75% or higher adherence with four or more select quality measures in heart failure (HF)

GOLD ACHIEVEMENT
These hospitals are recognized for two or more consecutive years of 85% or higher adherence on all achievement measures applicable to heart failure (HF)

SILVER PLUS ACHIEVEMENT
These hospitals are recognized for 12 consecutive months of 85% or higher adherence on all achievement measures applicable and 75% or higher adherence with four or more select quality measures in heart failure (HF)

SILVER ACHIEVEMENT
These hospitals are recognized for 12 consecutive months of 85% or higher adherence on all achievement measures applicable to heart failure (HF)

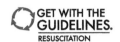
GET WITH THE GUIDELINES. RESUSCITATION

GOLD ACHIEVEMENT
These hospitals are recognized for two or more consecutive years of 85% or higher adherence to designated achievement measures applicable to resuscitation (R)

SILVER ACHIEVEMENT
These hospitals are recognized for one calendar year of 85% or higher adherence to designated achievement measures applicable to resuscitation (R)

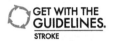
GET WITH THE GUIDELINES. STROKE

GOLD PLUS ACHIEVEMENT
These hospitals are recognized for two or more consecutive years of 85% or higher adherence on all achievement measures applicable and at least 75% or higher adherence with five or more select quality measures in stroke (S)

GOLD ACHIEVEMENT
These hospitals are recognized for two or more consecutive years of 85% or higher adherence on all achievement measures applicable to strokee (S)

SILVER PLUS ACHIEVEMENT
These hospitals are recognized for 12 consecutive months of 85% or higher adherence on all achievement measures applicable and at least 75% or higher adherence with five or more select quality measures in stroke (S)

SILVER ACHIEVEMENT
These hospitals are recognized for 12 consecutive months of 85% or higher adherence on all achievement measures applicable to stroke (S)

MISSION: LIFELINE

GOLD PLUS RECEIVING
These hospitals meet Gold Receiving Center criteria and in addition are recognized for 75% or higher achievement of First Door-to-Device time of 120 minutes or less for transferred STEMI patients

GOLD RECEIVING
These hospitals are recognized for consecutive 24-month intervals of 85% or higher composite adherence to all STEMI Receiving Center Performance Achievement indicators and 75% or higher compliance on each performance measure

GOLD REFERRING
These hospitals are recognized for consecutive 24-month intervals of 85% or higher composite adherence to all STEMI Referring Center Performance Achievement indicators and 75% or higher compliance on each performance measure

SILVER PLUS RECEIVING
These hospitals meet Silver Receiving Center criteria and in addition are recognized for 75% or higher achievement of First Door-to-Device time of 120 minutes or less for transferred STEMI patients

SILVER RECEIVING
These hospitals are recognized for consecutive 12-month intervals of 85% or higher composite adherence to all STEMI Receiving Center Performance Achievement indicators and 75% or higher compliance on each performance measure

SILVER REFERRING
These hospitals are recognized for consecutive 12-month intervals of 85% or higher composite adherence to all STEMI Referring Center Performance Achievement indicators and 75% or higher compliance on each performance measure

TARGET: HF

HONOR ROLL
These hospitals are recognized for at least one calendar quarter of 50% or higher adherence to all relevant Target: Heart Failure measures in addition to current Bronze, Silver or Gold Get With The Guidelines-Heart Failure recognition status

TARGET: STROKE

HONOR ROLL ELITE PLUS
These hospitals are recognized for at least four consecutive quarters of 75% or higher achievement of door-to-needle times within 60 minutes AND 50% achievement of door-to-needle times within 45 minutes in applicable stroke patients in addition to currtent Silver or Gold Get With The Guidelines-Stroke recognition status.

HONOR ROLL ELITE
These hospitals are recognized for at least four consecutive quarters of 75% or higher achievement of door-to-needle times within 60 minutes in applicable stroke patients in addition to current Silver or Gold Get With The Guidelines-Stroke recognition status.

HONOR ROLL
These hospitals are recognized for one calendar quarter of 50% or higher achievement of door-to-needle times within 60 minutes in applicable stroke patients in addition to current Bronze, Silver or Gold Get With The Guidelines-Stroke recognition status.

A BIG THANKS TO OUR SPONSORS.

We appreciate these sponsors for funding our healthcare quality programs and for respecting our clinical independence.

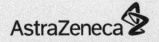 AstraZeneca

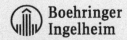 Boehringer Ingelheim

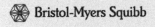 Medtronic

 Bristol-Myers Squibb

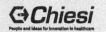 Pfizer

 Chiesi — People and ideas for innovation in healthcare

 Daiichi-Sankyo

AMGEN Cardiovascular

Find your hospital listed alphabetically by state!

For a searchable map of hospitals within this region and across the U.S. visit heart.org/myhealthcare

ALABAMA

- Baptist Medical Center South, Montgomery, AL
- Brookwood Medical Center, Birmingham, AL
- Coosa Valley Medical Center, Sylacauga, AL
- Crestwood Medical Center, Huntsville, AL
- Eliza Coffee Memorial Hospital, Florence, AL
- Flowers Hospital, Dothan, AL
- Gadsden Regional Medical Center, Gadsden, AL
- Grandview Medical Center, Birmingham, AL
- Huntsville Hospital, Huntsville, AL
- Mobile Infirmary, Mobile, AL
- Princeton Baptist Medical Center, Birmingham, AL
- Providence Hospital, Mobile, AL
- South Baldwin Regional Medical Center, Foley, AL
- Southeast Alabama Medical Center, Dothan, AL
- St. Vincent's Birmingham, Birmingham, AL
- Stringfellow Memorial Hospital, Anniston, AL
- Trinity Medical Center, Birmingham, AL
- UAB Hospital, Birmingham, AL
- University of South Alabama Medical Center, Mobile, AL
- Walker Baptist Medical Center, Jasper, AL

ALASKA

- Alaska Regional Hospital, Anchorage, AK
- Providence Alaska Medical Center, Anchorage, AK

ARIZONA

- Abrazo Arizona Heart Hospital, Phoenix, AZ
- Abrazo Arrowhead Campus, Glendale, AZ
- Abrazo Central Campus, Phoenix, AZ
- Abrazo Maryvale Campus, Phoenix, AZ
- Abrazo Scottsdale Campus, Phoenix, AZ
- Banner Baywood Medical Center, Mesa, AZ
- Banner Boswell Medical Center, Sun City, AZ
- Banner Del E. Webb Medical Center, Sun City West, AZ
- Banner Desert Medical Center, Mesa, AZ
- Banner Estrella Medical Center, Phoenix, AZ
- Banner Thunderbird Medical Center, Glendale, AZ
- Banner University Medical Center Phoenix, Phoenix, AZ
- Banner University Medical Center Tucson, Tucson, AZ
- Carondelet Neurological Institute at St. Joseph's Hospital, Tucson, AZ
- Carondelet St. Mary's Hospital, Tucson, AZ
- Dignity Health - Chandler Regional Medical Center, Chandler, AZ
- Dignity Health - Mercy Gilbert Medical Center, Gilbert, AZ
- Dignity Health St. Joseph's Hospital & Medical Center, Phoenix, AZ
- HonorHealth Deer Valley Medical Center, Phoenix, AZ
- HonorHealth John C. Lincoln Medical Center, Phoenix, AZ
- HonorHealth Scottsdale Osborn Medical Center, Scottsdale, AZ
- Mayo Clinic Hospital, Phoenix, AZ
- Mountain Vista Medical Center, Mesa, AZ
- Tucson Medical Center, Tucson, AZ

ARKANSAS

- Baptist Health Medical Center, Little Rock, AR
- CHI St. Vincent Hot Spings, Hot Springs, AR
- Mercy Hospital Rogers, Rogers, AR
- Sparks Health System, Fort Smith, AR
- St. Bernards Medical Center, Jonesboro, AR
- University of Arkansas for Medical Sciences, Little Rock, AR
- Washington Regional Medical Center, Fayetteville, AR

CALIFORNIA

- Alameda Hospital, Alameda, CA
- Alta Bates Summit Medical Center, Berkeley and Oakland, CA
- Arrowhead Regional Medical Center, Colton, CA
- California Hospital Medical Center, Los Angeles, CA
- California Pacific Medical Center, San Francisco, CA
- Cedars-Sinai Medical Center, Los Angeles, CA
- CHA Hollywood Presbyterian Medical Center, Los Angeles, CA
- CITRUS VALLEY MEDICAL CENTER Inter-Community Campus, Covina, CA
- CITRUS VALLEY MEDICAL CENTER Queen of the Valley Campus, West Covina, CA
- Community Hospital of the Monterey Peninsula, Monterey, CA
- Community Memorial Health System, Ventura, CA
- Desert Regional Medical Center, Palm Springs, CA
- Dignity Health Bakersfield Memorial Hospital, Bakersfield, CA
- Dignity Health Dominican Hospital, Santa Cruz, CA
- Dignity Health Mercy General Hospital, Sacramento, CA
- Dignity Health Mercy San Juan Medical Center, Carmichael, CA
- Dignity Health Methodist Hospital of Sacramento, Sacramento, CA
- Dignity Health Northridge Hospital Medical Center, Northridge, CA
- Dignity Health Sequoia Hospital, Redwood City, CA
- Dignity Health St Bernardine Medical Center, San Bernardino, CA
- Dignity Health St. John's Regional Medical Center, Oxnard, CA
- Doctors Hospital of Manteca, Manteca, CA
- Doctors Medical Center, Modesto, CA
- El Camino Hospital, Mountain View, CA
- Emanuel Medical Center, Turlock, CA
- Encino Hospital Medical Center, Encino, CA
- Enloe Medical Center, Chico, CA
- Fountain Valley Regional Hospital and Medical Center, Fountain Valley, CA
- French Hospital Medical Center, San Luis Obispo, CA
- Garfield Medical Center, Monterey Park, CA
- Glendale Adventist Medical Center, Glendale, CA
- Good Samaritan Hospital - San Jose, San Jose, CA
- Henry Mayo Newhall Hospital, Valencia, CA
- Hoag Memorial Hospital Presbyterian, Newport Beach, CA
- Huntington Hospital, Pasadena, CA
- John F. Kennedy Memorial Hospital, Indio, CA
- John Muir Medical Center - Concord, Concord, CA
- John Muir Medical Center- Walnut Creek, Walnut Creek, CA
- Kaiser Foundation Hospital - Antioch, Antioch, CA
- Kaiser Foundation Hospital - Sacramento, Sacramento, CA
- Kaiser Foundation Hospital - San Diego, San Diego, CA
- Kaiser Foundation Hospital - San Francisco, San Francisco, CA
- Kaiser Foundation Hospital - Santa Clara, Santa Clara, CA
- Kaiser Foundation Hospital - Vacaville, Vacaville, CA
- Kaiser Foundation Hospital - Walnut Creek, Walnut Creek, CA
- Kaiser Foundation Hospital and Rehabilitation Center - Vallejo, Vallejo, CA
- Kaiser Foundation Hospital Roseville, Roseville, CA
- Kaiser Foundation Hospital- Redwood City, Redwood City, CA
- Kaiser Foundation Hospital, Downey, Downey, CA
- Kaiser Foundation Hospital, South San Francisco, South San Francisco, CA
- Kaiser Foundation Hospitals Manteca/Modesto, Manteca and Modesto, CA
- Kaiser Permanente - Fresno, Fresno, CA
- Kaiser Permanente - Los Angeles Medical Center, Los Angeles, CA
- Kaiser Permanente Baldwin Park Medical Center, Baldwin Park, CA
- Kaiser Permanente East Bay Oakland and Richmond Medical Centers, Oakland, CA
- Kaiser Permanente Fontana Medical Center, Fontana, CA
- Kaiser Permanente Fremont Medical Center, Fremont, CA
- Kaiser Permanente Hospital San Jose, San Jose, CA
- Kaiser Permanente Medical Center: San Rafael, San Rafael, CA
- Kaiser Permanente Moreno Valley Medical Center, Moreno Valley, CA
- Kaiser Permanente Ontario Medical Center, Ontario, CA
- Kaiser Permanente Riverside Medical Center, Riverside, CA
- Kaiser Permanente Santa Rosa Hospital, Santa Rosa, CA
- Kaiser Permanente South Bay Medical Center, Harbor City, CA
- Kaiser Permanente South Sacramento, Sacramento, CA
- Kaiser Permanente Woodland Hills Medical Center, Woodland Hills, CA
- Kaweah Delta, Visalia, CA
- Lakewood Regional Medical Center, Lakewood, CA
- Loma Linda University Health, Loma Linda, CA
- Long Beach Memorial, Long Beach, CA
- Los Alamitos Medical Center, Los Alamitos, CA
- Los Robles Hospital & Medical Center, Thousand Oaks, CA
- Marin General Hospital, Greenbrae, CA
- Marshall Medical Center, Placerville, CA
- Mercy Hospital of Folsom, Folsom, CA
- Mercy Hospitals, Bakersfield, CA
- Mercy Medical Center, Merced, CA
- Mercy Medical Center - Redding, Redding, CA
- Methodist Hospital of Southern California, Arcadia, CA
- Mills-Peninsula Health Services, Burlingame, CA
- NorthBay Healthcare, Fairfield, CA
- O'Connor Hospital, San Jose, CA
- Oroville Hospital, Oroville, CA
- PIH Health Hospital, Whittier, CA
- Placentia-Linda Hospital, Placentia, CA
- Pomona Valley Hospital Medical Center, Pomona, CA
- Providence Holy Cross Medical Center, Mission Hills, CA
- Providence Little Company of Mary Medical Center - San Pedro, San Pedro, CA
- Providence St. Joseph Medical Center, Burbank, CA
- Providence Tarzana Medical Center, Tarzana, CA
- Redlands Community Hospital, Redlands, CA
- Regional Medical Center of San Jose, San Jose, CA
- Riverside Community Hospital, Riverside, CA

American Heart Association | American Stroke Association.
life is why™

Riverside University Health System - Medical Center, Moreno Valley, CA
Ronald Reagan UCLA Medical Center, Los Angeles, CA
Saddleback Memorial Medical Center, Laguna Hills, CA
Saint Francis Memorial Hospital, San Francisco, CA
Saint Louise Regional Hospital, Gilroy, CA
Salinas Valley Memorial Healthcare System, Salinas, CA
San Antonio Regional Hospital, Upland, CA
San Joaquin Community Hospital, Bakersfield, CA
San Joaquin General Hospital, French Camp, CA
San Ramon Regional Medical Center, San Ramon, CA
Scripps Encinitas Memorial Hospital, Encinitas, CA
Scripps Green Hospital, La Jolla, CA
Scripps Memorial Hospital La Jolla, La Jolla, CA
Scripps Mercy Hospital San Diego and Chula Vista, San Diego, CA
Seton Medical Center - Daly City, Daly City, CA
Sharp Chula Vista Medical Center, Chula Vista, CA
Sharp Grossmont Hospital, La Mesa, CA
Sharp Memorial Hospital, San Diego, CA
Sherman Oaks Hospital, Sherman Oaks, CA
Sierra Nevada Memorial Hospital, Grass Valley, CA
Sierra Vista Regional Medical Center, San Luis Obispo, CA
Simi Valley Hospital, Simi Valley, CA
Southwest Healthcare System, Wildomar, CA
Southwest Healthcare System, Murrieta, CA
St Jude Medical Center, Fullerton, CA
St. Francis Medical Center, Lynwood, CA
St. John's Pleasant Valley Hospital, Camarillo, CA
St. Mary's Medical Center, San Francisco, CA
Sutter Health Eden Medical Center, Castro Valley, CA
Sutter Health Memorial Medical Center, Modesto, CA
Sutter Novato Community Hospital, Novato, CA
Temecula Valley Hospital, Temecula, CA
Torrance Memorial Medical Center, Torrance, CA
Tri-City Medical Center, Oceanside, CA
Twin Cities Community Hospital, Templeton, CA
UC San Diego Health System, La Jolla, CA
UC San Diego Health System, San Diego, CA
Ukiah Valley Medical Center, Ukiah, CA
University of California Irvine Medical Center, Orange, CA
University of California, Davis Medical Center, Sacramento, CA
USC Norris Cancer Hospital, Los Angeles, CA
USC Verdugo Hills Hospital, Glendale, CA
Ventura County Medical Center/Santa Paula Hospital, Ventura, CA
Washington Hospital Healthcare System, Fremont, CA
White Memorial Medical Center, Los Angeles, CA
Woodland Memorial Hospital - Woodland Healthcare, Woodland, CA

COLORADO

Boulder Community Health Foothills Hospital, Boulder, CO
Denver Health Medical Center, Denver, CO
Good Samaritan Medical Center, Lafayette, CO
Littleton Adventist Hospital, Littleton, CO
Lutheran Medical Center, Wheat Ridge, CO
Medical Center of the Rockies, Loveland, CO
Memorial Health System, Colorado Springs, CO
North Colorado Medical Center, Greeley, CO
Parker Adventist Hospital, Parker, CO
Parkview Medical Center, Pueblo, CO
Penrose-St. Francis Health Services, Colorado Springs, CO
Platte Valley Medical Center, Brighton, CO
Porter Adventist Hospital- Centura Health, Denver, CO
Presbyterian/St. Luke's Medical Center, Denver, CO
Rose Medical Center, Denver, CO
Sky Ridge Medical Center, Lone Tree, CO
St. Anthony Hospital, Lakewood, CO
St. Anthony North Hospital, Westminster, CO
St. Mary - Corwin Medical Center, Pueblo, CO
St. Mary's Hospital and Medical Center, Grand Junction, CO
Swedish Medical Center, Englewood, CO
The Medical Center of Aurora, Aurora, CO
University of Colorado Hospital, Aurora, CO

CONNECTICUT

Bridgeport Hospital, Bridgeport, CT
Connecticut Children's Medical Center, Hartford, CT
Eastern Connecticut Health Network, Manchester and Rockville, Manchester, CT
Greenwich Hospital, Greenwich, CT
Griffin Hospital, Derby, CT
Hartford Hospital, Hartford, CT
John Dempsey Hospital/UCONN Health Center, Farmington, CT
Lawrence + Memorial Hospital, New London, CT
MidState Medical Center, Meriden, CT
Norwalk Hospital, Norwalk, CT
Saint Francis Hospital and Medical Center, Hartford, CT

Saint Mary's Health System, Waterbury, CT
St. Vincent's Medical Center, Bridgeport, CT
Stamford Hospital, Stamford, CT
The Hospital of Central Connecticut, New Britain, CT
The William W. Backus Hospital, Norwich, CT
Waterbury Hospital, Waterbury, CT
Yale - New Haven Hospital, New Haven, CT

DELAWARE

Beebe Healthcare, Lewes, DE
Christiana Care Health System, Newark, DE
Nanticoke Memorial Hospital, Seaford, DE
Saint Francis Hospital, Wilmington, DE

DISTRICT OF COLUMBIA

MedStar Washington Hospital Center, Washington, DC
Providence Hospital, Washington, DC
Sibley Memorial Hospital, Washington, DC
The George Washington University Hospital, Washington, DC

FLORIDA

Arnold Palmer Hospital for Children, Orlando, FL
Aventura Hospital and Medical Center, Aventura, FL
Baptist Hospital of Miami, Miami, FL
Baptist Medical Center - Beaches (Baptist Health), Jacksonville Beach, FL
Baptist Medical Center - Jacksonville (Baptist Health), Jacksonville, FL
Baptist Medical Center - South (Baptist Health), Jacksonville, FL
Baptist Medical Center of Nassau, Inc., Fernandina Beach, FL
Bayfront Health St. Petersburg, St. Petersburg, FL
Boca Raton Regional Hospital, Boca Raton, FL
Brandon Regional Hospital, Brandon, FL
Broward Health Coral Springs, Coral Springs, FL
Broward Health Medical Center, Fort Lauderdale, FL
Broward Health North, Pompano Beach, FL
Cape Coral Hospital, Cape Coral, FL
Capital Regional Medical Center, Tallahassee, FL
Central Florida Regional Hospital, Sanford, FL
Cleveland Clinic Florida, Weston, FL
Delray Medical Center, Delray Beach, FL
Doctors Hospital of Sarasota, Sarasota, FL
Englewood Community Hospital, Englewood, FL
Flagler Hospital, Inc., Saint Augustine, FL
Florida Hospital Altamonte, Altamonte Springs, FL
Florida Hospital Apopka, Apopka, FL
Florida Hospital Celebration Health, Celebration, FL
Florida Hospital DeLand, DeLand, FL
Florida Hospital East Orlando, Orlando, FL
Florida Hospital Fish Memorial, Orange City, FL
Florida Hospital Flagler, Palm Coast, FL
Florida Hospital Kissimmee, Kissimmee, FL
Florida Hospital Memorial Medical Center, Daytona Beach, FL
Florida Hospital New Smyrna, New Smyrna Beach, FL
Florida Hospital North Pinellas, Tarpon Springs, FL
Florida Hospital Orlando, Orlando, FL
Florida Hospital Tampa, Tampa, FL
Florida Hospital Wesley Chapel, Wesley Chapel, FL
Florida Hospital Zephyrhills, Zephyrhills, FL
FLORIDA MEDICAL CENTER a campus of North Shore, Fort Lauderdale, FL
Fort Walton Beach Medical Center, Fort Walton Beach, FL
Good Samaritan Medical Center, West Palm Beach, FL
Gulf Coast Medical Center, Fort Myers, FL
Halifax Health, Daytona Beach, FL
Health Park Medical Center, Fort Myers, FL
Hialeah Hospital, Hialeah, FL
Holmes Regional Medical Center , Melbourne, FL
Holy Cross Hospital, Fort Lauderdale, FL
Indian River Medical Center, Vero Beach, FL
Jackson Memorial Hospital, Miami, FL
Jackson North Medical Center, North Miami Beach, FL
James A. Haley Veterans' Hospital, Tampa, FL
Jupiter Medical Center, Jupiter, FL
Lakeland Regional Health, Lakeland, FL
Largo Medical Center, Largo, FL
Lee Memorial Hospital, Fort Myers, FL
Manatee Memorial Hospital, Bradenton, FL
Mease Countryside Hospital, Safety Harbor, FL
Memorial Hospital, Jacksonville, FL
Memorial Hospital Pembroke, Pembroke Pines, FL
Memorial Hospital West, Pembroke Pines, FL
Memorial Regional Hospital, Hollywood, FL
Mercy Hospital, Miami, FL
Miami Childrens Hospital, Miami, FL

Morton Plant Hospital, Clearwater, FL
Morton Plant North Bay Hospital, New Port Richey, FL
Mount Sinai Medical Center, Miami Beach, FL
NCH Healthcare System, Naples, FL
North Shore Medical Center, Miami, FL
Northside Hospital and Tampa Bay Heart Institute, Saint Petersburg, FL
Ocala Health, Ocala, FL
Orange Park Medical Center, Orange Park, FL
Orlando Regional Medical Center, Orlando, FL
Osceola Regional Medical Center, Kissimmee, FL
Palm Beach Gardens Medical Center, Palm Beach Gardens, FL
Palmetto General Hospital, Hialeah, FL
Palms of Pasadena Hospital, South Pasadena, FL
Physicians Regional Medical Center – Pine Ridge, Naples, FL
Sacred Heart Health System, Pensacola, FL
Sarasota Memorial Health Care System, Sarasota, FL
South Florida Baptist Hospital, Plant City, FL
St. Joseph's Hospital, Tampa, FL
St. Joseph's Hospital- North, Lutz, FL
St. Mary's Medical Center, West Palm Beach, FL
St. Vincent's Medical Center Riverside, Jacksonville, FL
St. Vincent's Medical Center Southside, Jacksonville, FL
Tallahassee Memorial HealthCare, Tallahassee, FL
Tampa General Hospital, Tampa, FL
UF Health Shands Hospital, Gainesville, FL
University of Miami Hospital, Miami, FL
Venice Regional Bayfront Health, Venice, FL
Wellington Regional Medical Center, Wellington, FL
West Boca Medical Center, Boca Raton, FL
West Florida Hospital, Pensacola, FL
Winter Haven Hospital, Winter Haven, FL
Wuesthoff Medical Center Rockledge, Rockledge, FL

GEORGIA

Atlanta Medical Center, Atlanta, GA
Cartersville Medical Center, Cartersville, GA
Coliseum Medical Centers, Macon, GA
DeKalb Medical Center, Inc., Decatur, GA
Emory Johns Creek Hospital, Duluth, GA
Emory Saint Joseph's Hospital, Atlanta, GA
Emory University Hospital, Atlanta, GA
Emory University Hospital Midtown, Atlanta, GA
Fairview Park Hospital, Dublin, GA
Floyd Medical Center, Rome, GA
Grady Health System, Atlanta, GA
Gwinnett Hospital System, Lawrenceville, GA
Habersham Medical Center, Demorest, GA
Hamilton Medical Center, Dalton, GA
Memorial Health University Medical Center, Savannah, GA
Midtown Medical Center, Columbus, GA
Northside Hospital Atlanta, Atlanta, GA
Northside Hospital Cherokee, Canton, GA
Northside Hospital Forsyth, Cumming, GA
Phoebe Putney Memorial Hospital, Albany, GA
Piedmont Fayette Hospital, Fayetteville, GA
Piedmont Henry Hospital, Stockbridge, GA
Piedmont Hospital, Atlanta, GA
Piedmont Newnan Hospital, Newnan, GA
Redmond Regional Medical Center, Rome, GA
South Georgia Medical Center, Valdosta, GA
Southern Regional Health System, Riverdale, GA
St. Francis Hospital, Inc., Columbus, GA
St. Joseph's Hospital, Savannah, GA
St. Mary's Health Care System, Athens, GA
The Medical Center Navicent Health, Macon, GA
University Hospital, Augusta, GA
Wellstar Cobb Hospital, Austell, GA
WellStar Douglas Hospital, Douglasville, GA
WellStar Kennestone Hospital, Marietta, GA
WellStar North Fulton Hospital, Roswell, GA
WellStar Spalding Regional Hospital, Griffin, GA

HAWAII

Castle Medical Center, Kailua, HI
Hilo Medical Center, Hilo, HI
Kaiser Foundation Hospital - Moanalua, Honolulu, HI
Maui Memorial Medical Center, Wailuku, HI
Pali Momi Medical Center, Aiea, HI
Straub Clinic & Hospital, Honolulu, HI
The Queen's Medical Center, Honolulu, HI
The Queen's Medical Center West Oahu, Ewa Beach, HI
Wahiawa General Hospital, Wahiawa, HI
Wilcox Memorial Hospital, Lihue, HI

IDAHO

Eastern Idaho Regional Medical Center- EIRMC, Idaho Falls, ID
St. Luke's Health System, Treasure Valley, Boise, ID
West Valley Medical Center, Caldwell, ID

ILLINOIS

Advocate BroMenn Medical Center, Normal, IL
Advocate Christ Medical Center, Oak Lawn, IL
Advocate Condell Medical Center, Libertyville, IL
Advocate Good Samaritan Hospital, Downers Grove, IL
Advocate Good Shepherd Hospital, Barrington, IL
Advocate Illinois Masonic Medical Center, Chicago, IL
Advocate Lutheran General Hospital, Park Ridge, IL
Advocate Sherman Hospital, Elgin, IL
Advocate South Suburban Hospital, Hazel Crest, IL
Alexian Brothers Medical Center, Elk Grove Village, IL
Carle Foundation Hospital, Urbana, IL
Centegra Hospital -Woodstock, Woodstock, IL
Centegra Hospital- McHenry, McHenry, IL
Copley Memorial Hospital, Aurora, IL
Decatur Memorial Hospital, Decatur, IL
Edward Hospital, Naperville, IL
Elmhurst Hospital, Elmhurst, IL
FHN Memorial Hospital, Freeport, IL
Galesburg Cottage Hospital, Galesburg, IL
Holy Cross Hospital, Chicago, IL
Loyola University Medical Center, Maywood, IL
MacNeal Hospital, Berwyn, IL
Memorial Hospital of Carbondale, Carbondale, IL
Memorial Medical Center, Springfield, IL
Mercy Hospital & Medical Center, Chicago, IL
Mount Sinai Hospital, Chicago, IL
Northwest Community Hospital, Arlington Heights, IL
Northwestern Lake Forest Hospital, Lake Forest, IL
Northwestern Medicine- Central Dupage Hospital, Winfield, IL
Northwestern Medicine- Delnor Hospital, Geneva, IL
Northwestern Memorial Hospital, Chicago, IL
Northwestern Memorial Hospital, Chicago, IL
OSF Saint Anthony Medical Center, Rockford, IL
OSF Saint Francis Medical Center, Peoria, IL
OSF St. Joseph Medical Center, Bloomington, IL
Presence Saint Francis Hospital, Evanston, IL
Presence Saint Joseph Hospital-Elgin, Elgin, IL
Presence Saint Joseph Medical Center, Joliet, IL
Rush University Medical Center, Chicago, IL
Silver Cross Hospital, New Lenox, IL
SIU Herrin Hospital, Herrin, IL
St. Alexius Medical Center, Hoffman Estates, IL
St. Elizabeth's Hospital, Belleville, IL
St. John's Hospital-Prairie Heart, Springfield, IL
Swedish Covenant Hospital, Chicago, IL
UnityPoint Methodist, Peoria, IL
University of Chicago Medical Center, Chicago, IL
University of Illinois Hospital and Health Sciences Systems, Chicago, IL
Vista Medical Center East, Waukegan, IL

INDIANA

Columbus Regional Hospital, Columbus, IN
Community Hospital, Munster, IN
Community Hospital of Anderson, Anderson, IN
Floyd Memorial Hospital and Health Services, New Albany, IN
Franciscan St. Anthony Health – Michigan City, Michigan City, IN
Franciscan St. Elizabeth Health- Lafayette East, Lafayette, IN
Franciscan St. Francis Health - Indianapolis, Indianapolis, IN
Indiana University Health Ball Memorial Hospital, Muncie, IN
Indiana University Health Methodist Hospital, Indianapolis, IN
IU Health Bloomington Hospital, Bloomington, IN
IU Health West Hospital, Avon, IN
Lutheran Hospital, Fort Wayne, IN
Methodist Hospitals, Inc., Gary, IN
Parkview Health, Fort Wayne, IN
Porter Regional Hospital, Valparaiso, IN
St. Catherine Hospital, Inc., East Chicago, IN
St. Mary Medical Center, Hobart, IN
St. Mary's Medical Center, Evansville, IN
St. Vincent Heart Center of Indiana, Indianapolis, IN
St. Vincent Heart Center of Indiana on the St. Vincent Indianapolis Hospital Campus, Indianapolis, IN

IOWA

Hancock County Memorial Hospital, Britt, IA
Iowa City VA Health Care System, Iowa City, IA
Mercy Iowa City, Iowa City, IA

Mercy Medical Center - Des Moines, Des Moines, IA
Mercy Medical Center - Dubuque, Dubuque, IA
Mercy Medical Center - Sioux City, Sioux City, IA
Mercy West Lakes Hospital, West Des Moines, IA
St. Luke's Regional Medical Center, Sioux City, IA
University of Iowa Hospitals and Clinics, Iowa City, IA

KANSAS

Hays Med, Hays, KS
Menorah Medical Center, Overland Park, KS
Olathe Medical Center, Olathe, KS
Overland Park Regional Medical Center, Overland Park, KS
Saint Catherine Hospital, Garden City, KS
Saint Francis Health Center, Topeka, KS
Saint Luke's South Hospital, Overland Park, KS
Shawnee Mission Medical Center, Shawnee Mission, KS
Stormont-Vail HealthCare, Topeka, KS
The University of Kansas Hospital, Kansas City, KS
Via Christi Hospital St. Francis, Wichita, KS
Wesley Medical Center, Wichita, KS

KENTUCKY

Baptist Health LaGrange, LaGrange, KY
Baptist Health Lexington, Lexington, KY
Baptist Health Louisville, Louisville, KY
Baptist Health Paducah, Paducah, KY
Caldwell County Hospital, Princeton, KY
Fleming County Hospital, Flemingsburg, KY
Hardin Memorial Health, Elizabethtown, KY
Jewish Hospital, Louisville, KY
King's Daughters Medical Center, Ashland, KY
Lake Cumberland Regional Hospital, Somerset, KY
Norton Brownsboro Hospital, Louisville, KY
Norton Hospital, Louisville, KY
Norton Women's and Kosair Children's Hospital, Louisville, KY
Our Lady of Bellefonte Hospital Bon Secours KY Health System, Ashland, KY
Paul B Hall Regional Medical Hospital, Paintsville, KY
Pikeville Medical Center, Pikeville, KY
Saint Joseph Hospital, Lexington, KY
Sts. Mary and Elizabeth Hospital, Louisville, KY
The Medical Center at Bowling Green, Bowling Green, KY
University of Kentucky Hospital, Lexington, KY
University of Louisville Hospital, Louisville, KY

LOUISIANA

CHRISTUS St. Frances Cabrini Hospital, Alexandria, LA
CHRISTUS St. Patrick Hospital, Lake Charles, LA
East Jefferson General Hospital, Metairie, LA
Lakeview Regional Medical Center, Covington, LA
Louisiana Heart Hospital, Lacombe, LA
Ochsner Medical Center - New Orleans, New Orleans, LA
Our Lady of Lourdes Regional Medical Center, Lafayette, LA
Our Lady of the Lake Regional Medical Center, Baton Rouge, LA
Rapides Regional Medical Center, Alexandria, LA
St. Francis Medical Center, Monroe, LA
Terrebonne General Medical Center, Houma, LA
Tulane University Hospital and Clinic, New Orleans, LA
West Jefferson Medical Center, Marrero, LA

MAINE

Central Maine Medical Center, Lewiston, ME
Eastern Maine Medical Center, Bangor, ME
Maine Medical Center, Portland, ME
Mercy Hospital, Portland, ME
Pen Bay Medical Center, Rockport, ME
York Hospital, York, ME

MARYLAND

Adventist HealthCare Shady Grove Medical Center, Rockville, MD
Anne Arundel Medical Center, Annapolis, MD
Atlantic General Hospital, Berlin, MD
Calvert Memorial Hospital, Prince Frederick, MD
Doctor's Community Hospital, Lanham, MD
Frederick Memorial Hospital, Frederick, MD
Greater Baltimore Medical Center, Baltimore, MD
Holy Cross Hospital, Silver Spring, MD
Howard County General Hospital, Columbia, MD
Johns Hopkins Bayview Medical Center, Baltimore, MD
MedStar Franklin Square Medical Center, Baltimore, MD
MedStar Good Samaritan Hospital, Baltimore, MD
MedStar Harbor Hospital, Baltimore, MD
MedStar Montgomery Medical Center, Olney, MD
MedStar Southern Maryland Hospital Center, Clinton, MD
MedStar Union Memorial Hospital, Baltimore, MD
Mercy Medical Center, Baltimore, MD
Meritus Medical Center, Hagerstown, MD
Northwest Hospital, Randallstown, MD
Peninsula Regional Medical Center, Salisbury, MD
Prince George's Hospital Center, Cheverly, MD
Saint Agnes Hospital, Baltimore, MD
Sinai Hospital, Baltimore, MD
Suburban Hospital Johns Hopkins Medicine, Bethesda, MD
The Johns Hopkins Hospital, Baltimore, MD
Union Hospital of Cecil County, Elkton, MD
University of Maryland Baltimore Washington Medical Center, Glen Burnie, MD
University of Maryland Charles Regional Medical Center, La Plata, MD
University of Maryland Medical Center, Baltimore, MD
University of Maryland Medical Center Midtown Campus, Baltimore, MD
University of Maryland Shore Medical Center at Easton, Easton, MD
University of Maryland St. Joseph Medical Center, Towson, MD
University of Maryland Upper Chesapeake Medical Center, Bel Air, MD
Washington Adventist Hospital, Takoma Park, MD
Western Maryland Health System, Cumberland, MD

MASSACHUSETTS

Addison Gilbert Hospital, Gloucester, MA
Baystate Franklin Medical Center, Greenfield, MA
Baystate Mary Lane Hospital, Ware, MA
Baystate Wing Hospital, Palmer, MA
Berkshire Medical Center, Pittsfield, MA
Beth Israel Deaconess Hospital - Needham, Needham, MA
Beth Israel Deaconess Hospital-Plymouth, Plymouth, MA
Beth Israel Deaconess Medical Center, Boston, MA
Beverly Hospital, Beverly, MA
Boston Medical Center, Boston, MA
Brigham and Women's Faulkner Hospital, Boston, MA
Brigham and Women's Hospital, Boston, MA
Cooley Dickinson Hospital, Northampton, MA
Emerson Hospital, Concord, MA
Fairview Hospital, Great Barrington, MA
Falmouth Hospital/Cape Cod Healthcare, Falmouth, MA
Hallmark Health - Lawrence Memorial Hospital, Medford, MA
Harrington Hospital, Southbridge, MA
Heywood Hospital, Gardner, MA
Holyoke Medical Center, Holyoke, MA
Lahey Hospital & Medical Center, Burlington, Burlington, MA
Lowell General Hospital - Main Campus, Lowell, MA
Lowell General Hospital - Saints Campus, Lowell, MA
Massachusetts General Hospital, Boston, MA
Melrose Wakefield Hospital, Melrose, MA
Mercy Medical Center, Springfield, MA
MetroWest Medical Center - Framingham Union Hospital, Framingham, MA
MetroWest Medical Center - Leonard Morse Hospital, Natick, MA
Milford Regional Medical Center, Milford, MA
Mount Auburn Hospital, Cambridge, MA
Nashoba Valley Medical Center, Ayer, MA
Newton-Wellesley Hospital, Newton, MA
Noble Hospital, Westfield, MA
North Shore Medical Center, Lynn, MA
North Shore Medical Center - Salem, Salem, MA
Norwood Hospital, Norwood, MA
Saint Anne's Hospital, Fall River, MA
Saint Vincent Hospital, Worcester, MA
Signature Healthcare Brockton Hospital, Brockton, MA
South Shore Hosptial, South Weymouth, MA
Southcoast Hospitals, St. Luke's Site, New Bedford, MA
St. Elizabeth's Medical Center, Brighton, MA
Sturdy Memorial Hospital, Attleboro, MA
Tufts Medical Center, Boston, MA
UMass Memorial Medical Center, Worcester, MA
UMass Memorial Medical Center – Memorial Campus, Worcester, MA

MICHIGAN

Beaumont Hospital, Grosse Pointe, Grosse Pointe, MI
Beaumont Hospital, Troy, Troy, MI
Borgess Medical Center, Kalamazoo, MI
Covenant HealthCare, Saginaw, MI
Detroit Receiving Hospital, Detroit, MI
DMC Harper University Hospital, Detroit, MI
DMC Huron Valley Hospital, Commerce Township, MI
DMC Sinai Grace Hospital, Detroit, MI
Garden City Hospital, Garden City, MI
Genesys Regional Medical Center, Grand Blanc, MI
Henry Ford Hospital and Health Network, Detroit, MI
Henry Ford Macomb Hospital, Clinton Township, MI
Holland Hospital, Holland, MI
Lakeland Healthcare, Saint Joseph, MI

McLaren - Flint, Flint, MI
McLaren Bay Region, Bay City, MI
McLaren Greater Lansing, Lansing, MI
McLaren Northern Michigan, Petoskey, MI
McLaren Oakland, Pontiac, MI
McLaren Port Huron Hospital, Port Huron, MI
Mercy Health Saint Mary's, Grand Rapids, MI
Metro Health Hospital, Wyoming, MI
MidMichigan Medical Center-Midland an affiliate of MidMichigan Health System, Midland, MI
Munson Medical Center, Traverse City, MI
ProMedica Bixby Hospital, Adrian, MI
Promedica Herrick Hospital, Tecumseh, MI
Sparrow Hospital, Lansing, MI
St. Joseph Mercy Hospital Ann Arbor, Ypsilanti, MI
St. Joseph Mercy Livingston Hospital, Ypsilanti, MI
St. Joseph Mercy Oakland, Pontiac, MI
St. Mary Mercy Hospital, Livonia, MI
St. Mary's of Michigan, Saginaw, MI
University of Michigan Health System, Ann Arbor, MI

MINNESOTA

CentraCare Health St. Cloud Hospital, Saint Cloud, MN
Essentia Health East. St. Mary's Medical Center, Duluth, MN
Fairview Southdale Hospital, Edina, MN
Mayo Clinic Health System in Mankato, Mankato, MN
Mayo Clinic Hospital, Saint Marys Campus, Rochester, MN
Mercy Hospital, Coon Rapids, MN
North Memorial Medical Center, Robbinsdale, MN
Regions Hospital, Saint Paul, MN
St. Luke's, Duluth, MN
University of Minnesota Heart Care at Fairview Ridges Hospital, Burnsville, MN
University of Minnesota Medical Center, Minneapolis, MN

MISSISSIPPI

Baptist Memorial Hospital - DeSoto, Southaven, MS
Baptist Memorial Hospital - -Golden Triangle, Columbus, MS
Baptist Memorial Hospital - North Mississippi, Oxford, MS
Forrest General Hospital, Hattiesburg, MS
Magnolia Regional Health Center, Corinth, MS
Merit Health Wesley, Hattiesburg, MS
MS Baptist Medical Center, Jackson, MS
Ocean Springs Hospital (Singing River Health System), Ocean Springs, MS
River Oaks Hospital, Jackson, MS
Singing River Hospital (Singing River Health System), Pascagoula, MS
St. Dominic Memorial Hospital, Jackson, MS
University of Mississippi Health Care, Jackson, MS

MISSOURI

Barnes-Jewish Hospital, Saint Louis, MO
Boone Hospital, Columbia, MO
Centerpoint Medical Center, Independence, MO
Christian Hospital, Saint Louis, MO
Citizens Memorial Health Care, Bolivar, MO
Cox Medical Center Branson, Branson, MO
CoxHealth, Springfield, MO
Des Peres Hospital, Saint Louis, MO
Freeman Health System, Joplin, MO
Lake Regional Hospital, Osage Beach, MO
Lee's Summit Medical Center, Lees Summit, MO
Liberty Hospital, Liberty, MO
Mercy Hospital Jefferson, Crystal City, MO
Mercy Hospital Springfield, Springfield, MO
Mercy Hospital St. Louis, Saint Louis, MO
Mosaic Life Care, Saint Joseph, MO
North Kansas City Hospital, North Kansas City, MO
Parkland Health Center, Farmington, MO
Progress West Hospital, O Fallon, MO
Research Medical Center, Kansas City, MO
Saint Luke's East Hospital, Lees Summit, MO
Saint Luke's Hospital of Kansas City, Kansas City, MO
Saint Luke's North Hospital, Kansas City, MO
Southeast Health, Cape Girardeau, MO
SSM DePaul Health Center, Bridgeton, MO
SSM Health Saint Louis University Hospital, Saint Louis, MO
SSM St. Clare Health Center, Fenton, MO
SSM St. Joseph Health Center, Saint Charles, MO
SSM St. Joseph Hospital West, Lake St Louis, MO
SSM. St. Mary's Health Center, Richmond Heights, MO
St. Anthony's Medical Center, Saint Louis, MO
St. Joseph Medical Center, Kansas City, MO
St. Luke's Hospital, Chesterfield, MO
St. Mary's Medical Center, Blue Springs, MO
University of Missouri Health Care, Columbia, MO

MONTANA

Bozeman Health Deaconess Hospital, Bozeman, MT
Benefis Health System, Great Falls, MT
Billings Clinic, Billings, MT
Kalispell Regional Medical Center, Kalispell, MT
Providence St. Patrick Hospital, Missoula, MT
St. Peter's Hospital, Helena, MT

NEBRASKA

BryanLGH Medical Center, Lincoln, NE
CHI Health Creighton University Medical Center, Omaha, NE
Good Samaritan Health System, Kearney, NE
Great Plains Health, North Platte, NE
Nebraska Medicine, Omaha, NE
Nebraska Methodist Hospital, Omaha, NE
Saint Elizabeth Regional Medical Center, Lincoln, NE

NEVADA

Centennial Hills Hospital Medical Center, Las Vegas, NV
Desert Springs Hospital Medical Center, Las Vegas, NV
MountainView Hospital, Las Vegas, NV
Northern Nevada Medical Center, Sparks, NV
Renown Regional Medical Center, Reno, NV
Saint Mary's Regional Medical Center, Reno, NV
Southern Hills Hospital and Medical Center, Las Vegas, NV
Spring Valley Hospital Medical Center, Las Vegas, NV
St. Rose Dominican - Rose de Lima Campus, Henderson, NV
St. Rose Dominican - Siena Campus, Henderson, NV
St. Rose Dominican- San Martin Campus, Las Vegas, NV
Summerlin Hospital Medical Center, Las Vegas, NV
Sunrise Hospital and Medical Center, Las Vegas, NV
University Medical Center of Southern Nevada, Las Vegas, NV
Valley Hospital Medical Center, Las Vegas, NV

NEW HAMPSHIRE

Catholic Medical Center, Manchester, NH
Exeter Hospital, Exeter, NH
Southern New Hampshire Medical Center, Nashua, NH
St. Joseph Hospital, Nashua, NH
Wentworth-Douglass Hospital, Dover, NH

NEW JERSEY

Bayshore Community Hospital, Holmdel, NJ
Capital Health Medical Center - Hopewell, Pennington, NJ
Capital Health Regional Medical Center, Trenton, NJ
CarePoint Health - Bayonne Medical Center, Bayonne, NJ
CarePoint Health - Christ Hospital, Jersey City, NJ
CarePoint Health - Hoboken University Medical Center, Hoboken, NJ
CentraState Medical Center, Freehold, NJ
Chilton Medical Center, Pompton Plains, NJ
Cooper University Hospital, Camden, NJ
Englewood Hospital and Medical Center, Englewood, NJ
Hackensack University Medical Center, Hackensack, NJ
HackensackUMC Mountainside, Montclair, NJ
HackensackUMC Palisades, North Bergen, NJ
Holy Name Medical Center, Teaneck, NJ
Inspira Medical Center Elmer, Elmer, NJ
Inspira Medical Center Vineland, Vineland, NJ
Inspira Medical Center Woodbury, Woodbury, NJ
Jersey City Medical Center – Barnabas Health, Jersey City, NJ
Jersey Shore University Medical Center, Neptune, NJ
JFK Medical Center, Edison, NJ
Kennedy University Hospital- Cherry Hill, Cherry Hill, NJ
Kennedy University Hospital- Stratford, Stratford, NJ
Kennedy University Hospital- Washington Township, Turnersville, NJ
Monmouth Medical Center, Long Branch, NJ
Morristown Medical Center, Morristown, NJ
Newton Medical Center, Newton, NJ
Ocean Medical Center, Brick, NJ
Our Lady of Lourdes Medical Center, Camden, NJ
Overlook Medical Center, Summit, NJ
Riverview Medical Center, Red Bank, NJ
Robert Wood Johnson University Hospital, New Brunswick, NJ
Robert Wood Johnson University Hospital Hamilton, Hamilton, NJ
Robert Wood Johnson University Hospital Somerset, Somerville, NJ
RWJ University Hospital Rahway, Rahway, NJ
Saint Peter's University Hospital, New Brunswick, NJ
Southern Ocean Medical Center, Manahawkin, NJ
St. Francis Medical Center, Trenton, NJ
St. Joseph's Regional Medical Center, Paterson, NJ
St. Luke's Warren Hospital, Phillipsburg, NJ
The Valley Hospital, Ridgewood, NJ

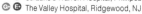

G+ HH G+ E University Hospital, Newark, NJ
G+ Virtua Memorial Hospital, Mt. Holly, NJ

NEW MEXICO

S+ Lea Regional Medical Center, Hobbs, NM
S G+ G+ Lovelace Medical Center, Albuquerque, NM
G San Juan Regional Medical Center, Farmington, NM
G+ HH S+ E University of New Mexico Hospitals, Albuquerque, NM

NEW YORK

G G G+ Albany Medical Center, Albany, NY
G+ E Arnot Ogden Medical Center, Elmira, NY
G+ E Auburn Community Hospital, Auburn, NY
S G+ E Bassett Medical Center, Cooperstown, NY
G+ G+ Bronx-Lebanon Hospital Center, Bronx, NY
G+ HH Brookdale University Hospital Medical Center, Brooklyn, NY
G+ HH Brookhaven Memorial Hospital Medical Center, Patchogue, NY
G+ G+ G+ Catholic Health - Kenmore Mercy Hospital, Buffalo, NY
G+ HH G+ E Catholic Health - Mercy Hospital of Buffalo, Buffalo, NY
G+ HH G+ Catholic Health - Sisters of Charity Hospital, Sisters of Charity St. Joseph Campus, Buffalo, NY
S+ Cayuga Medical Center at Ithaca, Ithaca, NY
S Cohen Children's Medical Center, New Hyde Park, NY
G+ G G+ Crouse Hospital, Syracuse, NY
G+ HH DeGraff Memorial Hospital, Buffalo, NY
G+ HH Ellis Hospital, Schenectady, NY
G+ HH G+ Erie County Medical Center, Buffalo, NY
S F.F. Thompson Hospital, Canandaigua, NY
G+ E+ Faxton St. Luke's Healthcare, Utica, NY
G+ E Flushing Hospital Medical Center, Flushing, NY
G+ E Forest Hills Hospital, Forest Hills, NY
G G+ HH Gates Vascular Institute / Buffalo General Medical Center, Buffalo, NY
G+ Glen Cove Hospital, Glen Cove, NY
G+ Good Samaritan Hospital Medical Center, West Islip, NY
G+ E Guthrie Corning Hospital, Corning, NY
G+ HealthAlliance Hospital: Broadway Campus, Kingston, NY
S G+ HH Highland Hospital, Rochester, NY
G+ E Huntington Hospital, Huntington, NY
G+ HH Jamaica Hospital Medical Center, Richmond Hill, NY
G+ E John T. Mather Memorial Hospital, Port Jefferson, NY
G+ HH Kingsbrook Jewish Medical Center, Brooklyn, NY
G+ HH Lenox Hill Hospital, New York, NY
G+ HH LIJ Valley Stream, Valley Stream, NY
G+ HH Long Island Jewish Medical Center, New Hyde Park, NY
G+ E Maimonides Medical Center, Brooklyn, NY
G+ Mercy Medical Center, Rockville Centre, NY
S MidHudson Regional Hospital, Poughkeepsie, NY
G+ S Millard Fillmore Suburban Hospital, Williamsville, NY
G+ Montefiore Mount Vernon Hospital, Mount Vernon, NY
S Montefiore New Rochelle Hospital, New Rochelle, NY
G+ HH S G+ E Mount Sinai Beth Israel, New York, NY
G Mount Sinai Beth Israel Brooklyn, Brooklyn, NY
G+ E Mount Sinai Queens, Astoria, NY
G+ E Mount Sinai St. Luke's, New York, NY
G+ HH Mount Sinai St. Luke's & Mount Sinai West, New York, NY
G+ HH Mount St. Mary's Hospital, Lewiston, NY
G+ HH G+ E Nassau University Medical Center, East Meadow, NY
G+ E New York Community Hospital, Brooklyn, NY
G+ E New York Methodist Hospital, Brooklyn, NY
G+ E Newark–Wayne Community Hospital, Newark, NY
G+ E NewYork-Presbyterian/Columbia University Medical Center, New York, NY
G+ HH NewYork-Presbyterian/Hudson Valley Hospital, Cortlandt Manor, NY
G+ G HH NewYork-Presbyterian/Lawrence Hospital, Bronxville, NY
G+ E NewYork-Presbyterian/Lower Manhattan Hospital, New York, NY
G+ E NewYork-Presbyterian/Queens, Flushing, NY
G+ E NewYork-Presbyterian/The Allen Hospital, New York, NY
G+ E NewYork-Presbyterian/Weill Cornell Medical Center, New York, NY
G+ Niagara Falls Memorial Medical Center, Niagara Falls, NY
G+ E North Shore University Hospital, Manhasset, NY
G+ Northern Dutchess Hospital, Rhinebeck, NY
G+ HH Northern Westchester Hospital, Mount Kisco, NY
S Noyes Health, Dansville, NY
G+ E Nyack Hospital, Nyack, NY
G+ HH G G+ E NYC Health + Hospitals/Bellevue, New York, NY
S NYC Health + Hospitals/Coney Island, Brooklyn, NY
G+ E NYC Health + Hospitals/Elmhurst, Flushing, NY
S HH NYC Health + Hospitals/Harlem, New York, NY
G+ E NYC Health + Hospitals/Jacobi, Bronx, NY
G+ E NYC Health + Hospitals/Kings County, Brooklyn, NY
G+ E NYC Health + Hospitals/Lincoln, Bronx, NY
G+ NYC Health + Hospitals/Metropolitan, New York, NY
G+ NYC Health + Hospitals/Woodhull, Brooklyn, NY
G+ G+ E NYU Langone Medical Center, New York, NY

G+ E NYU Lutheran Medical Center, Brooklyn, NY
S+ Olean General Hospital, Olean, NY
G+ E Orange Regional Medical Center, Middletown, NY
G+ Our Lady of Lourdes Memorial Hospital, Binghamton, NY
G+ Peconic Bay Medical Center, Riverhead, NY
G+ HH Phelps Hospital, Sleepy Hollow, NY
G+ E Plainview Hospital, Plainview, NY
G+ E Richmond University Medical Center, Staten Island, NY
G+ E Rochester General Hospital, Rochester, NY
S Saint Joseph's Medical Center, Yonkers, NY
G+ SBH Health System, Bronx, NY
G+ HH G+ E South Nassau Communities Hospital, Oceanside, NY
G+ E Southampton Hospital, Southampton, NY
S G+ E Southside Hospital, Bay Shore, NY
G+ E St. Catherine of Siena Medical Center, Smithtown, NY
G+ E St. Charles Hospital, Port Jefferson, NY
G+ G+ HH St. Francis Hospital, The Heart Center, Roslyn, NY
G+ St. John's Episcopal Hospital, Far Rockaway, NY
S E St. John's Riverside Hospital, Yonkers, NY
S G+ E St. Joseph Hospital, Bethpage, NY
G+ St. Luke's Cornwall Hospital, Newburgh and Cornwall Campuses, Newburgh, NY
G+ St. Mary's Hospital, Troy, NY
S G+ S G+ HH St. Peter's Hospital, Albany, NY
G+ E Staten Island University Hospital, Staten Island, NY
G+ G+ E Stony Brook University Hospital, Stony Brook, NY
G+ Syosset Hospital, Syosset, NY
S+ HH G+ E The Brooklyn Hospital Center, Brooklyn, NY
S+ E The Mount Sinai Hospital, New York, NY
G+ E UHS Wilson Medical Center, Johnson City, NY
G+ E Unity Hospital, Rochester, NY
G+ HH University Hospital of Brooklyn - SUNY Downstate Medical Center, Brooklyn, NY
G+ HH S G G+ E University of Rochester Medical Center, Strong Memorial Hospital, Rochester, NY
G+ G+ E Upstate University Hospital, Syracuse, NY
G+ HH Vassar Brothers Medical Center, Poughkeepsie, NY
S+ HH Westchester Medical Center, Valhalla, NY
G+ HH White Plains Hospital, White Plains, NY
G+ G+ E Winthrop University Hospital, Mineola, NY
G+ HH Wyckoff Heights Medical Center, Brooklyn, NY

NORTH CAROLINA

G G G+ HH Cape Fear Valley Medical Center, Fayetteville, NC
G+ HH Carolinas HealthCare System Cleveland, Shelby, NC
G+ G+ E Carolinas HealthCare System NorthEast, Concord, NC
G+ S+ HH Carolinas HealthCare System Pineville, Charlotte, NC
G+ Carolinas HealthCare System Stanly, Albemarle, NC
G+ Carolinas HealthCare System Union, Monroe, NC
G+ G+ E Carolinas Medical Center, Charlotte, NC
G+ HH G+ E CaroMont Regional Medical Center, Gastonia, NC
S G+ HH S S+ HH Carteret Health Care Medical Center, Morehead City, NC
G+ HH G+ Central Carolina Hospital, Sanford, NC
G+ E Cone Health, Greensboro, NC
G+ HH Duke Raleigh Hospital, Raleigh, NC
G+ E Duke Regional Hospital, Durham, NC
G+ HH G+ S+ E Duke University Hospital, Durham, NC
G+ G G Frye Regional Medical Center, Hickory, NC
S High Point Regional UNC Health Care, High Point, NC
G+ E Hugh Chatham Memorial Hospital, Elkin, NC
G+ HH Iredell Memorial Hospital, Statesville, NC
G G G+ E Mission Hospitals, Inc., Asheville, NC
G+ G+ E New Hanover Regional Medical Center, Wilmington, NC
G+ G Novant Health Brunswick Medical Center, Bolivia, NC
G+ HH G+ G+ E Novant Health Forsyth Medical Center, Winston-Salem, NC
G G G Novant Health Huntersville Medical Center, Huntersville, NC
G+ G+ G+ E Novant Health Matthews Medical Center, Matthews, NC
G+ HH G+ G+ E Novant Health Presbyterian Medical Center, Charlotte, NC
G+ G+ Novant Health Rowan Medical Center, Salisbury, NC
G+ HH G+ Novant Health Thomasville Medical Center, Thomasville, NC
S Onslow Memorial Hospital, Jacksonville, NC
S Southeastern Regional Medical Center, Lumberton, NC
G+ G+ E UNC Hospitals, Chapel Hill, NC
G S HH UNC REX Healthcare, Raleigh, NC
G+ Vidant Medical Center, Greenville, NC
S G+ E Wake Forest Baptist Medical Center, Winston-Salem, NC
S G+ HH G+ HH WakeMed Cary Hospital, Cary, NC
G+ G+ E WakeMed Health & Hospitals - Raleigh Campus, Raleigh, NC

NORTH DAKOTA

G+ E Altru Health System, Grand Forks, ND
G+ HH CHI St. Alexius Health, Bismarck, ND
G+ G+ E Essentia Health, Fargo, ND
G+ E Sanford Medical Center Fargo, Fargo, ND
G+ Trinity Health, Minot, ND

OHIO

- Affinity Medical Center, Massillon, OH
- Ashtabula County Medical Center, Ashtabula, OH
- Atrium Medical Center, Franklin, OH
- Aultman Hospital, Canton, OH
- Cleveland Clinic, Cleveland, OH
- Euclid Hospital, Euclid, OH
- Fairfield Medical Center, Lancaster, OH
- Fairview Hospital - A Cleveland Clinic Hospital, Cleveland, OH
- Genesis Healthcare System, Zanesville, OH
- Good Samaritan Hospital, Dayton, OH
- Hillcrest Hospital - A Cleveland Clinic Hospital, Mayfield Heights, OH
- Kettering Medical Center, Dayton, OH
- Knox Community Hospital, Mount Vernon, OH
- Licking Memorial Hospital, Newark, OH
- Lima Memorial Health System, Lima, OH
- Louis Stokes Cleveland VA Medical Center, Cleveland, OH
- Marymount Hospital, Garfield Heights, OH
- Medina Hospital, Medina, OH
- Mercy Medical Center, Canton, OH
- Mercy St. Vincent Medical Center, Toledo, OH
- Mercy Youngstown, Youngstown, OH
- Miami Valley Hospital, Dayton, OH
- Mount Carmel East, Columbus, OH
- Mount Carmel Health System, Columbus, OH
- Mount Carmel St. Ann's, Westerville, OH
- OhioHealth Doctors Hospital, Columbus, OH
- OhioHealth Grant Medical Center, Columbus, OH
- OhioHealth Marion General Hospital, Marion, OH
- OhioHealth Riverside Methodist Hospital, Columbus, OH
- ProMedica Flower Hospital, Sylvania, OH
- ProMedica Toledo Hospital, Toledo, OH
- Salem Regional Medical Center, Salem, OH
- South Pointe Hospital, Warrensville Heights, OH
- Southwest General Health Center, Middleburg Heights, OH
- St. John Medical Center, Cleveland, OH
- St. Rita's Medical Center, Lima, OH
- St. Vincent Charity Medical Center, Cleveland, OH
- Summa Akron City Hospital, Akron, OH
- Sycamore Medical Center, Miamisburg, OH
- The Christ Hospital, Cincinnati, OH
- The MetroHealth System, Cleveland, OH
- The Ohio State University Wexner Medical Center, Columbus, OH
- The University of Toledo Medical Center, Toledo, OH
- UH Regional Hospitals, Bedford Medical Center and Richmond Medical Center, Richmond Heights, OH
- Union Hospital, Dover, OH
- University Hospitals Ahuja Medical Center, Beachwood, OH
- University Hospitals Case Medical Center, Cleveland, OH
- University Hospitals Elyria Medical Center, Elyria, OH
- University Hospitals Geauga Medical Center, Chardon, OH
- University Hospitals Parma Medical Center, Parma, OH
- University of Cincinnati Medical Center, Cincinnati, OH
- Upper Valley Medical Center, Troy, OH
- West Hospital, Cincinnati, OH
- Western Reserve Hospital, Cuyahoga Falls, OH
- Wooster Community Hospital, Wooster, OH

OKLAHOMA

- INTEGRIS Baptist Medical Center, Oklahoma City, OK
- INTEGRIS Southwest Medical Center, Oklahoma City, OK
- Jane Phillips Medical Center, Bartlesville, OK
- Mercy Hospital Oklahoma City Comprehensive Stroke Center, Oklahoma City, OK
- Norman Regional HealthPlex Heart Hospital, Norman, OK
- Oklahoma Heart Institute at Hillcrest Medical Center, Tulsa, OK
- St. Anthony Hospital, Oklahoma City, OK
- St. John Medical Center, Tulsa, OK

OREGON

- Asante Rogue Regional Medical Center, Medford, OR
- Good Samaritan Regional Medical Center, Corvallis, OR
- Kaiser Foundation Hospital-Westside, Hillsboro, OR
- Kaiser Sunnyside Medical Center, Clackamas, OR
- Legacy Emanuel Medical Center, Portland, OR
- Legacy Meridian Park Medical Center, Tualatin, OR
- Legacy Mount Hood Medical Center, Gresham, OR
- Oregon Health & Science University, Portland, OR
- Peacehealth Sacred Heart Medical Center at RiverBend, Springfield, OR
- Providence Medford Medical Center, Medford, OR
- Providence Milwaukie Hospital, Milwaukie, OR
- Providence Newberg Medical Center, Newberg, OR
- Providence Portland Medical Center, Portland, OR
- Providence Seaside Hospital, Seaside, OR
- Providence St. Vincent Medical Center, Portland, OR
- Providence Willamette Falls Medical Center, Oregon City, OR
- Salem Hospital, Salem, OR
- Sky Lakes Medical Center, Klamath Falls, OR
- St Charles Health System - Bend, Bend, OR
- Tuality Healthcare, Hillsboro, OR

PENNSYLVANIA

- Abington Health - Abington Memorial Hospital, Abington, PA
- Albert Einstein Medical Center, Philadelphia, PA
- Allegheny General Hospital, Pittsburgh, PA
- Allegheny Health Network Forbes Hospital, Monroeville, PA
- Allegheny Valley Hospital, Natrona Hts, PA
- Aria Health - Frankford Campus, Philadelphia, PA
- Bryn Mawr Hospital, Bryn Mawr, PA
- Butler Memorial Hospital, Butler, PA
- Canonsburg Hospital, Canonsburg, PA
- Carlisle Regional Medical Center, Carlisle, PA
- Chestnut Hill Hospital, Philadelphia, PA
- Conemaugh Valley Memorial Hospital, Johnstown, PA
- Crozer-Chester Medical Center, Upland, PA
- Delaware County Memorial Hospital, Drexel Hill, PA
- Doylestown Hospital, Doylestown, PA
- Einstein Medical Center Montgomery, East Norriton, PA
- Evangelical Community Hospital, Lewisburg, PA
- Geisinger Community Medical Center, Scranton, PA
- Geisinger Medical Center, Danville, PA
- Geisinger Wyoming Valley Medical Center, Wilkes Barre, PA
- Grand View Hospital, Sellersville, PA
- Hahnemann University Hospital, Philadelphia, PA
- Hanover Hospital, Hanover, PA
- Heritage Valley Beaver, Beaver, PA
- Heritage Valley Sewickley, Sewickley, PA
- Holy Redeemer Hospital, Meadowbrook, PA
- Holy Spirit Hospital: A Geisinger Affiliate, Camp Hill, PA
- Jameson Hospital, New Castle, PA
- Jeanes Hospital - Temple University Health System, Philadelphia, PA
- Jefferson Hospital, Clairton, PA
- Jefferson Hospital, Philadelphia, PA
- Jennersville Regional Hospital, West Grove, PA
- Lancaster General Hospital, Lancaster, PA
- Lankenau Medical Center, Wynnewood, PA
- Lansdale Hospital, Lansdale, PA
- Lehigh Valley Health Network Cedar Crest, Allentown, PA
- Lehigh Valley Health Network Muhlenberg, Bethlehem, PA
- Lehigh Valley Hospital- Hazleton, Hazleton, PA
- Mercy Fitzgerald Hospital, Darby, PA
- Mercy Philadelphia Hospital, Philadelphia, PA
- Mercy Suburban Hospital, Norristown, PA
- Monongahela Valley Hospital, Monongahela, PA
- Moses Taylor Hospital, Scranton, PA
- Mount Nittany Medical Center, State College, PA
- Nazareth Hospital, Philadelphia, PA
- Penn Highlands DuBois, Du Bois, PA
- Penn Medicine Chester County Hospital, West Chester, PA
- Penn Presbyterian Medical Center, Philadelphia, PA
- Penn State Hershey Medical Center, Hershey, PA
- Pennsylvania Hospital, Philadelphia, PA
- Phoenixville Hospital, Phoenixville, PA
- Pinnacle Health System - Harrisburg Hospital, Harrisburg, PA
- Pinnacle Health System - Harrisburg Hospital, Mechanicsburg, PA
- Pocono Medical Center, East Stroudsburg, PA
- Pottstown Memorial Medical Center, Pottstown, PA
- Reading Hospital, West Reading, PA
- Riddle Memorial Hospital, Media, PA
- Roxborough Memorial Hospital, Philadelphia, PA
- Sacred Heart Hospital, Allentown, PA
- Saint Vincent Health System, Erie, PA
- Schuylkill Medical Center East Norwegian Street, Pottsville, PA
- Schuylkill Medical Center South Jackson, Pottsville, PA
- St. Joseph Regional Health Network, Reading, PA
- St. Luke's Hospital-Miners Campus, Coaldale, PA
- St. Luke's University Hospital, Bethlehem, PA
- St. Mary Medical Center, Langhorne, PA
- Temple University Hospital, Philadelphia, PA
- The Chambersburg Hospital, Chambersburg, PA
- The Children's Hospital of Philadelphia, Philadelphia, PA
- The Good Samaritan Health System, Lebanon, PA
- The Hospital of the University of Pennsylvania, Philadelphia, PA
- UMPC Hamot, Erie, PA
- Uniontown Hospital, Uniontown, PA
- UPMC Altoona, Altoona, PA
- UPMC Hamot, Erie, PA
- UPMC Horizon, Greenville, PA
- UPMC McKeesport, McKeesport, PA
- UPMC Mercy Pittsburgh, Pittsburgh, PA

American Heart Association | American Stroke Association.
life is why™

UPMC Northwest, Seneca, PA
UPMC Presbyterian, Pittsburgh, PA
UPMC Shadyside, Pittsburgh, PA
UPMC St. Margaret, Pittsburgh, PA
Washington Health System, Washington, PA
Waynesboro Hospital, Waynesboro, PA
Wellspan Ephrata Community Hospital, Stevens, PA
WellSpan Health - York Hospital, York, PA

PUERTO RICO

Administracion De Servicios Medicos, San Juan, PR
Hospital HIMA - San Pablo - Caguas, Caguas, PR
Hospital HIMA San Pablo Bayamon, Bayamon, PR
Hospital HIMA San Pablo Fajardo, Fajardo, PR

RHODE ISLAND

Kent Hospital, Warwick, RI
Landmark Medical Center, Woonsocket, RI
Memorial Hospital of Rhode Island, Pawtucket, RI
Rhode Island Hospital, Providence, RI
South County Hospital Health Care System, Wakefield, RI

SOUTH CAROLINA

AnMed Health, Anderson, SC
Beaufort Memorial Hospital, Beaufort, SC
Bon Secours St. Francis Health System, Greenville, SC
Bon Secours St. Francis Hospital, Charleston, SC
Coastal Carolina Hospital, Hardeeville, SC
East Cooper Medical Center, Mount Pleasant, SC
Georgetown Memorial Hospital, Georgetown, SC
Grand Strand Medical Center, Myrtle Beach, SC
Greenville Memorial Hospital, Greenville, SC
Greer Memorial Hospital, Greer, SC
Hilton Head Hospital, Hilton Head, SC
Lexington Medical Center, West Columbia, SC
Mary Black Health System, Spartanburg, SC
McLeod Regional Medical Center, Florence, SC
Medical University of South Carolina Medical Center, Charleston, SC
Palmetto Health Baptist, Columbia, SC
Palmetto Health Baptist Parkridge, Columbia, SC
Palmetto Health Richland, Columbia, SC
Piedmont Medical Center, Rock Hill, SC
Regional Medical Center of Orangeburg & Calhoun Counties, Orangeburg, SC
Roper St. Francis Hospital, Charleston, SC
Self Regional Healthcare, Greenwood, SC
Spartanburg Regional Healthcare System, Spartanburg, SC
Springs Memorial Hospital, Lancaster, SC
Summerville Medical Center, Summerville, SC
Trident Medical Center, Charleston, SC
Waccamaw Community Hospital, Murrells Inlet, SC

SOUTH DAKOTA

Avera Heart Hospital of South Dakota, Sioux Falls, SD
Rapid City Regional Hospital, Rapid City, SD
Sanford USD Medical Center, Sioux Falls, SD

TENNESSEE

Baptist Memorial Hospital Memphis, Memphis, TN
Blount Memorial, Maryville, TN
Bristol Regional Medical Center, Bristol, TN
CHI Memorial Hospital, Chattanooga, TN
Erlanger Health System, Chattanooga, TN
Fort Sanders Regional Medical Center, Knoxville, TN
Holston Valley Medical Center, Kingsport, TN
Johnson City Medical Center, Johnson City, TN
NorthCrest Medical Center, Springfield, TN
Parkridge Medical Center, Chattanooga, TN
Parkwest Medical Center, Knoxville, TN
Saint Francis Hospital - Memphis, Memphis, TN
St. Francis Hospital Bartlett, Bartlett, TN
Tennova Healthcare Harton, Tullahoma, TN
The University of Tennessee Medical Center, Knoxville, TN
TriStar Centennial Medical Center, Nashville, TN
Vanderbilt University Medical Center, Nashville, TN

TEXAS

Baptist Health System, San Antonio, TX
Baylor Jack and Jane Hamilton Heart and Vascular Hospital, Dallas, TX
Baylor Medical Center at Irving, Irving, TX
Baylor Medical Center at McKinney, McKinney, TX
Baylor Regional Medical Center at Grapevine, Grapevine, TX
Baylor Scott & White Hillcrest Medical Center, Waco, TX

Baylor Scott & White Medical Center - Round Rock, Round Rock, TX
Baylor University Medical Center at Dallas, Dallas, TX
Bayshore Medical Center, Pasadena, TX
Centennial Medical Center, Frisco, TX
CHI St. Luke's Health Memorial Lufkin, Lufkin, TX
CHI St. Luke's Health – Baylor St. Luke's Medical Center, Houston, TX
CHI St. Luke's Health–The Woodlands Hospital, The Woodlands, TX
CHRISTUS Hospital St. Elizabeth & St. Mary, Port Arthur, TX
CHRISTUS Spohn Hospital Corpus Christi - Shoreline, Corpus Christi, TX
CHRISTUS St. Michael Health System, Texarkana, TX
Citizens Medical Center, Victoria, TX
Clear Lake Regional Medical Center, Webster, TX
Connally Memorial Medical Center, Floresville, TX
Conroe Regional Medical Center, Conroe, TX
Corpus Christi Medical Center, Corpus Christi, TX
Covenant Medical Center, Lubbock, TX
Cypress Fairbanks Medical Center, Houston, TX
Dallas Regional Medical Center, Mesquite, TX
Del Sol Medical Center, El Paso, TX
DeTar Healthcare System, Victoria, TX
Doctors Hospital at Renaissance, Edinburg, TX
Doctors Hospital at White Rock Lake, Dallas, TX
East Texas Medical Center, Tyler, TX
Good Shepherd Medical Center, Longview, TX
Good Shepherd Medical Center - Marshall, Marshall, TX
Harris Health System- Ben Taub General Hospita, Houston, TX
HCA- West Houston Medical Center, Houston, TX
Hendrick Medical Center, Abilene, TX
Houston Methodist Hospital, Houston, TX
Houston Methodist San Jacinto Hospital, Baytown, TX
Houston Methodist Sugar Land Hospital, Sugar Land, TX
Houston Methodist West Hospital, Houston, TX
Houston Methodist Willowbrook Hospital, Houston, TX
Houston Northwest Medical Center, Houston, TX
JPS Health Network, Fort Worth, TX
Kingwood Medical Center Hospital, an HCA Affiliated Hospital, Kingwood, TX
Lake Pointe Medical Center, Rowlett, TX
Las Palmas Medical Center, El Paso, TX
Medcial City Dallas Hospital, Dallas, TX
Medical Center Hospital, Odessa, TX
Memorial Hermann - Texas Medical Center, Houston, TX
Memorial Hermann Greater Heights Hospital, Houston, TX
Memorial Hermann Katy Hospital, Katy, TX
Memorial Hermann Memorial City Medical Center, Houston, TX
Memorial Hermann Northeast Hospital, Humble, TX
Memorial Hermann Southeast Hospital, Houston, TX
Memorial Hermann Southwest Hospital, Houston, TX
Memorial Hermann The Woodlands, The Woodlands, TX
Methodist Charlton Medical Center, Dallas, TX
Methodist Dallas Medical Center, Dallas, TX
Methodist Hospital, San Antonio, TX
Methodist Mansfield Medical Center, Mansfield, TX
Methodist Richardson Medical Center, Richardson, TX
Methodist Stone Oak Hospital, San Antonio, TX
Metroplex Hospital, Killeen, TX
Midland Memorial Hospital, Midland, TX
Nacogdoches Medical Center, Nacogdoches, TX
North Central Baptist Hospital, San Antonio, TX
North Cypress Medical Center, Cypress, TX
Northwest Texas Healthcare System, Amarillo, TX
OakBend Medical Center, Richmond, TX
Park Plaza Hospital, Houston, TX
Parkland Health & Hospital System, Dallas, TX
Providence Health Center, Waco, TX
Scott & White Medical Center - Temple, Temple, TX
Seton Medical Center Austin, Austin, TX
Seton Medical Center Hays, Kyle, TX
Seton Medical Center Williamson, Round Rock, TX
Shannon Medical Center, San Angelo, TX
Southwest General Hospital, San Antonio, TX
St. David's Georgetown, Georgetown, TX
St. David's Medical Center, Austin, TX
St. David's North Austin Medical Center, Austin, TX
St. David's Round Rock Medical Center, Round Rock, TX
St. Joseph Medical Center, Houston, TX
St. Joseph Regional Health Center, Bryan, TX
Texas Health Arlington Memorial Hospital, Arlington, TX
Texas Health Denton, Denton, TX
Texas Health Heart and Vascular Hospital, Arlington, TX
Texas Health Hurst Euless Bedford, Bedford, TX
Texas Health Presbyterian Hospital Dallas, Dallas, TX
The Heart Hospital Baylor Plano, Plano, TX
The Hospitals of Providence East Campus, El Paso, TX

The Hospitals of Providence Memorial Campus, El Paso, TX
The Hospitals of Providence Sierra Campus, El Paso, TX
The Medical Center of Plano, Plano, TX
The University of Texas Medical Branch - Galveston Campus, Galveston, TX
Tomball Regional Medical Center, Tomball, TX
United Regional Healthcare System, Wichita Falls, TX
University Health System, San Antonio, TX
University Medical Center Brackenridge, Austin, TX
University Medical Center of El Paso, El Paso, TX
UT Southwestern Medical Center, Dallas, TX
Valley Baptist Medical Center-Brownsville, Brownsville, TX
Valley Baptist Medical Center-Harlingen, Harlingen, TX
Valley Regional Medical Center, Brownsville, TX
Wadley Regional Medical Center, Texarkana, TX
Wise Health System, Decatur, TX

UTAH

American Fork Hospital, American Fork, UT
Davis Hospital and Medical Center, Layton, UT
Dixie Regional Medical Center, Saint George, UT
Intermountain Medical Center, Murray, UT
Jordan Valley Medical Center/Jordan Valley Medical Center-West Valley Campus, West Jordan, UT
Lakeview Hospital, Bountiful, UT
McKay-Dee Hospital, Ogden, UT
Mountain View Hospital - Payson, Payson, UT
Ogden Regional Medical Center, Ogden, UT
St. Mark's Hospital, Salt Lake City, UT
Timpanogos Regional Hospital, Orem, UT
University of Utah Health Care, Salt Lake City, UT
Utah Valley Regional Medical Center, Provo, UT

VERMONT

The University of Vermont Medical Center, Burlington, VT

VIRGINIA

Augusta Health, Fishersville, VA
Bon Secours DePaul Medical Center, Norfolk, VA
Bon Secours Maryview Medical Center, Portsmouth, VA
Bon Secours Memorial Regional Medical Center, Mechanicsville, VA
Bon Secours Rappahannock General Hospital, Kilmarnock, VA
Bon Secours Richmond Community Hospital, Richmond, VA
Bon Secours St. Francis Medical Center, Midlothian, VA
Bon Secours St. Mary's Hospital, Richmond, VA
Carilion Roanoke Memorial Hospital, Roanoke, VA
Centra Lynchburg General Hospital, Lynchburg, VA
Centra Southside Community Hospital, Farmville, VA
Chesapeake Regional Medical Center, Chesapeake, VA
Inova Alexandria Hospital, Alexandria, VA
Inova Fair Oaks Hospital, Fairfax, VA
Inova Fairfax Hospital, Falls Church, VA
Inova Loudoun Hospital, Leesburg, VA
Inova Mount Vernon Hospital, Alexandria, VA
John Randolph Medical Center, Hopewell, VA
Mary Washington Hospital, Fredericksburg, VA
Novant Health Prince William Medical Center, Manassas, VA
Reston Hospital Center, Reston, VA
Riverside Regional Medical Center, Newport News, VA
Sentara CarePlex Hospital, Hampton, VA
Sentara Leigh Hospital, Norfolk, VA
Sentara Norfolk General Hospital/Sentara Heart Hospital, Norfolk, VA
Sentara Northern Virginia Medical Center, Woodbridge, VA
Sentara Virginia Beach General Hospital, Virginia Beach, VA
Sentara Williamsburg Regional Medical Center, Williamsburg, VA
Southside Regional Medical Center, Petersburg, VA
Twin County Regional Healthcare, Galax, VA
University of Virginia Health System, Charlottesville, VA
VCU Community Memorial Hospital, South Hill, VA
Virginia Commonwealth University Medical Center, Richmond, VA
Virginia Hospital Center, Arlington, VA
Winchester Medical Center, Winchester, VA

WASHINGTON

Capital Medical Center, Olympia, WA
Confluence Health-Central Washington Hospital, Wenatchee, WA
Deaconess Hospital, Spokane, WA
EvergreenHealth, Kirkland, WA
Harborview Medical Center, Seattle, WA
Harrison Medical Center, Bremerton, WA
Jefferson Healthcare, Port Townsend, WA
Kittitas Valley Healthcare, Ellensburg, WA
Legacy Salmon Creek Medical Center, Vancouver, WA

MultiCare Auburn Medical Center, Auburn, WA
MultiCare Good Samaritan Hospital, Puyallup, WA
MultiCare Tacoma General Allenmore Hospital, Tacoma, WA
Northwest Hospital & Medical Center, Seattle, WA
Ocean Beach Hospital, Ilwaco, WA
Overlake Medical Center, Bellevue, WA
PeaceHealth St. Joseph Medical Center, Bellingham, WA
Providence Holy Family Hospital, Spokane, WA
Providence Regional Medical Center Everett, Everett, WA
Providence Sacred Heart Medical Center & Children's Hospital, Spokane, WA
Providence St. Peter Hospital, Olympia, WA
Skagit Valley Hospital, Mount Vernon, WA
St. Clare Hospital, Lakewood, WA
St. Joseph Medical Center, Tacoma, WA
Swedish Edmonds, Edmonds, WA
Swedish Medical Center - Issaquah Campus, Issaquah, WA
Swedish Medical Center, Cherry Hill, Seattle, WA
Trios Health, Kennewick, WA
University of Washington Medical Center, Seattle, WA
UW Medicine Valley Medical Center, Renton, WA
Virginia Mason Hospital and Medical Center, Seattle, WA
Yakima Regional Medical and Cardiac Center, Yakima, WA
Yakima Valley Memorial Hospital, Yakima, WA

WEST VIRGINIA

Cabell Huntington Hospital, Huntington, WV
CAMC General Hospital, Charleston, WV
Camden Clark Medical Center, Parkersburg, WV
Davis Medical Center, Elkins, WV
Mongongalia General Hospital, Morgantown, WV
Ohio Valley Medical Center, Inc., Wheeling, WV
St. Mary's Medical Center, Huntington, WV
United Hospital Center, Bridgeport, WV
West Virginia University Hospital, Inc., Morgantown, WV
Wheeling Hospital, Wheeling, WV

WISCONSIN

Aspirus Wausau Hospital, Wausau, WI
Aurora BayCare Medical Center, Green Bay, WI
Aurora Lakeland Medical Center, Elkhorn, WI
Aurora Medical Center - Grafton, Grafton, WI
Aurora Medical Center - Kenosha, Kenosha, WI
Aurora Medical Center Manitowoc County, Two Rivers, WI
Aurora Medical Center Summit, Oconomowoc, WI
Aurora Medical Center Washington County, Hartford, WI
Aurora Medical Center- Oshkosh, Oshkosh, WI
Aurora Memorial Hospital Burlington, Burlington, WI
Aurora Sheboygan Memorial Medical Center, Sheboygan, WI
Aurora Sinai Medical Center, Milwaukee, WI
Aurora St. Luke's Medical Center, Milwaukee, WI
Aurora St. Luke's South Shore, Cudahy, WI
Aurora West Allis Medical Center, West Allis, WI
Bellin Memorial Hospital, Green Bay, WI
Beloit Memorial Hospital, Beloit, WI
Columbia - St. Mary's Hospital, Milwaukee, WI
Columbia-St. Mary's Hospital - Ozaukee, Mequon, WI
Froedtert Hospital, Milwaukee, WI
Gundersen Lutheran Medical Center, La Crosse, WI
Mayo Clinic Health System in Eau Claire, Eau Claire, WI
Mayo Clinic Health System LaCrosse, La Crosse, WI
Mercy Hospital and Trauma Center, Janesville, WI
Meriter-UnityPoint Health, Madison, WI
Ministry Saint Clare's Hospital, Weston, WI
Ministry Saint Joseph's Hospital, Marshfield, WI
Oconomowoc Memorial Hospital, Oconomowoc, WI
Sacred Heart Hospital, Eau Claire, WI
St. Agnes Hospital, Fond Du Lac, WI
St. Clare Hospital and Health Services, Baraboo, WI
St. Mary's Hospital, Madison, WI
St. Mary's Hospital Medical Center, Green Bay, WI
St. Vincent Hospital, Green Bay, WI
Theda Clark Medical Center, Neenah, WI
University of Wisconsin Hospital and Clinics, Madison, WI
Waukesha Memorial Hospital, Waukesha, WI
Wheaton Franciscan Healthcare - Elmbrook, Brookfield, WI
Wheaton Franciscan Healthcare - St. Joseph, Milwaukee, WI
Wheaton Franciscan Healthcare – St. Francis, Milwaukee, WI
Wheaton Franciscan Healthcare All Saints, Racine, WI
William S. Middleton Memorial Veterans Hospital, Madison, WI

WYOMING

Cheyenne Regional Medical Center, Cheyenne, WY
Wyoming Medical Center, Casper, WY

American Heart Association | American Stroke Association.
life is why™

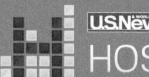
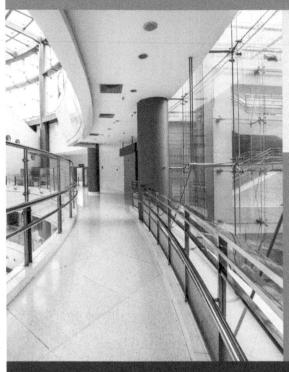

A QUESTION OF
IDENTITY

Before treatment, make sure the doctor knows you're you

BY ELIZABETH GARDNER

margaret A. McGiffen is used to getting mail intended for her sister-in-law, Margaret L. McGiffen. But she was quite dismayed that a similar mix-up happened at the hospital back in 2012 when she needed surgery. The Indiana resident requested sleep medication her doctor had ordered, and a nurse couldn't find the order in her record. Then she checked her wristband: Margaret L. McGiffen. "She takes 19 pills a day, and I take two," McGiffen says. "I don't know what would have happened if they had brought me her insulin."

Staffers hurried to correct the error. But as recently as last December, Margaret A. was asked to complete a patient satisfaction survey concerning a test given to Margaret L. For her part, Margaret L. hasn't experienced confusion. But "I always make sure they know which one I am," she says.

PATIENT IDENTIFICATION errors plague all health care providers, and they only promise to propagate more quickly with the rise of electronic health records and the spread of data sharing. "Maybe no one in your community has your name, but now you have to think about everyone else in the whole world," says Lesley Kadlec, director of practice excellence at the American Health Information Management Association (whose doctor's office once confused her with her husband's late first wife). ECRI Institute, a nonprofit focused on improving health

care, included ID errors in its most recent annual top-10 list of patient safety concerns along with health IT that's a mismatch with workflow and inadequate test-result reporting and follow-up, for example. Bill Marella, ECRI's executive director of patient safety operations, says patient ID errors can run the gamut from getting

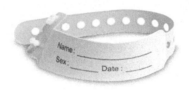

PATIENT ID **ERRORS** WILL **PROPAGATE** MORE *QUICKLY* WITH THE RISE OF *ELECTRONIC RECORDS* AND *DATA SHARING.*

someone else's medication at a pharmacy to being assigned someone else's records during a hospital admission.

Reliably identifying a patient is more difficult than it might seem, and busy staffers often don't take the necessary steps, says Charles Christian, vice president of technology and engagement at the Indiana Health Information Exchange, which helps providers in Indiana share data on patients. A 2012 report from the Bipartisan Policy Center noted that in a single Texas county, there were 2,488 people named Maria Garcia, and 231 of

them shared a birthdate with at least one other Maria Garcia. Confusion can arise when names, addresses, phone numbers and even genders change.

Meanwhile, fear of identity theft has curbed the use of Social Security numbers, which are not intended for identification anyway. Some EHR systems let the provider add a photo of the patient, but that feature isn't universally available or always used. A few hospitals are starting to rely on biometrics like fingerprints or iris scans to verify identities at registration. McGiffen's hospital now checks name (including middle initial), date of birth, address and phone number; photo ID provides backup when there's any doubt. And a "name alert" is generated when someone who registers has a name similar to one already in the system.

A national health ID system would be the simplest solution, but Congress has so far blocked funding for development of such a system. AHIMA is currently working to persuade the government a discussion is needed. Meantime, the College of Healthcare Information Management Executives is offering a million-dollar prize for the best national health ID strategy. Over 100 entries have been submitted, and the winner will be announced in early 2017.

How can patients protect themselves? Make sure your providers verify your identity at every visit and before every test and procedure. At a minimum, they should request name and birthdate; extra identifiers like address and phone number add protection. If someone starts to give you a test or a medication you're not expecting, be sure you're not getting care intended for someone else. ●

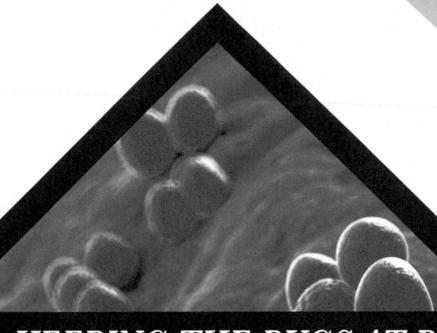

KEEPING THE BUGS AT BAY

Hospitals still have work to do to bring their rates of infection down

BY KATHERINE HOBSON

I n 2012, Jerolyn Ireland had a benign brain tumor removed. "The operation was a breeze," she says, but back at home, the surgical site became red and irritated. As she waited to get in to see her doctor, the infection worsened. Finally, she found out it was caused by the dreaded MRSA bacterium, a form of staphylococcus resistant to many antibiotics that Ireland, a reg-

istered nurse, believes she contracted during her hospital stay. Now 76 and living in Houlton, Maine, Ireland has needed multiple surgeries to repair the damage to her head. "I still have pain because of nerve damage," she says. And even with health coverage, her out-of-pocket costs have been crippling, especially since she had to stop working. "When I get a phone call, I think it's a collection agency," she says.

Recent statistics from the Centers for Disease Control and Prevention confirm what Ireland suspects that she illustrates: Medicine still has quite a long way to go to eliminate infections acquired via contact with the very health care system that is supposed to make people better. This type of infection affected about 722,000 people in acute care hospitals in 2011, more than 10 percent of whom died. Significant progress has been made on some fronts; central line infections, for example, are way down. But there's been a smaller decline – just 17 percent – in surgical site infections and little movement at all in problems associated with urinary catheters.

Meantime, concern has been growing about the frightening prevalence of bacteria that are resistant to many antibiotics, thus rendering them potentially untreatable (box, Page 62). The CDC says that in 2014, the chance that a health care-associated infection was caused by any of six key resistant bacteria, including MRSA and vancomycin-resistant Enterococcus, was 1 in 7 in short-term acute care hospitals and 1 in 4 in long-term acute care facilities. These are figures CDC director Thomas Frieden called "deeply concerning" and "chilling" respectively.

As for the scope of sepsis, the life-threatening organ dysfunction that can occur with any type of infection, hospital-acquired or otherwise, the CDC's data suggest that all told nearly 2.5 million people died at least in part due to sepsis from 1999 to 2014.

So what has been working and what further can be done? "The crown jewel" of prevention efforts to date is the one aimed at bloodstream infections associated with central lines, says Arjun Srinivasan, the associate director for healthcare-associated infection prevention programs at the CDC. At short-term acute care hospitals, the numbers were down by 50 percent in 2014 from 2008.

That's the result of a big push to implement such steps as a simple checklist reminding clinicians to wash their hands, replace soiled dressings, and properly clean the patient's skin. Peter Pronovost, who directs the Armstrong Institute for Patient Safety and Quality at Johns Hopkins School of Medicine and who developed the checklist, says success also has depended on a culture of high expectations emanating from the C-suite. "If the goal was 'zero,' even if they didn't achieve it, institutions did better," he says. Successful leaders have made reporting of infections transparent and established some kind of feedback loop so staffers can see how they're doing, he says.

The same enthusiasm could be deployed in other trouble spots, such as that of catheter-associated urinary tract infections, called CAUTIs, where the numbers haven't budged. Those infections extend hospital stays, require antibiotics, and cause an estimated 13,000 deaths per year. They call for more extensive efforts, since urinary catheters are widely used and are placed by a larger group of people, Srinivasan says.

But it can be done. "The recipe is very clear," says Marvin Moe Bell, a family medicine physician at HonorHealth Scottsdale in Arizona. "Basically it's to use urinary catheters less or to use them for shorter periods of time." In 2012 the intensive care unit at his hospital, the Scottsdale Osborn Medical Center, had a high CAUTI rate, with 54 infections – about 60 percent higher than the expected number. Bell and his team implemented a system that educates clinicians about when catheters are and aren't indicated, asks for justification

METHICILLIN-RESISTANT STAPHYLOCOCCUS AUREUS, OR MRSA (AT LEFT), AND VANCOMYCIN-RESISTANT ENTEROCOCCUS

in the patient's electronic medical record if a catheter is ordered, and presents a daily reminder in the health record to consider whether it's time to discontinue the catheter. As catheter use decreased, so did infections. In the ICU, rates dropped by 25 percent in 2014 and by 88 percent in 2015. (A change in the definition of CAUTI was responsible for about a quarter of the latter year's decline).

While commonsense basics such as hand hygiene and keeping surfaces clean have long been recognized as powerful and important tools, many facilities are still falling far short. According to the CDC, health care providers follow proper hand-cleaning procedures less than half of the time. And only about half of surfaces in hospitals are properly cleaned, says John Boyce, an infection control consultant who recently served as head of infection control at Yale-New Haven Hospital.

INTERNAL AUDITS AT SENTARA HEALTHCARE, based in Norfolk, Virginia, have shown a much more impressive record on meeting hand hygiene guidelines, with 94 to 95 percent compliance at the end of 2014. Still, "it wasn't at 100 percent," says Jennifer Kreiser, vice president and nurse executive at Sentara Leigh Hospital. "We needed to set up a mechanism so we didn't allow anyone to do the wrong thing." The system changed its approach from individual to team accountability with a program called All Hands on Deck that encourages personnel to use that phrase if they see someone fail to wash. Those who don't speak up are held accountable for the lapse.

The goal, says Scott Miller, an infectious disease physician who is vice president of medical affairs at Sentara Leigh, is to mimic the atmosphere of the operating room at the patient's bedside. "If I walked into the OR and hadn't scrubbed in, there would be people all over me pushing me out the door, asking why not." At the end of 2015, audits showed the compliance rate had risen to 99 percent, with some units consistently hitting 100 percent, Kreiser says. Better hand hygiene along with other efforts have brought infection rates at Sentara lower.

As with hand-washing, proper surface cleaning is straightforward in theory, but not in practice. Some harmful bugs, like MRSA and

> ## PROPER *HAND-CLEANING* HAPPENS *LESS THAN HALF* OF THE TIME.

E. COLI

the diarrhea-causing C. difficile, when shed from one patient, can survive long enough to infect the next patient who occupies the room. Regular disinfectant, properly applied, can kill the bacteria, but "properly applied" means covering every surface and keeping it wet for at least a few minutes to do the job. Such procedures have to be followed all the time, since even patients who show no symptoms can leave harmful bacteria on surfaces around them.

Boyce says change requires involving the housekeeping staff in quality improvement campaigns and giving them ongoing feedback about how well they're doing. Hospitals are also looking to new technologies to help with improvement. Spraying hydrogen peroxide vapor into a room after a patient carrying antibiotic-resistant bacteria had moved out, for example, reduced the chances that the next occupant would acquire the bug by 64 percent, according to a 2013 study conducted at Johns Hopkins. The downside: The room has to be unoccupied for up to three hours.

ANOTHER PROMISING METHOD uses ultraviolet light on top of the normal cleaning process to irradiate any remaining bacteria. Last year, researchers at Duke Medicine found that adding the light reduced by one-third the chance that patients staying overnight in a room previously occupied by a carrier of antibiotic-resistant bacteria would get sick. A third approach uses copper's antimicrobial properties. Researchers at Sentara are investigating whether copper-coated surfaces and copper-infused bed linens will reduce infections.

Health care organizations are also working to fight antibiotic-resistant bacteria by curbing the use of the drugs in the first place. Whenever antibiotics are called upon, some strains of bacteria don't die off, and those resistant strains can survive and multiply. The more antibiotics are used without sufficient caution, the more resistance becomes a problem. Besides working to prevent infections that would trigger a prescription, the government and health systems aim to manage antibiotics better, using microbial cultures to pinpoint which

drug should be prescribed and to reassess the need as time goes on, and by keeping a course of treatment as short as possible. Any patient who is prescribed an antibiotic should ask what's being treated and whether the drug will actually benefit that condition, advises Trevor Van Schooneveld, an infectious disease physician at the University of Nebraska Medical Center and medical director of the hospital's antimicrobial stewardship program.

And that's not all patients can do to protect themselves. Kathy Day, a registered nurse in Bangor, Maine, who became a patient advocate after her father died from hospital-acquired MRSA pneumonia, says she recommends a MRSA screening test ahead of any but the most minor surgery. If you're a carrier, you can be decolonized with some easy measures, helping to prevent infections in yourself or other patients. Some hospitals already perform this type of testing, but there's an ongoing debate over which patient groups should be screened.

Day also recommends that family members keep bleach-based wipes next to the bedside and use them to keep "anything that's touched by patient or caregiver" clean. Encourage any visitors to use hand sanitizer, too. ●

A SUPERBUG SCARE

I n May, doctors in Pennsylvania sent samples from a woman's urinary tract infection to the Walter Reed National Military Medical Center in Bethesda, Maryland. Because the infection was drug resistant, they needed help finding an antibiotic that would work. The alarming news that the samples contained a strain of E. coli resistant to colistin, a powerful antibiotic that

is a last resort against several diseases and had not been known to fail, quickly made headlines. Luckily for the patient, her infection reacted to other antibiotics. But the discovery of a colistin-resistant gene in the bacterium, known as mcr-1, is very worrying, researchers say.

The mcr-1 gene resides in DNA fragments in the bacterium that can replicate and exchange genetic information with neighboring bacteria, in a process called "horizontal" gene transfer. "Mcr-1 is the missing piece"

that could lead to total resistance to drugs now available, says Alexander Kallen, the team lead for antimicrobial resistance and emerging pathogens at the Centers for Disease Control and Prevention. If the gene spreads to other dangerous bacteria that are already resistant to most antibiotics, he says, the result could potentially be an incurable superbug.

The CDC is ramping up efforts to prevent mcr-1 from becoming widespread, says Kallen. Every lab in the agency's nationwide Antibiotic Resistance Lab Network will be better armed to detect and isolate mcr-1 and other newly discovered resistance genes. –Peter Rathmell

CHAPTER

3

PATIENT POWER

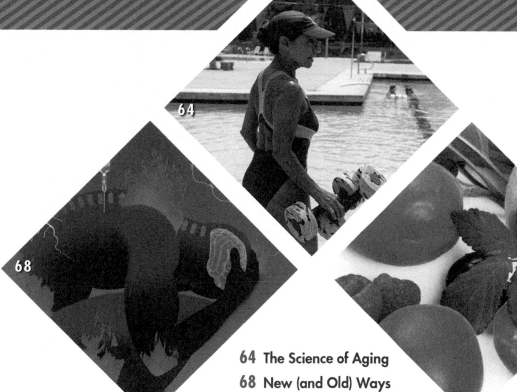

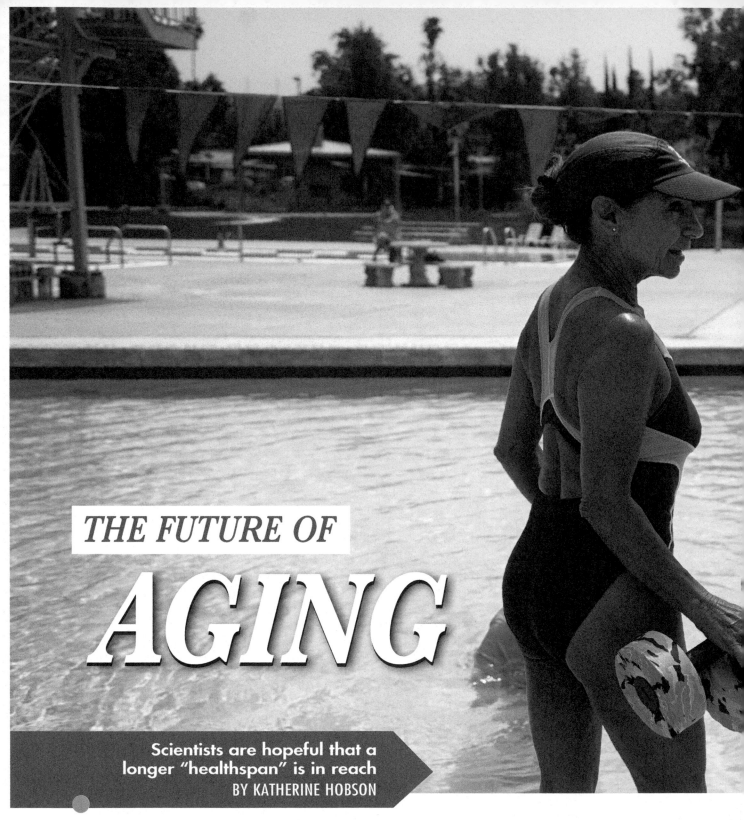

THE FUTURE OF
AGING

Scientists are hopeful that a
longer "healthspan" is in reach
BY KATHERINE HOBSON

Imagine a day in the not-too-distant future. You're in your late 40s, and it's time for a special doctor's visit. The physician reviews your lifestyle, sleep habits and health history and orders some blood work to compare certain biomarkers with baseline measures taken when you were in your 20s. Then she gives you a personalized prescription for change that includes a diet that mimics the effects of fasting and a drug that helps your cells clear out malfunctioning proteins. The goal? To make you age more slowly and lengthen your "healthspan."

If it sounds like science fiction, you're right – for now. But researchers in the field of geroscience, which explores the relationship between aging and diseases like cancer, heart disease and Alzheimer's, see that day coming. They are marshalling evidence that the same cellular processes that drive aging also result in those diseases, and that it's possible to slow the damage down. "The idea is that if you can treat the underlying causes of aging, you can delay all of these things as a group," says Steven Austad, scientific director of the American Federation for Aging Research

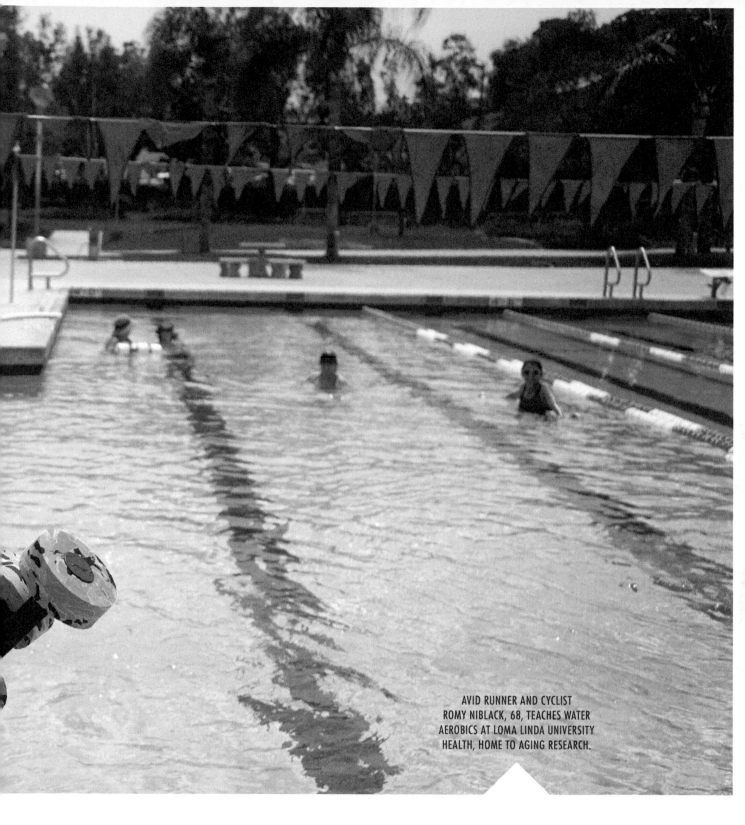

AVID RUNNER AND CYCLIST
ROMY NIBLACK, 68, TEACHES WATER
AEROBICS AT LOMA LINDA UNIVERSITY
HEALTH, HOME TO AGING RESEARCH.

and a professor at the University of Alabama–Birmingham. "That's a whole different way of thinking about medicine."

THE GOAL IS NOT TO EXTEND LIFESPAN, though that may indeed happen. Instead it's to extend the length of time you're healthy and active. "We want people to be in their 80s and feel like they're in their 50s and 60s," says Brian Kennedy, president and CEO at the Buck Institute for Research on Aging in Novato, California. That's not far-fetched, according to The New England Centenarian Study at Boston Medical Center, whose current subjects range in age from 100

to 115 and have been followed in some cases for 10 years to get a sense of what underlies the longest lives and healthy aging. People who make it to 109 and beyond have generally been independent and quite healthy well into their 90s and even past 100, says Thomas Perls, founder of the study and professor of medicine. One 106-year-old participant maintains her own garden and does her own canning; a 110-year-old still plays the piano.

Evelyn Folstrom, 109, uses a walker to get around and lives with her daughter and son-in-law in Northfield, Minnesota, but she can still read her daily devotionals and Bible (with her glasses), write letters to her 13 great-grandchildren, and occasionally get to church. She says she hasn't had any major health issues, other than two bouts of colon cancer in 1986 and 2003 that were "taken care of promptly."

THAT KIND OF "COMPRESSION OF MORBIDITY" would be good not only for individuals (who wouldn't like more time to volunteer or play with grandchildren?) but also for society, says Kennedy. A projected one-fifth of Americans will be 65 or older by 2030, and their health care costs will be overwhelming if they have multiple chronic diseases and cope with disability.

Working with a range of organisms from yeast to worms to rodents, scientists have homed in on several interrelated processes they suspect drive aging. These probably differ in their effect between people, says Felipe Sierra, director of the division of aging biology at the National Institute on Aging. (Thus that personalized aging strategy at your future physical.)

Proteostasis, for one, is a fancy name for the quality-control system at work in your cells. Like a factory, a cell has ways to ensure the proteins it makes are up to snuff, says Ana Maria Cuervo, co-director of the Institute for Aging Research at Albert Einstein College of Medicine in New York. If they're not, the malfunctioning proteins are supposed to be broken down and used to build new proteins or as energy. Cuervo's lab specializes in autophagy, one part of that system that works less well with age and is linked to Alzheimer's and Parkinson's disease. Her lab is looking for interventions, whether lifestyle or drugs, that might repair this age-related quality-control decline.

ANOTHER AREA OF EXPLORATION IS INFLAMMATION. Low-grade, chronic systemic inflammation in the absence of an infection is a factor in most age-related diseases; it's even known as "inflammaging." The sources of it aren't well known, but scientists are investigating possible contributors, including a state called cellular senescence. When cells undergo mutations or other damaging disruptions, normally the defect is fixed or the cell dies. But sometimes it slips into a kind of twilight zone, no longer dividing but not dying, either. Senescent cells can sometimes produce pro-inflammatory proteins that can damage other cells, says James Kirkland, a professor of aging research and director of the Kogod Center on Aging at the Mayo Clinic in Minnesota. And they're strongly associated with diseases of aging like cancer, atherosclerosis, diabetes and dementia.

Kirkland and his colleagues wondered what would happen if senescent cells were removed. In mice, they've shown that certain drugs called senolytics can do just that – and slow the progression of age-related changes and even partially reverse them. In a study published last year, the researchers found that a commercially available cancer drug and the supplement quercetin, an antioxidant, improved cardiovascular function, exercise endurance, and osteoporosis and increased healthspan when used together.

Kirkland cautions that it's not yet clear whether the benefits will carry over into humans. The abandoned medicine cabinet of history is full of drugs that cured diseases in rodents but didn't pan out in human beings. But often those diseases – take Alzheimer's, for example – must be engineered into the lab animals since they don't occur naturally. Since aging is a process that seems to happen similarly across species, researchers are cautiously optimistic that the research will translate.

Other drugs, too, are being eyed for their potential. A top contender, which has increased both lifespan and healthspan in mice by targeting a protein that controls key cellular functions, is rapamycin, used in people to prevent rejection of transplanted organs. Matt Kaeberlein, a professor of pathology at the University of Washington Medical Center in Seattle, is now studying whether rapamycin has a similar effect in pet dogs, which he thinks might be great models for aging research because they share an environment with humans and are genetically varied.

Kaeberlein and his team have so far put 25 healthy dogs through a 10-week trial of rapamycin; while he can't yet talk specifics, changes in cardiac function show a trend similar to the benefits seen in mice. He is planning a larger study that would follow 600 dogs randomized to either the drug or a placebo for at least three years to see whether the drug impacts vulnerability to cancer and cardiovascular disease, immune function, mobility, and cognitive function. "We want to really assess whether aging has been delayed," he says.

ONE DRUG STUDY IS ACTUALLY APPROACHING the human stage. Nir Barzilai, director of the Institute for Aging Research at Einstein, is spearheading an effort to test metformin, a diabetes drug, as a bulwark against a host of common age-related diseases. That's a very different strategy from the usual one of matching a drug to a single disease. The researchers settled on metformin as the first candidate for this type of study because it has a long track record of safety, and epidemiological evidence in humans suggests it might lower the risk for several different diseases. Now

{ WHAT CAN YOU DO NOW? *EAT A HEALTHY* DIET AND EXERCISE. }

the search is on for necessary funding – some $64 million to track 3,000 people over six years, says Barzilai. The start date of the trial will depend on funding, with a goal of beginning within a year, he says.

WHAT, IF ANYTHING, CAN PEOPLE DO NOW to lengthen their healthspan? Some clues come from studies of members of the Seventh-day Adventist Church, which recommends members exercise regularly, eat a well-balanced vegetarian diet, and avoid tobacco and alcohol. That advice seems to have paid off in Loma Linda, California, which has a significant concentration of Adventists and has been identified as the only U.S. "Blue Zone," an area recognized by researchers as a place where people tend to "live measurably longer, better." (The other Blue Zones are Sardinia, Italy; Okinawa, Japan; Costa Rica's Nicoya Peninsula; and the Greek island of Ikaria.)

Researchers at Loma Linda University have for decades studied the lifestyle habits of church members, with 96,000 people in the U.S. and Canada currently enrolled. A study published in 2001 of more than 34,000 non-Hispanic white Adventists in California found that a 30-year-old female participant could expect to live 7.3 years longer and a male could expect to live 4.4 years longer than other white Californians. Besides exercise and the vegetarian diet, regular consumption of nuts and being careful about body weight were factors making a difference.

Studies like this can't determine whether lifestyle behaviors actually led to longevity. But the evidence "is about as good as you can get," says Gary Fraser, principal investigator of the ongoing Adventist Health Study-2 and a professor of medicine and epidemiology at Loma Linda. The findings suggest that while genetics are likely heavily involved in living past 90, most people are equipped to reach that age if they make the right choices, says Perls.

Some researchers are also focusing on when, as opposed to what, you eat. Intermittent fasting, which involves periods of little or no food, have shown benefits in mice. Valter Longo, director of the University of Southern California Longevity Institute, is studying a diet that mimics fasting, with five consecutive days of a low protein and low sugar diet amounting to 800 to 1,100 calories per day. For most healthy people, that could be done once every three to six months, he says. Animal studies suggest that starting to eat normally again after a period of food scarcity can regenerate organs by turning on stem cells. And a small pilot study found that a similar diet in humans improved such markers for age-related diseases as trunk fat, glucose and C-reactive protein, a measure of inflammation. A larger trial of 100 people is finished but the results haven't yet been published, says Longo.

Importantly, the diet is safer than outright fasting, says Longo, who, along with his lab members and family members, follows the regimen. But he warns that people who want to try it should speak with their physicians, and that it isn't appropriate for diabetics taking medications. Nor are the long-term effects known (though data from clinics that supervise fasting for 10 to 21 days indicate periodic fasting is safe). Other researchers are looking at variations on this theme, such as restricting food consumption to an eight-hour window in the day.

Research also suggests that stress management plays a role. Prolonged psychological stress seems to promote many hallmarks of aging, including inflammation and the shortening of the protective caps on the end of chromosomes known as telomeres, according to Elissa Epel, a professor of psychiatry at the University of California–San Francisco. Short telomeres are associated with the early onset of disease, though it's not known whether they actually cause aging. But she and her colleagues, led by Eli Puterman at UCSF, have found that a diet of healthful foods like fruits, vegetables and nuts and fewer unhealthful ones like fried foods and soda, along with regular exercise and quality sleep, can counteract those effects. Separately, she also recommends fostering social connections and relationships, and purpose in life.

FOLSTROM, WHO WILL BECOME A "SUPERCENTENARIAN" when she turns 110 this year, would seem to be evidence supporting much of this advice. She's had a "normal, happy life," growing up on a farm and living mostly in her beloved Minnesota with her husband, a pastor, until he died in 1999. Along the way she worked in various jobs, including as a country schoolteacher and a switchboard operator. She never drank or smoked. "We have to take care of our bodies," she says. She's always been religious and credits God's plan for her longevity.

Will geroscience help more people follow in her footsteps? The research is very exciting, says the NIA's Sierra, though "we are really in the infancy of this." So stay tuned. ●

NEW (AND OLD) WAYS TO BATTLE PAIN

Concerns about opioids are leading to an expanded arsenal

BY COURTNEY RUBIN

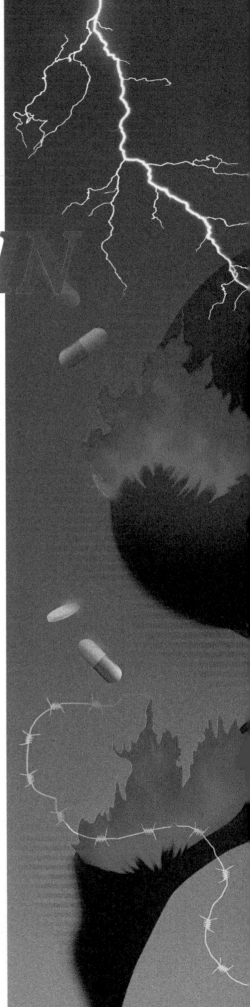

One day in early 2008, Israel Andrade, a department manager at a home store in Dallas, was helping to move a heavy carpet when he herniated all the lumbar discs in his back. Thus began a seven-year search for relief from chronic pain.

Andrade tried several medications, including the opioid hydrocodone, which left him "too doped up to do anything." Then there was a morphine patch, a lidocaine patch, steroid injections in his back, nerve blocks, and three procedures using radiofrequency to destroy pain-carrying nerve fibers. While these treatments do the job for some people, they left Andrade still in so much distress that he couldn't stay in any one position for very long, and a 30-yard walk to the mailbox required medication and hours of rest.

Finally, last year, a doctor recommended a surgical procedure that interferes with nerve signals between the spinal cord and brain. "It's been a godsend," says Andrade, 61, who now walks two miles several times a week. "My pain is nearly gone."

With 1 in 5 Americans suffering from chronic pain, the race is on to rediscover and invent alternatives to opioids. Overdose deaths from all opioids have nearly quadrupled since 1999, to more than 28,000 in 2014, according to the Centers for Disease Control and Prevention. Over half of those deaths were due to prescription

medications. Doctors were "giving pain medication for every little sniffle," says Charles Kim, an assistant professor in the department of rehabilitation medicine and anesthesiology at NYU Langone Medical Center in New York. "We've realized now we can't do that anymore."

The push for alternatives has led to new interest in treatments often neglected in the opioid era. Acupuncture, for one, was shown in a 2012 Archives of Internal Medicine study involving some 18,000 patients to provide significant relief for osteoarthritis, headaches, and back and neck pain. In the two-hour procedure that helped Andrade, which can alter how the body perceives pain, doctors implanted a device about the size of a deck of cards under his skin and tiny insulated wires on his spine that use low-frequency electricity to interrupt the pain signal. And researchers are also hard at work searching for new and better treatments. Here's a look at some of the most promising nonopioid options, old and new:

NEUROSTIMULATION. The technique that helped Andrade has been around since 1967, and can be enlisted almost anywhere in the body to help manage everything from migraines to pain that persists after a person has had shingles.

Probably the most prevalent type relies on devices that stimulate nerves in the spine to treat pain in the back and in the legs and arms, often substitut-

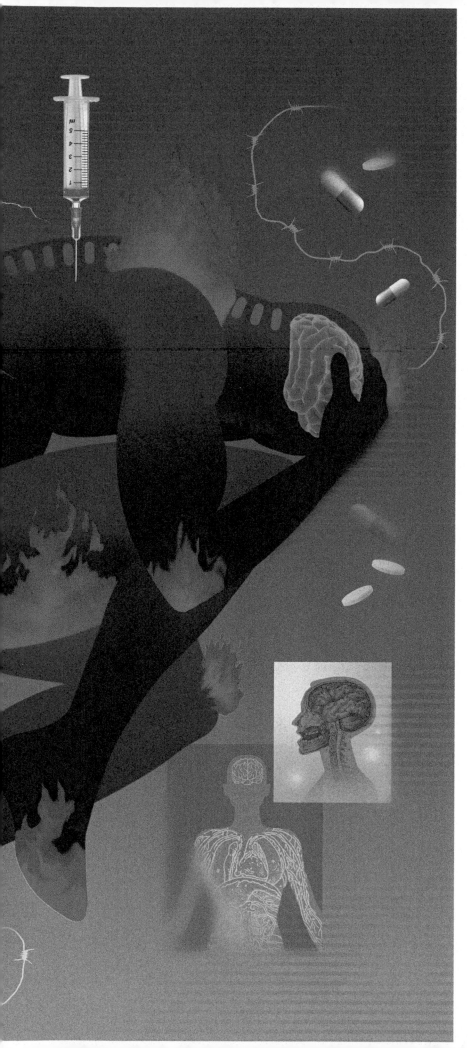

ing a gentle tingling called paresthesia. (For headaches, neurostimulation devices might be implanted in the neck or even in the gums.)

Though the technology has been on the market for several decades, the recent surge of innovation in pain management has improved it significantly. The devices are smaller, for example, and battery life has been extended from just a couple of years to as long as 10. Andrade's implant, whose electrical flow he can turn off and adjust via a remote controller, has a sensor that "remembers" what level of stimulation is needed in various body positions and automatically adjusts for movement.

The latest wrinkle: In 2015, the Food and Drug Administration approved the first such device that delivers high frequency stimulation – up to 10,000 hertz – instead of the traditional 50 hertz. The high frequency eliminates the tingling feeling associated with these devices, and according to a 2015 study published in the journal Anesthesiology is nearly twice as effective as low frequency in dealing with chronic back and limb pain.

People who have not responded well to traditional spinal cord stimulation might want to investigate a new variation that specifically works on the dorsal root ganglion, a small bundle of nerves connected to every vertebra in the spine. The FDA just gave it the green light earlier this year. These nerves act like traffic lights, controlling what sensations enter the spine, and electric stimulation can switch on the red light for pain. Because the leads are smaller and can be positioned more precisely, research has indicated that the devices are particularly helpful in treating pain that's hard to target with traditional spinal cord stimulation, such as in the groin, foot or lower limbs.

Next up is a not-yet-approved stimulator that delivers "burst stimulation," instead of a constant flow. The theory is that the intermittent pulsing mimics nerve cells, providing better relief. A 2015 study published in the Clini-

MIGHT EXERCISE HELP? MAYBE

Should you try exercise for your persistent aching knee or shoulder? Physical activity may be just what the doctor ordered, but first you should see a doctor.

"Before you treat a symptom you need to figure out what's causing it," cautions Seth Leopold, a University of Washington School of Medicine professor of orthopaedics and sports medicine. If exercise is appropriate, your doctor may decide the best first step is to refer you to a physical therapist.

For joint pain, David Reavy, a Chicago PT, often recommends any type of activity that is low impact, such as riding a bike, swimming, or taking part in water aerobics. "These exercises decrease stress to the joint and allow it to move without the impact and force you might get in other types of exercise," he says. He particularly likes anything aquatic, because the water resistance involved forces patients to use their core and also allows them to strengthen their hips.

Strength training is often prescribed, because strengthening the muscles around the joint allows them to absorb the force in the area, rather than the joint itself. Stretching and releasing also can work to relieve pain because it increases the range of motion, so you're able to use more muscles more efficiently. The more muscles you can use when you move, Reavy says, the less stress you'll put on your joints.

Iyengar yoga, a type that uses props such as belts, blocks and blankets to help students reach positions correctly, is also often suggested. University of Pennsylvania researchers found a "statistically significant" reduction in pain for osteoarthritis patients with 90-minute Iyengar sessions once a week for eight weeks. Sharon Kolasinski, the director of rheumatology at the Penn Musculoskeletal Center and the study's lead author, hypothesizes that the practice increases a person's confidence in moving and using the joints and improves range of motion, strength and balance. –C.R.

cal Journal of Pain found that burst stimulation "was significantly better" than the constant kind, and that nearly two-thirds of patients who weren't helped by standard stimulation responded.

IMPLANTED PUMP. The titanium pump, like the stimulator device, is enjoying new life. Implanted pumps deliver medications (including opioids) in a targeted way to the fluid surrounding the spinal cord, which means they can be given at a fraction of the dose received orally. "If you're giving a dose of 300 milligrams of a drug orally, like morphine, you can give 1 milligram of that drug to the spinal fluid and have an approximately equal effect," says Lance Roy, an assistant professor of anesthesia at Duke University Medical Center. "The tiny doses minimize some of the side effects and really improve quality of life." Implanted pumps are frequently used in people for whom oral medications or injections haven't worked or for whom the side effects were intolerable.

The devices deliver medicine to the spinal cord via a catheter, and are refilled every one to three months at the doctor's office through a needle. Technological advances have made the pumps safer and more convenient; they can now be programmed by remote control to release the proper dose, for example.

Still, pumps are by no means a sure bet. A 2014 review of studies published in the Journal of Pain Research suggested that while they're useful for treating cancer pain, it's hard to draw conclusions about how well they relieve other types, in part because of the lack of randomized trials.

BIACUPLASTY. One new option for treating chronic pain of the neck or back resulting from herniated or bulging disks is a 30-minute outpatient procedure that uses X-ray guidance and two electrodes to create lesions along the disc nerves. The nerves are thus

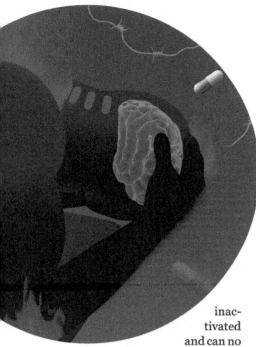

inactivated and can no longer transmit pain signals to the brain. Research presented at last year's American Academy of Pain Medicine meeting suggested that the procedure, which is less invasive and less risky than the surgical procedures, worked better than so-called "conservative" back pain therapies, which include weight loss, acupuncture and anti-inflammatory drugs.

The procedure is "something that can help with one of the most common disabilities in the Western world: low back pain," says Paul Christo, an associate professor in the division of pain medicine at Johns Hopkins who is also the host of "Aches and Gains," a five-year-old radio show on Sirius XM about overcoming pain. Biacuplasty coagulates the nerves in the discs, he says, and there's a chance it may even help heal fissures or cracks in degenerated discs. "We just don't know yet, but I think there's great potential there." Biacuplasty is still too new to be covered by most insurers.

DRUG THERAPY. Drugs other than opioids have been around to treat pain for years, too; there's a focus now on trying them before moving on to the more problematic painkillers. Anticonvulsants such as Lyrica can lessen neuropathic pain, though doctors aren't sure how. Antidepressants are sometimes prescribed for musculoskeletal pain and diabetic neuropathy; they work by increasing the neurotransmitters serotonin and norepinephrine, which reduce pain.

Botulinum toxin, aka Botox, is also being recruited. It blocks the release of the neurotransmitter acetycholine, forcing muscles to relax. The drug has been approved to treat migraines. A 2013 review of studies found that a single injection could relieve pain and improve function and quality of life in people with arthritis, though the paper noted that the studies were small.

Researchers are also investigating new drugs, one of the most promising being injections of a compound called resiniferatoxin found in a cactus-like Moroccan plant that works by blocking the transmission of pain signals. Essentially, the substance – 1,000

"ABOUT 1 IN 5 AMERICANS *SUFFERS* FROM *CHRONIC PAIN.*"

times hotter than capsaicin, the chemical in hot peppers – destroys the neurons responsible for inflammatory pain by burning them.

Anti-nerve growth factor modulators, a class of drugs that excites Christo, prevent the protein from binding to its receptor on neurons, thus blocking pain transmission. And cannabinoid receptor agonists – which, as their name suggests, are a derivative of cannabis – may have potential, too. These drugs target cannabinoid receptors, which are located throughout the body and play a role in pain.

STEM CELL THERAPY. In this controversial procedure, doctors take bone marrow from the hip, remove stem cells and inject them into areas plagued by pain. The idea is that the stem cells may turn into new cartilage and tissue. A 2014 international clinical trial found that a single injection into degenerated discs reduced low back pain for at least a year. But "we're still really in the infancy stages with this," cautions NYU Langone's Kim.

Stem cell therapy is often performed in conjunction with another experimental procedure using platelet-rich plasma, or PRP. Blood is drawn and plasma is extracted by spinning the blood in a centrifuge. Concentrated platelets and other nutrients are added in, and the mixture is injected near the pain site. Theoretically, the PRP promotes healing. The treatment has a long (though inconclusive) history of use to treat injured professional athletes.

Some doctors see promise; plenty are skeptical. "There's more evidence to back up acupuncture" than PRP, Kim says. According to the American Academy of Orthopaedic Surgeons, it so far seems most effective for chronic tendonitis of the elbow or Achilles tendon.

One happy customer is Dean Scarpa, 56, a business owner from Voorhees, New Jersey, who suffered from arthritic pain in his knees, then tore his anterior cruciate ligament and meniscus in his right knee skiing. Scarpa says he was told he'd need surgery, but he was disturbed when he read that few skiers get back to their previous levels after an operation. So instead he went to a Philadelphia-area sports medicine doctor, who performed the stem cell procedure over a month. Within three months, Scarpa's knee felt better, and within six months, he could jump on it. He then had the PRP treatment on his left knee. The pain there, too, has gone away. "I knew there was a chance these things might not work" and surgery might become necessary, Scarpa says. So far, it hasn't been. ●

LET THE GAMES BEGIN!

The principles of game theory can inspire you to walk more, eat better, and even quit smoking | BY COURTNEY RUBIN

Sitting all day is not a great way to stay heathy, as Debi Bisnette had long known. But in spite of all the articles she'd read about the health benefits of taking a walk at lunchtime, somehow the accounts payable clerk from Orlando, Florida, always ended up sitting in the break room with her colleagues.

Then, in January, Bisnette signed up for a special clip-on gadget – a "Trio Tracker" she wears on her waistband – customized for her by UnitedHealthcare, her company's insurer. It buzzes if she sits for more than an hour, and little trophies pop up on its face for each of three goals she seeks to meet daily: six sessions of 300 steps within five minutes, separated by an hour; 3,000 steps in 30 minutes; and 10,000 steps total for the day. Now Bisnette does get moving at lunchtime.

"It's fun to see the trophies appear," says Bisnette, 59, who has lost 12 pounds. It also doesn't hurt that meeting the challenges earns her up to $4 per day in health care reimbursement, which can add up to $1,460 per year toward her deductible.

BISNETTE IS AMONG the millions of Americans experiencing the gamifying of health care, the application of game principles like competition or cooperation that play to such motivations as desire for mastery, all in the service of inspiring people to make better decisions. It's a trend that's only taken off recently, with the widespread use of

smartphones, wearable devices and wireless technology.

Game theory has been applied to everything from getting the best price on a car to political machinations to suggestions by some German academics for how to break through the impasses on climate talks. "Games activate certain very deep and core aspects of our psychology, which is why every civilization has had them," says Kevin Werbach, an associate professor of legal studies and business ethics at the University of Pennsylvania's Wharton School and a leader in the emerging field of gamification. Werbach's class on the topic, which teaches the mechanisms and how to use them effectively, is one of Coursera's most popular massive open online courses, or MOOCs.

In health, designers are creating apps that nudge people along in all sorts of ways. They use the intrinsic sense of accomplishment and the extrinsic unlocking of achievements (and gifts) to encourage pregnant women on Medicaid to keep their doctors' appointments, for example. Or to get young cystic fibrosis patients to do their breathing exercises by puffing into a tube controller to speed an on-screen pirate ship. Insurance companies,

of course, have embraced games because they can promote better lifestyle habits, such as walking or eating more vegetables. Minnesota-based United-Healthcare, for example, even has a full-time games producer.

You don't have to be a video game fan to see the appeal; anyone who's ever played tag or hide-and-seek can get the idea. Arrianne Hoyland, that United-Healthcare games producer, notes that "If I asked my dad, "Are you a gamer?" he'd say no way. But he plays solitaire. Solitaire is, like, his sport."

One quick and easy way to turn an activity into a game is to award points, badges or financial incentives. But the best attempts to gamify go beyond that, says Frank Lee, associate professor of digital media and director of Drexel University's

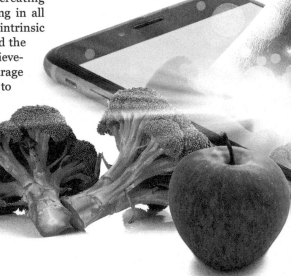

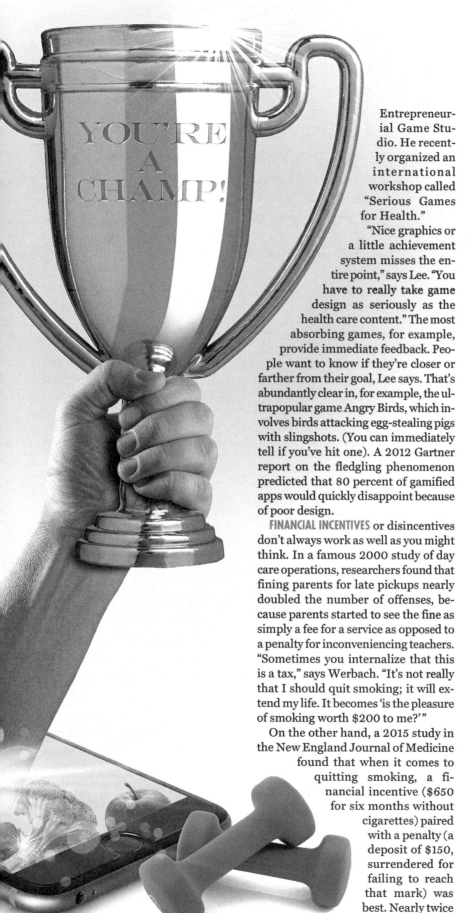

Entrepreneurial Game Studio. He recently organized an international workshop called "Serious Games for Health."

"Nice graphics or a little achievement system misses the entire point," says Lee. "You have to really take game design as seriously as the health care content." The most absorbing games, for example, provide immediate feedback. People want to know if they're closer or farther from their goal, Lee says. That's abundantly clear in, for example, the ultrapopular game Angry Birds, which involves birds attacking egg-stealing pigs with slingshots. (You can immediately tell if you've hit one). A 2012 Gartner report on the fledgling phenomenon predicted that 80 percent of gamified apps would quickly disappoint because of poor design.

FINANCIAL INCENTIVES or disincentives don't always work as well as you might think. In a famous 2000 study of day care operations, researchers found that fining parents for late pickups nearly doubled the number of offenses, because parents started to see the fine as simply a fee for a service as opposed to a penalty for inconveniencing teachers. "Sometimes you internalize that this is a tax," says Werbach. "It's not really that I should quit smoking; it will extend my life. It becomes 'is the pleasure of smoking worth $200 to me?'"

On the other hand, a 2015 study in the New England Journal of Medicine found that when it comes to quitting smoking, a financial incentive ($650 for six months without cigarettes) paired with a penalty (a deposit of $150, surrendered for failing to reach that mark) was best. Nearly twice as many people succeeded compared to those offered the $650 carrot alone. Typically financial disincentives are administered by charging the credit card number you've given at sign-up.

PACT IS AN APP THAT grew out of a behavioral economics class its co-founders took as undergraduates at Harvard. It debuted in 2012 as GymPact, asking users to commit to a certain number of gym visits per week and using GPS to track their check-ins at sports facilities. Users were charged penalties for not reaching their goals, but also received cash if they did.

The app has since evolved to include goals like eating more vegetables (users upload pictures of what they're eating; technology verifies that the pictures actually have been taken with the user's phone, as opposed to being "borrowed" from somewhere on the Internet). Anyone can use the app, though the company also works with some businesses to allow employees to collect cash rewards and offset health care expenses, such as deductibles.

A game available to everyone that takes aim at mental as well as physical health, called SuperBetter, was designed by Jane McGonigal, the director of games research and development at the nonprofit Institute for the Future in Palo Alto, out of personal need. McGonigal had sustained a head injury in 2009 that had left her feeling depressed, hopeless and lethargic – until she decided to turn her recovery into a game. The result, a free app, was released in 2012.

The game encourages people to be their own superheroes, renaming long-term goals (such as quitting smoking, exercising more, lowering stress and combating anxiety) "epic wins." These are broken down into daily "quests" such as, in the case of exercise, walking around the block or dancing to a favorite song. Along the way, players also work on four kinds of resilience (physical, emotional, social and mental) by completing "Power Ups," activities that help them in day-to-day life such as making contact with a friend. Players strive to defeat the "bad guys" standing in their way – procrastination, say, or short car trips that could just as easily be walked. Research at the University of Pennsylvania found that playing SuperBetter for 30 days reduced symptoms of anxiety and depression and increased a player's belief in his or her own ability to succeed and achieve goals.

LIKE SUPERBETTER, Rally Health offers help making small daily changes, though the online and mobile platforms call them "missions" instead of quests. Rally, so far available to some 23 million Americans through their health insurers or employer groups, suggests missions based on a survey users fill out. Users can also choose their own from four different categories: eat, move, feel and care.

Missions can range from turning off the computer and TV early (in the "feel" category, relating to stress) to swapping a sugary drink for water. Completing missions earns you virtual coins that can be used in sweepstakes and auctions that are dangling goods like an Apple TV or an Apple watch.

The platform's core customer is a fortysomething female – these women tend to be "the stewards of health care for the family," says Rhett Woods, Rally's chief creative officer. Rally subscribes to the positive affirmation model. There's no loss aversion (as in penalties) here. "We want people always to feel like they're earning or moving forward," Woods says. More than 40 percent of users are actively involved in earning rewards, according to company figures.

As any good game does, Rally is evolving based on people's experience using it. An early iteration offered multiple types of currency, with different colored coins that could be earned in various categories. "We learned that things need to be as simple as humanly possible," Woods says. "And when we simplified to a single currency, we found engagement went up significantly." That counts as a win. ●

THE CALORIE CONUNDRUM

Is your low-fat, low-cal diet actually working against you?

BY MARGARET LOFTUS

heather Reyes has spent the better part of the last decade struggling to lose the 40 extra pounds she gained in her early 20s and the weight she put on during her pregnancies. The Aurora, Illinois, mother of two counted calories ad nauseum, at one point losing 30 pounds during a stint on Weight Watchers. But inevitably her willpower would fade. As soon as she strayed from her diet, she says, "the floodgates would open," and the pounds would creep back on. "As much as I wanted to lose weight, I wanted to eat."

Last winter, Reyes, now 34, embarked on yet another weight-loss plan based on the recently published book "Always Hungry?" by David Ludwig, an endocrinologist and obesity expert at Boston Children's Hospital who directs the weight management clinic there (story, Page 120) and is also a professor of nutrition at the Harvard School of Public Health. His research into the biology of metabolism supports a weight-loss message quite different from the one she'd been getting: Don't count calories. Fat is your friend. Whole milk and full-fat yogurt are fine. Since starting the regime in February, Reyes has shed 40 pounds and six inches from her waist, and her cholesterol, blood pressure and resting heart rate have dropped – all without worrying about the calorie count. "My doctor is thrilled. She told me to keep doing what I'm doing," Reyes says. What's more, she reports, she "feels amazing."

YOU NEED ONLY peruse the "Always Hungry?" Facebook page to find hundreds of testimonials like Reyes'. But the notion that a calorie-restricting approach to weight loss might actually be a bad idea – Ludwig makes the case that it's the type of calorie you consume more than simply the number that makes you fat – has generated controversy. Most experts, including the U.S. Centers for Disease Control and Prevention, continue to emphasize the eat less, move more mantra that has been the prevailing advice for the last 40 years. "The ultimate goal for weight loss is to eat fewer calories than you burn," says Gary Foster, Weight Watchers' chief scientific officer and founder and former director of Temple University's Center for Obesity Research and Education.

The problem, Ludwig notes, is that

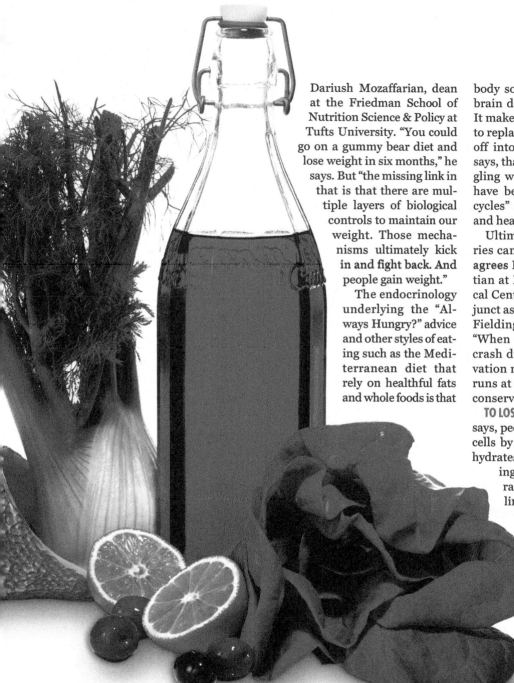

Dariush Mozaffarian, dean at the Friedman School of Nutrition Science & Policy at Tufts University. "You could go on a gummy bear diet and lose weight in six months," he says. But "the missing link in that is that there are multiple layers of biological controls to maintain our weight. Those mechanisms ultimately kick in and fight back. And people gain weight."

The endocrinology underlying the "Always Hungry?" advice and other styles of eating such as the Mediterranean diet that rely on healthful fats and whole foods is that

body soon runs low on fuel. "So the brain does what it's supposed to do: It makes us hungry, and [we] overeat to replace the calories being siphoned off into fat cells." Little wonder, he says, that "most people who are struggling with their weight or are obese have been through dozens of these cycles" and often end up defeated – and heavier.

Ultimately, simply restricting calories can make losing weight harder, agrees Dana Hunnes, a senior dietitian at Ronald Reagan UCLA Medical Center in Los Angeles and an adjunct assistant professor at the UCLA Fielding School of Public Health. "When we restrict calories or go on crash diets, our bodies go into starvation mode, where our metabolism runs at a significantly slower rate to conserve energy."

TO LOSE WEIGHT PERMANENTLY, Ludwig says, people can "reprogram" their fat cells by getting rid of refined carbohydrates and adding generous helpings of high fat foods that "don't raise insulin at all." With insulin levels stable, the cells store fewer calories and pounds drop off gradually as the body's "set point," or the weight it naturally gravitates toward, lowers. Good choices include nuts and nut butters, full-fat dairy, olive oil, rich sauces and spreads, and avocado. "Opposite to what we've been told for 40 years, these fats are extremely healthful," he says.

Even saturated fat has its place, he says. While overdoing it can adversely affect cholesterol levels and promote chronic inflammation, many foods "like full-fat yogurt and real dark chocolate are great for the heart, and there's no reason to avoid them." His plan emphasizes the "monos," monounsaturated fats like nuts and olive oil, and omega-3s found in fish.

As is true of many diet programs, the first two weeks of this plan are

the low-cal, low-fat approach of the past few decades ignores biology, and that the highly processed foods that many calorie-counters eat in place of fat in fact go a long way toward explaining why Americans are heavier than ever. (More than 70 percent of Americans age 20 or older are overweight and more than one-third of adults are obese, according to the CDC.) There's no question that a focus on cutting calories does work in the short term, says

highly processed carbohydrates like bread, crackers, cereal, chips, candy and sugary drinks send insulin levels in the bloodstream soaring as they quickly digest into sugar. Ludwig likens insulin to a sort of Miracle-Gro for fat cells, since the hormone's job is to guide calories into the fat cells for storage. "The type of calories you consume affects the number of calories you burn," he says. And when fat cells feast, the rest of the

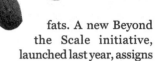

designed to jump-start weight loss. By cutting out sugar-laden and processed foods and getting half of your total daily intake from fat for that period, you get off the blood sugar rollercoaster and tame those junk-food cravings. The rest of the menu is equally split between protein and whole carbs such as fruit, beans and nonstarchy vegetables.

The second phase, which may last a few weeks to many months depending on your weight, calls for a slight decrease in fat intake and an uptick in carbs to include whole-kernel grains like brown rice, steel-cut oats and quinoa.

The final phase, intended to be a model for a lifelong approach to eating, calls for about 40 percent complex carbohydrates, 40 percent fat, and 20 percent protein, similar to versions of the Mediterranean diet. It even reintroduces a small amount of processed carbs. While the plan doesn't impose any calorie limitations, neither does it give you carte blanche to start bingeing. Weight loss is intended to happen slowly and naturally as you eat until you're satisfied.

WHILE NO DIET HAS BEEN PROVEN in a rigorous clinical trial, says Ludwig, the plan is based on dozens of studies by his group as well as hundreds of studies by others. In one pilot, 237 people who followed the program for 16 weeks, typically losing a pound or two a week, reported decreased hunger, increased energy, and improved well-being. And a study that he and his colleagues published in the Journal of the American Medical Association in 2012 supports the premise that the type of food you eat matters more than simply how much.

That work examined a group of adults who followed both a low-fat and a low-carb plan, each of which allowed for the same number of calories per day. While on the low-carb plan, participants burned an average of 325 more calories each day than they burned while eating minimal fat.

To be sure, this isn't the only diet that promises to cure your cupcake cravings. Susan Roberts, a professor of nutrition and psychiatry at Tufts, has developed an approach known as the "I" Diet (idiet. com) that is high in fiber, protein and high-volume foods such as vegetables that fill you up and is low in those "high-glycemic" foods that make blood sugar levels shoot up. Foods like macaroni and cheese and chocolate pudding are allowed but have been reformulated using whole grain rather than white pasta and sugar substitutes.

Ultimately, Roberts says, the plan can actually rewire the brain to crave healthy foods. In a 2014 study published in Nutrition & Diabetes, Tufts researchers gave subjects who had been on the diet for six months an MRI and found that the reward centers of the brains were excited when they viewed images of healthy foods, but not when they looked at images of junk food.

The Weight Watchers program, which performs well in the U.S. News Best Diets rankings (Page 78), is based on calorie-counting but also uses a point system to steer followers toward lean protein, fruits and veggies and away from sugar and saturated fats. A new Beyond the Scale initiative, launched last year, assigns each food and beverage a SmartPoints value, a single number calculated to reflect four components: calories, saturated fat, sugar and protein. So a yogurt parfait that has the same number of calories as two pancakes with maple syrup – 300 – would cost you only three of your daily SmartPoints allotment, compared to the pancakes' 12 points. Fruit and most vegetables cost zero points.

Weight Watchers' Foster believes one key reason dieters fail has less to do with hunger than with their environment – the many, many opportunities to eat – and choices. "We eat when we're bored, when we're driving, when we're texting, when we're procrastinating," he notes. Hence the company's built-in support system, which includes online chats with Weight Watchers coaches and the classic weekly meetings, where members dish about weight-loss tips, recipes, successes and plateaus.

Mozaffarian applauds Weight Watchers for recognizing that some foods are clearly more beneficial to weight loss than others. "Quality trumps quantity in the long term," he says.

That's something that Reyes has learned to appreciate. She can enjoy foods like whole-milk yogurt and red meat and no longer craves sweets. "It's helped me deal with the wanting," she says. She also no longer feels guilty about her choices. Her plans for her recent birthday, for example, involved making herself a cake, eating a little bit, and giving the rest away. ●

INSULIN ACTS SORT OF LIKE *PLANT FOOD* FOR FAT CELLS.

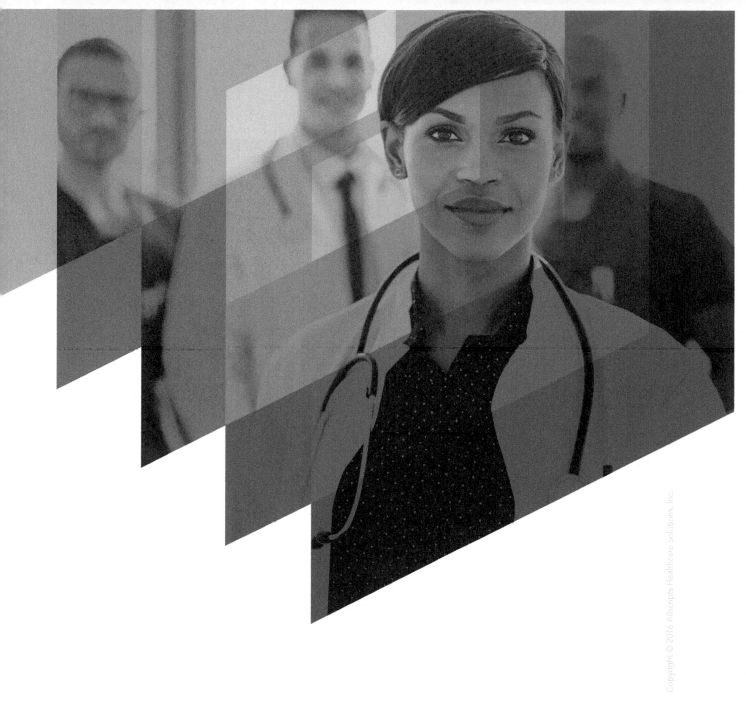

Congratulations

Allscripts clients make up 100% of U.S. News & World Report's
2016-2017 "Honor Roll" for Best Hospitals.

Learn more at www.allscripts.com   ⬡ Allscripts®

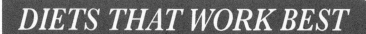

DIETS THAT WORK BEST

U.S. News puts 38 eating plans through their paces

HOW DOES A DIET WIN A PLACE in the Best Diets rankings? Cutting through the clutter of conflicting claims and hype can be a challenge, so U.S. News asked a panel of nationally recognized experts (Page 78) to assess how effective some of the best-known eating plans are, whether the goal is to lose weight, improve heart health, or manage diabetes. Our panelists reviewed the research, added their own fact-finding, and rated the diets from 1 to 5 (the top score) in a number of areas: short-term weight loss (the likelihood of losing significant weight dur-

ing the first 12 months); long-term weight loss (the likelihood of maintaining significant weight loss for two years or more); diabetes prevention and management; heart health (effectiveness at preventing cardiovascular disease and reducing risk for heart patients); ease of compliance; nutritional completeness (how well a plan conforms with federal dietary guidelines); and safety (whether, for example, it omits key nutrients). Which plan can help you meet your goals? Check out the results in these pages. For more on the plans, visit usnews.com/bestdiets.

HOW THE PLANS STACK UP OVERALL

Thirty-eight diets were rated from 1 to 5 on multiple measures. Rank is based on a score compiled from panelists' average scores for each measure. The results:

Rank	Diet	Overall score	Short-term weight loss	Long-term weight loss	For diabetes	For heart health	Nutrition	Safety	Ease of complying
1	DASH	4.1	3.2	3.0	3.6	4.3	4.7	4.9	3.1
2	Mind	4.0	3.1	2.9	3.5	4.1	4.3	4.7	3.7
2	TLC	4.0	3.2	2.8	3.2	4.5	4.6	4.8	3.0
4	Fertility	3.9	3.0	2.6	3.7	3.7	4.4	4.4	3.7
4	Mayo Clinic	3.9	3.3	2.9	3.5	3.6	4.3	4.7	3.1
4	Mediterranean	3.9	3.0	2.9	3.4	4.0	4.4	4.8	3.3
4	Weight Watchers	3.9	4.0	3.5	3.1	3.4	4.1	4.6	3.7
8	Flexitarian	3.8	3.4	3.3	3.5	3.8	4.0	4.4	3.3
8	Volumetrics	3.8	3.6	3.2	3.4	3.5	4.2	4.6	3.2
10	Jenny Craig	3.7	3.8	3.2	3.0	3.2	4.0	4.4	3.6
11	Biggest Loser	3.6	4.1	2.9	3.6	3.5	3.8	4.1	2.9
11	Ornish	3.6	3.1	2.8	3.5	4.6	3.8	4.2	1.9
13	Traditional Asian	3.5	2.9	2.7	3.2	3.3	3.9	4.2	2.8
13	Vegetarian	3.5	2.9	2.9	3.4	3.6	3.7	4.2	2.7
15	Anti-Inflammatory	3.3	2.6	2.6	3.4	3.6	3.4	3.9	2.7
15	Slim Fast	3.3	3.4	3.2	3.2	2.8	3.4	3.6	3.2
15	Spark Solution	3.3	3.6	2.8	2.9	2.9	3.6	4.0	2.3
18	Flat Belly	3.2	3.1	2.3	2.8	3.2	3.5	4.0	2.7
18	HMR	3.2	4.1	3.0	3.0	2.9	3.4	3.4	2.9
18	Nutrisystem	3.2	3.2	2.3	2.7	2.4	3.7	4.0	3.1
21	Abs	3.0	3.1	2.1	2.7	2.7	3.4	3.5	2.6
21	Engine 2	3.0	3.4	2.9	3.5	3.9	2.7	3.3	1.6
21	South Beach	3.0	3.7	2.3	2.5	2.9	3.2	3.4	2.8
21	Vegan	3.0	3.4	3.3	3.5	3.9	2.8	3.0	1.7
25	Eco-Atkins	2.9	3.8	2.5	2.5	3.3	2.8	3.3	2.1
25	Glycemic-Index	2.9	2.8	2.2	2.7	2.3	3.1	3.8	2.1
25	Zone	2.9	3.0	2.3	2.3	2.8	3.2	3.7	2.2
28	Macrobiotic	2.7	3.1	2.5	3.1	3.2	2.5	3.0	1.7
28	Medifast	2.7	3.5	2.0	2.6	2.7	3.1	3.0	2.4
30	Acid Alkaline	2.6	2.6	2.0	2.2	2.4	2.9	3.1	2.0
30	Supercharged Hormone	2.6	3.1	2.3	2.4	2.5	2.6	2.9	2.2
32	Body Reset	2.5	2.8	1.7	1.8	2.1	2.7	3.2	2.0
32	Fast	2.5	3.2	2.3	2.4	2.5	2.1	2.6	2.4
34	Atkins	2.3	4.0	2.5	2.5	2.1	1.8	2.2	2.3
34	Raw food	2.3	3.7	3.3	2.6	2.8	2.1	2.1	1.1
36	Dukan	2.0	3.0	2.0	2.0	1.7	1.9	2.3	1.5
36	Paleo	2.0	2.1	1.7	2.1	2.0	2.0	2.3	1.7
38	Whole 30	1.9	2.9	1.5	1.9	1.7	1.7	2.4	1.3

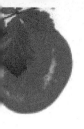

BEST WEIGHT-LOSS DIETS

Diets are ranked by the average of the scores experts assigned them for producing short- and long-term results.

Rank	Diet	Avg. score
1	Weight Watchers	3.8
2	HMR	3.6
3	Biggest Loser	3.5
3	Jenny Craig	3.5
3	Raw Food	3.5
6	Volumetrics	3.4
7	Atkins	3.3
7	Flexitarian	3.3
7	Slim Fast	3.3
7	Vegan	3.3

BEST DIABETES DIETS

These plans scored highest for both managing and preventing the condition.

Rank	Diet	Avg. score
1	Fertility	3.7
2	Biggest Loser	3.6
2	DASH	3.6
4	Engine 2	3.5
4	Flexitarian	3.5
4	Mayo Clinic	3.5
4	Mind	3.5
4	Ornish	3.5
4	Vegan	3.5
10	Anti-Inflammatory	3.4
10	Mediterranean	3.4
10	Vegetarian	3.4
10	Volumetrics	3.4

BEST COMMERCIAL DIETS

Nutritional value, ease of use and safety are counted, as well as weight-loss effectiveness.

Rank	Diet	Avg. score
1	Mayo Clinic	3.9
1	Weight Watchers	3.9
3	Jenny Craig	3.7
4	Biggest Loser	3.6
5	Slim Fast	3.3
5	Spark Solution	3.3
7	Flat Belly	3.2
7	HMR	3.2
7	Nutrisystem	3.2
10	Abs Diet	3.0
10	South Beach	3.0

BEST DIETS FOR THE HEART

With these plans, you take aim at cholesterol, blood pressure and triglycerides as well as weight.

Rank	Diet	Avg. score
1	Ornish	4.6
2	TLC	4.5
3	DASH	4.3
4	Mind	4.1
5	Mediterranean	4.0
6	Engine 2	3.9
6	Vegan	3.9
8	Flexitarian	3.8
9	Fertility	3.7
10	Anti-Inflammatory	3.6
10	Mayo Clinic	3.6
10	Vegetarian	3.6

BEST PLANT-BASED DIETS

These diets emphasize minimally processed foods from plants and are good bets for weight loss.

Rank	Diet	Avg. score
1	Mediterranean	3.9
2	Flexitarian	3.8
3	Ornish	3.6
4	Traditional Asian	3.5
4	Vegetarian	3.5
6	Anti-Inflammatory	3.3
7	Engine 2	3.0
7	Vegan	3.0
9	Eco-Atkins	2.9
10	Macrobiotic	2.7
11	Raw Food	2.3

EASIEST-TO-FOLLOW DIETS

The ranking is based on ease of use and a diet's ability to deliver weight loss and good nutrition.

Rank	Diet	Avg. score
1	Fertility	3.7
1	Mind	3.7
1	Weight Watchers	3.7
4	Jenny Craig	3.6
5	Flexitarian	3.3
5	Mediterranean	3.3
7	Slim Fast	3.2
7	Volumetrics	3.2
9	DASH	3.1
9	Mayo Clinic	3.1
9	Nutrisystem	3.1

THE DIET PANEL

Twenty-two experts reviewed detailed assessments of the U.S. News list of 38 diets and rated them on a number of key measures, described on Page 77.

Kathie Beals
Associate professor (clinical), division of nutrition, University of Utah

Amy Campbell
Nutrition and wellness consultant and writer

Lawrence Cheskin
Founder and director, Johns Hopkins Weight Management Center

Michael Davidson
Director of preventive cardiology, University of Chicago Medical Center

Marion Franz
Nutrition and health consultant, Nutrition Concepts by Franz Inc.

Teresa Fung
Professor of nutrition, Simmons College

Andrea Giancoli
Nutrition advocate, consultant and communicator

Carole V. Harris
Senior fellow, public health division, ICF International

David Katz
Director, Yale-Griffin Prevention Research Center

Penny Kris-Etherton
Distinguished professor of nutrition, Pennsylvania State University

Robert Kushner
Clinical director, Northwestern Comprehensive Center on Obesity

JoAnn Manson
Professor of women's health, Harvard Medical School

Lori Mosca
Director of preventive cardiology, New York-Presbyterian Hospital

Yasmin Mossavar-Rahmani
Associate professor of clinical epidemiology and population health, Albert Einstein College of Medicine

Elisabetta Politi
Nutrition director, Duke Diet and Fitness Center

Rebecca Reeves
Adjunct assistant professor, University of Texas School of Public Health

Michael Rosenbaum
Professor of clinical pediatrics and clinical medicine; associate director of the Clinical Research Resource at Columbia University Medical Center

Lisa Sasson
Clinical associate professor of nutrition, food studies and public health, New York University

Joanne Slavin
Professor, department of food science and nutrition, University of Minnesota

Laurence Sperling
Director of preventive cardiology, Emory Clinic

Sachiko St. Jeor
Professor emeritus of internal medicine, University of Nevada School of Medicine

Brian Wansink
Director, Food and Brand Lab, Cornell University

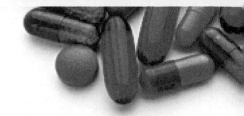

PHARMACIST FAVORITES

The pros suggest the best bets for your over-the-counter picks

When you've got a drippy nose or a monster headache, chances are you make a beeline for your local pharmacy in search of relief. Selecting one product from the dizzying array of brand names that greet you on the store shelves can be daunting. For some, the which-product-should-I-buy decision comes down to price. For others, it's brand loyalty ("Mom always went with ..."). For still others, it's whichever medication has the most convincing TV commercial. Often, it's a decision people have had to make alone. But no longer. Enter the pharmacists, who are tasked with instructing patients on how and when to take a prescribed medicine, to advise on potential side effects, and to stay alert for the possibility of risky drug interactions. For 20 years, the industry trade publication Pharmacy Times has surveyed thousands of pharmacists nationwide to pinpoint their top recommendations on a range of over-the-counter products. The results, published annually in its OTC Guide, are then widely circulated to pharmacists throughout the country to help them guide consumers' shopping decisions. And now this inside intel is available to you, too.

U.S. News and Pharmacy Times have combed through the survey responses to show how different brands stack up in more than 150 over-the-counter product categories. The tables that follow here reveal the top four or five brand-name picks (or more in crowded categories) for a number of popular product types, including antihistamines, cold remedies and sunscreen. Percentages have been rounded.

Though you should always read package labels for ingredients, directions and warnings, don't hesitate to check with your pharmacist as you navigate the drugstore aisles. For the full results in all 150-plus categories, visit **usnews.com/tophealthproducts**.

ACID REDUCERS

Product	% Pharmacists recommending
Prilosec OTC	36%
Zantac	23%
Pepcid	17%
Nexium 24HR	13%
Tums Dual Action	5%

ACNE TREATMENTS

Product	% Pharmacists recommending
Neutrogena	27%
Clearasil	21%
PanOxyl	20%
Oxy	9%
Proactiv	7%
Persa-Gel	7%
Clean & Clear Advantage	6%

ADHESIVE BANDAGES

Product	% Pharmacists recommending
Band-Aid	73%
Nexcare	16%
Curad	11%

ANTIBIOTICS/ ANTISEPTICS (TOPICAL)

Product	% Pharmacists recommending
Neosporin	74%
Polysporin	11%
Hibiclens	7%
Bacitraycin Plus	4%
Betadine	2%

ANTIHISTAMINES (ORAL)

Product	% Pharmacists recommending
Claritin	40%
Zyrtec	36%
Allegra Allergy	12%
Benadryl	6%
Chlor-Trimeton	5%

ARTHRITIS PAIN RELIEVERS (ORAL)

Product	% Pharmacists recommending
Aleve	35%
Advil	26%
Tylenol Arthritis Pain	23%
Motrin	16%

#1 PHARMACIST RECOMMENDED BRAND 2016-2017 **U.S.News** & WORLD REPORT *Pharmacy Times*

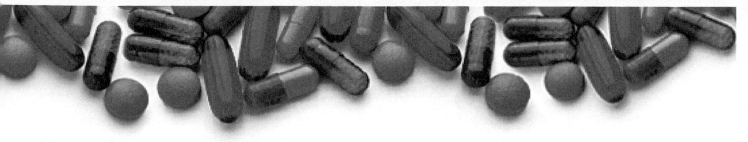

ARTIFICIAL TEARS

Product	% Pharmacists recommending
Refresh	32%
Systane	32%
Tears Naturale	13%
GenTeal	7%
Clear Eyes	4%

ATHLETE'S FOOT/ ANTIFUNGAL PRODUCTS

Product	% Pharmacists recommending
Lamisil	46%
Lotrimin	42%
Tinactin	7%
Micatin	2%
Zeasorb	2%

BLOOD PRESSURE MONITORS

Product	% Pharmacists recommending
Omron	83%
LifeSource	10%
HoMedics	7%

BURN TREATMENTS

Product	% Pharmacists recommending
Neosporin	36%
Dermoplast	21%
Lanacane Spray	14%
Curad Silver Solution	7%
A+D Ointment	7%
Bacitraycin Plus	5%
Polysporin	5%

CHOLESTEROL MANAGEMENT

Product	% Pharmacists recommending
Nature Made Fish Oil	31%
Nature's Bounty Fish Oil	17%
Metamucil	17%
Slo-Niacin	11%
Schiff MegaRed	9%

COLD REMEDIES

Product	% Pharmacists recommending
Cepacol	27%
Halls Defense	25%
Cold-eeze	24%
Zicam	17%
Sucrets	5%

CONTACT LENS SOLUTIONS

Product	% Pharmacists recommending
Opti-Free	42%
Renu multi-purpose solution	23%
Biotrue	13%
Complete Multi-Purpose Solution Easy Rub Formula	7%
Clear Care Cleaning & Disinfecting Solution	7%

COUGH SUPPRESSANTS

Product	% Pharmacists recommending
Delsym	41%
Mucinex DM	34%
Robitussin	21%
Tylenol Cold & Cough	2%
NyQuil	1%

DANDRUFF SHAMPOO

Product	% Pharmacists recommending
Head & Shoulders	29%
Nizoral	27%
Selsun Blue	27%
T/Gel	15%
Denorex	1%

DECONGESTANTS (ORAL)

Product	% Pharmacists recommending
Sudafed (pseudoephedrine)	47%
Claritin-D	13%
Mucinex D	12%
Sudafed PE (phenylephrine)	10%
Advil Cold & Sinus	8%
Zyrtec-D	6%

DIAPER RASH PRODUCTS

Product	% Pharmacists recommending
Desitin Diaper Rash	34%
A+D Diaper Rash Ointment	23%
Boudreaux's Butt Paste	14%
Triple Paste	8%
Balmex	7%
Calmoseptine	6%
Aquaphor Baby	5%

DIGITAL THERMOMETERS

Product	% Pharmacists recommending
Braun ThermoScan	28%
Omron	27%
Vicks	19%
3M Nexcare	6%
Nexcare	6%
LifeSource	5%

FIBER SUPPLEMENTS

Product	% Pharmacists recommending
Metamucil	40%
Benefiber	29%
FiberCon	13%
Citrucel	12%
Fiber Choice	3%

FLU TREATMENT PRODUCTS

Product	% Pharmacists recommending
TheraFlu	24%
Tylenol Cold & Flu Severe	24%
Coricidin HBP Cold & Flu	11%
DayQuil Cold & Flu	11%
NyQuil Cold & Flu	11%
Alka-Seltzer Plus Cold + Flu	10%

HAND SANITIZERS

Product	% Pharmacists recommending
Purell	71%
Germ-X	20%
Burt's Bees	4%
Gold Bond	2%
Nexcare	2%

INFANT FORMULAS

Product	% Pharmacists recommending
Enfamil	49%
Similac	37%
Gerber Good Start	7%
Isomil	5%
EleCare	2%

MIGRAINE HEADACHE RELIEVERS

Product	% Pharmacists recommending
Excedrin Migraine	74%
Advil Migraine	13%
Aleve	9%
Tylenol	2%
Bufferin	1%
Hyland's Migraine Headache	1%

MULTIVITAMINS

Product	% Pharmacists recommending
Centrum	57%
One A Day	18%
Nature Made	10%
Nature's Bounty	8%
Vitafusion Multivites	4%

PRENATAL VITAMINS

Product	% Pharmacists recommending
One A Day Prenatal	40%
Nature Made Multi Prenatal	18%
Centrum Specialist Prenatal	16%
Nature's Bounty Prenatal	12%
Vitafusion PreNatal	5%

SLEEP AIDS

Product	% Pharmacists recommending
Unisom	40%
Tylenol PM	23%
Advil PM	8%
Vicks ZzzQuil	8%
Sominex	7%
Simply Sleep	5%

SUNSCREEN

Product	% Pharmacists recommending
Neutrogena	35%
Coppertone	27%
Bullfrog	12%
Banana Boat	8%
CeraVe	7%
Hawaiian Tropic	5%

TOOTHPASTE

Product	% Pharmacists recommending
Crest	40%
Colgate	25%
Sensodyne	18%
Aquafresh	7%
Tom's of Maine	4%

UPSET STOMACH REMEDIES

Product	% Pharmacists recommending
Pepto-Bismol	54%
Emetrol	29%
Alka-Seltzer	10%
Kaopectate	7%

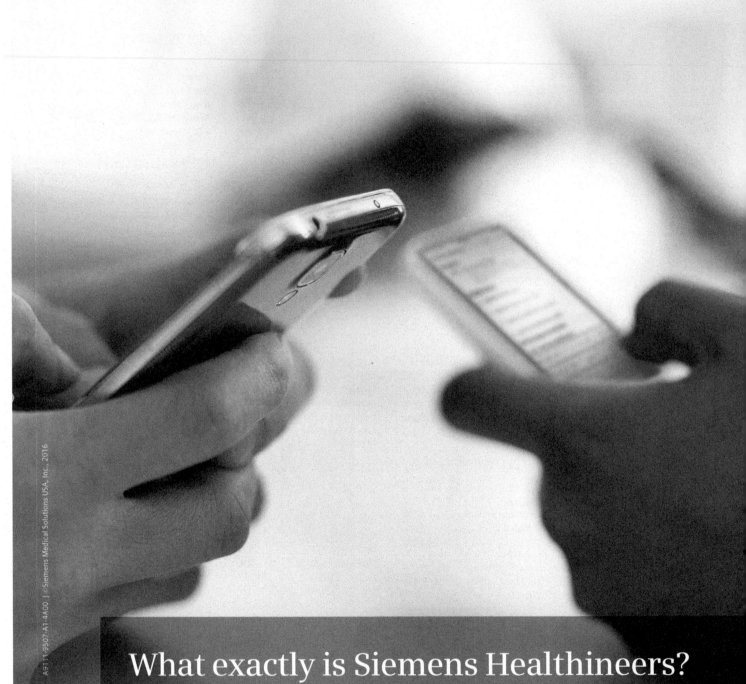

What exactly is Siemens Healthineers?

usa.siemens.com/healthineers

CHAPTER

4

BEST HOSPITALS

BEST
HOSPITALS
U.S.News & WORLD REPORT
2016–17

BEST HOSPITALS

THE HONOR ROLL

THE 20 MEDICAL CENTERS BELOW excel in both the complex and the routine. Starting this year, the Honor Roll recognizes hospitals that perform well with both kinds of patients. The 20 centers are nationally ranked in 10 or more of the 16 Best Hospitals specialties and are also rated "high performing" in all or most of nine relatively common types of care, from treating heart failure to colon cancer surgery, in our procedures and conditions ratings (found at usnews.com/best-hospitals). Honor Roll standing is based on points. A hospital that was top-ranked in all 16 specialties and rated high performing in all nine procedures and conditions would have received 448 points. The 20 highest scorers qualified for the Honor Roll.

BEST HOSPITALS
U.S.News & WORLD REPORT
HONOR ROLL 2016–17

1 **Mayo Clinic**
Rochester, Minn., 418 points

2 **Cleveland Clinic**
378 points

3 **Massachusetts General Hospital,** Boston, 371 points

4 **Johns Hopkins Hospital**
Baltimore, 349 points

5 **UCLA Medical Center**
Los Angeles, 331 points

6 **New York-Presbyterian University Hospital of Columbia and Cornell**
296 points

7 **UCSF Medical Center**
San Francisco, 273 points

8 **Northwestern Memorial Hospital**
Chicago, 266 points

9 **Hospitals of the University of Pennsylvania-Penn Presbyterian**
Philadelphia, 252 points

10 **NYU Langone Medical Center**
New York, 247 points

11 **Barnes-Jewish Hospital/ Washington University**
St. Louis, 241 points

12 **UPMC Presbyterian Shadyside**
Pittsburgh, 236 points

13 **Brigham and Women's Hospital,** Boston, 235 points

14 **Stanford Health Care-Stanford Hospital**
Stanford, Calif., 227 points

15 **Mount Sinai Hospital**
New York, 226 points

16 **Duke University Hospital**
Durham, N.C., 222 points

17 **Cedars-Sinai Medical Center**
Los Angeles, 220 points

18 **University of Michigan Hospitals and Health Centers**
Ann Arbor, 195 points

19 **Houston Methodist Hospital**
191 points

20 **University of Colorado Hospital,** Aurora, 190 points

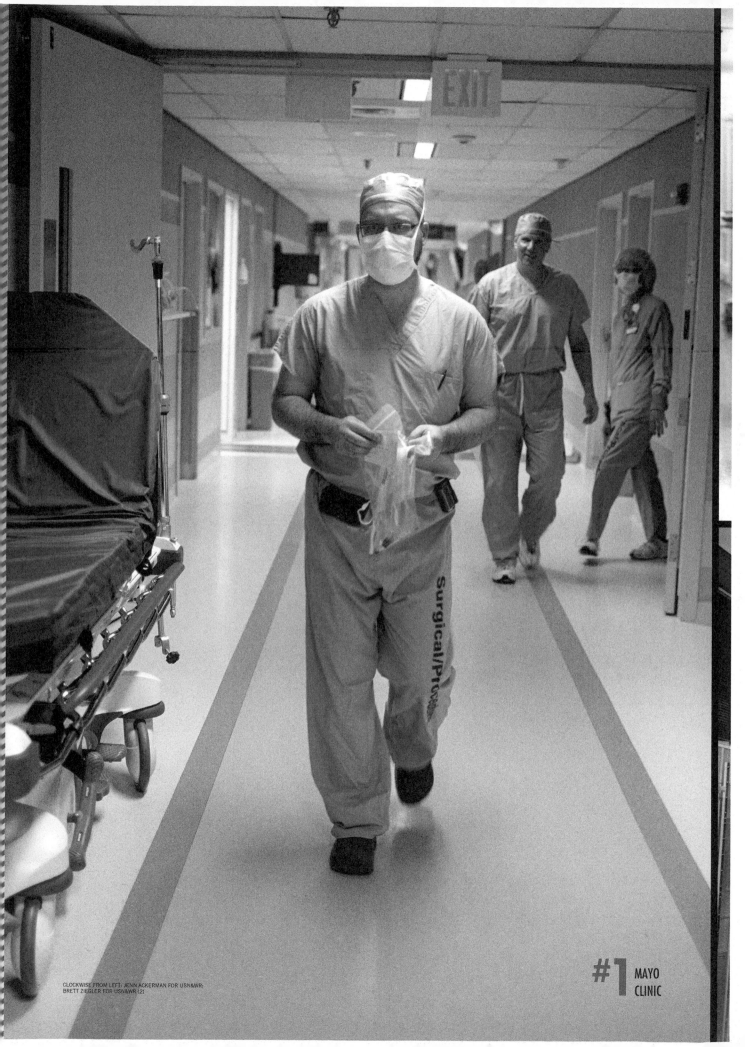

#1 MAYO
CLINIC

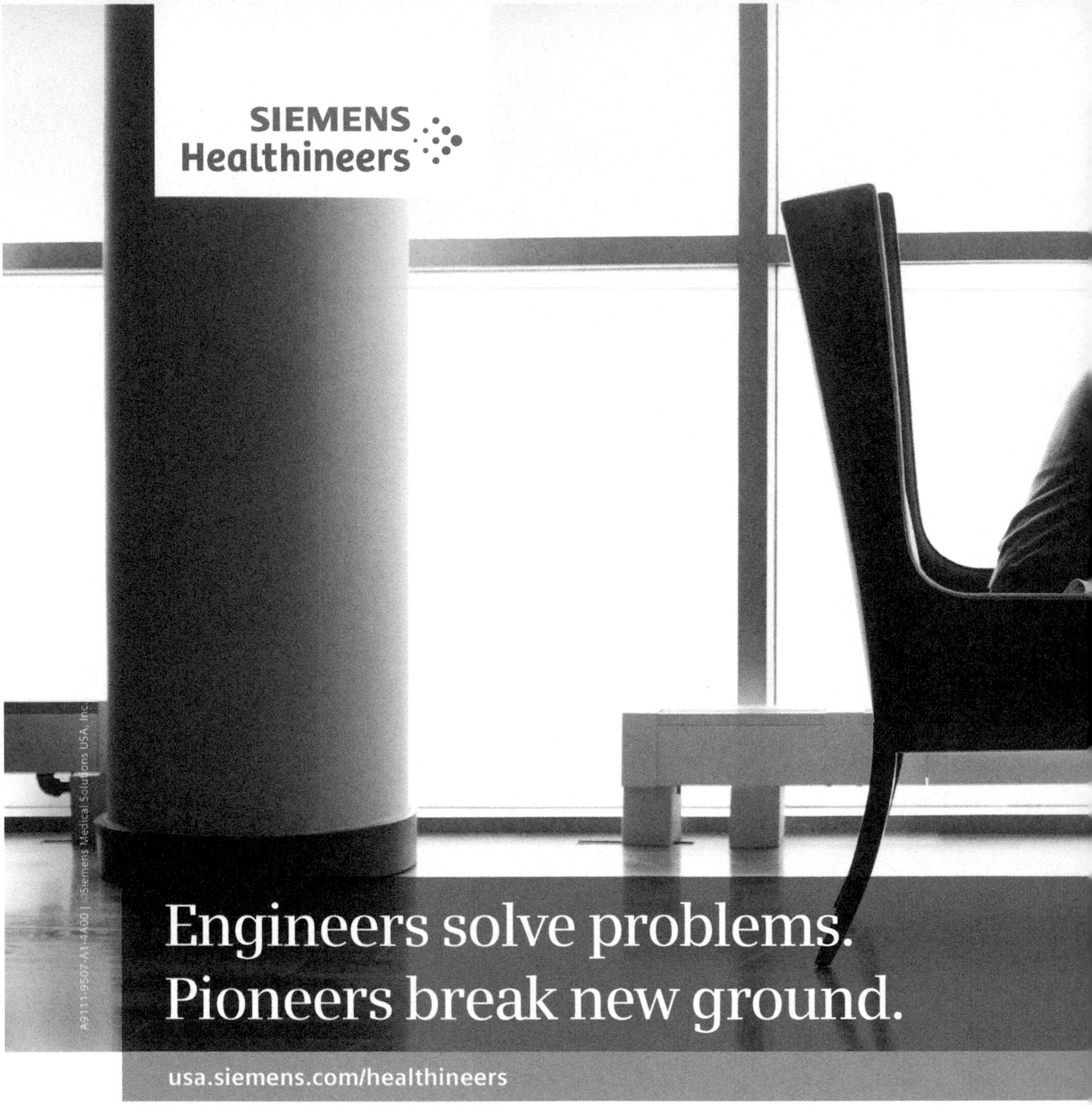

SIEMENS
Healthineers

Engineers solve problems.
Pioneers break new ground.

usa.siemens.com/healthineers

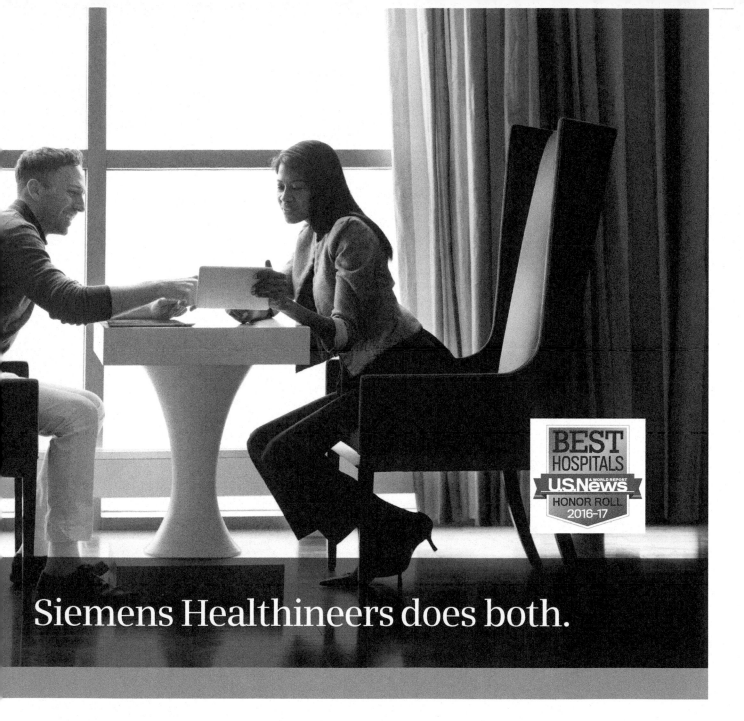

Siemens Healthineers does both.

Healthcare is changing, and change is full of opportunity. Our goal is to help you realize your full potential, and we've changed our name to underscore how. Introducing Siemens Healthineers—combining deep engineering know-how with a pioneering spirit that boldly embraces the future.

In addition to ground-breaking technologies in imaging, laboratory diagnostics, and clinical IT, we offer an expanding portfolio of advanced therapies and molecular diagnostics, as well as new enterprise services. All to help healthcare providers improve patient outcomes while reducing the cost of delivering them.

Perhaps that's why nine out of ten hospitals in the U.S. depend on our solutions, including all the hospitals on the U.S. News Honor Roll.[1,2]

Along with our new name comes a renewed commitment. More than ever, our focus is on forging true and lasting partnerships—based on risks that are shared, promises that are kept, and trust that is truly earned.

It comes down to this: we will do all we can to ensure our partners' success, because that is what partnership is all about.

[1]IMS Hospital Database and SAP Installed Base: May 2015. c2015.
[2]U.S. News & World Report: Best Hospitals 2016-17: Overview and Honor Roll [Internet]. Washington, D.C.: U.S. News & World Report; c2016.

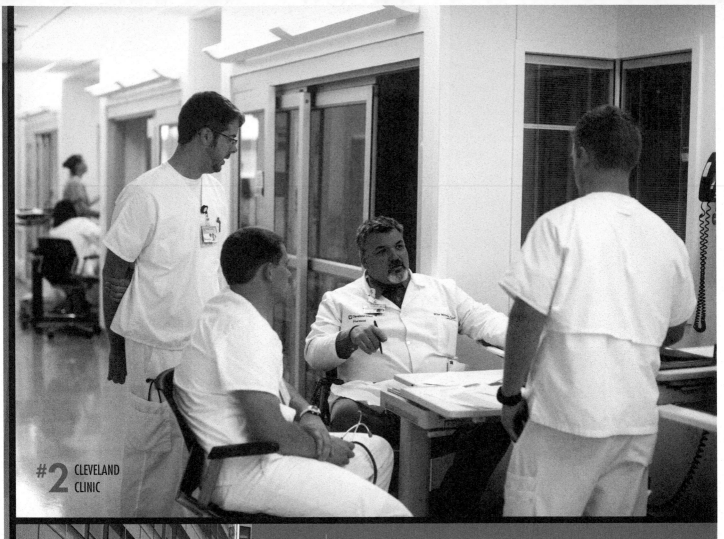

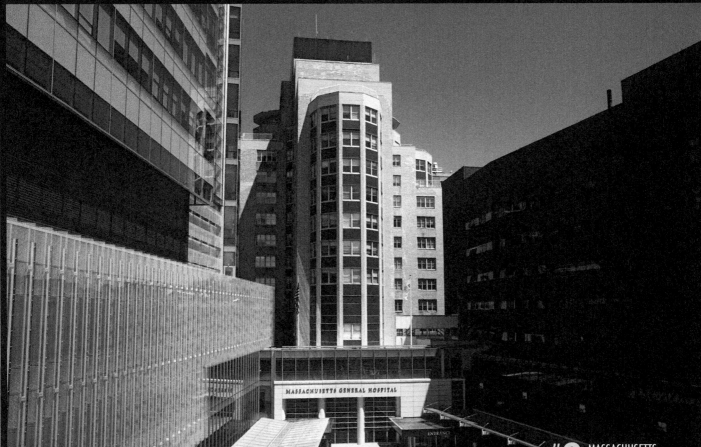

A GUIDE TO
THE RANKINGS

We screened 4,667 U.S. hospitals, and just 154 of them made the 2016-17 rankings

BY AVERY COMAROW

now in their 27th year, the Best Hospitals annual rankings have the same mission as they've had from the start: to help guide patients whose care is especially difficult to the right place. Their surgery or condition may be notably complex. Or their risk may be heightened by advanced age, physical infirmity or an existing medical condition.

Such patients account for just 2 or 3 percent of all hospital patients, but that adds up to millions of individuals and, for them, the majority of hospitals are the wrong choice. Community hospitals typically are not up to speed on the special techniques and precautions called for in treating a man of 85 or 90 with a leaky heart valve, for example. They should decline to admit him for care, and many do. But some would go ahead anyway. A hospital ranked by U.S. News in cardiology and heart surgery is likely to have the experience and expertise to operate safely.

The following pages list hospitals ranked in 16 specialties, from cancer to urology. Of 4,667 hospitals evaluated this year, only 154 performed well enough to rank in even one of them.

In 12 of 16 specialties, hard data,

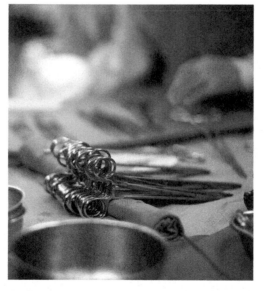

much of it from the federal government, mostly determined whether a hospital was ranked. Some kinds of data, such as death rates, are obviously connected with quality. Numbers of patients and the balance of nurses to patients are examples of data that are also important but the quality connection is less evident. We also factored in, as a form of peer review, results from annual surveys of physicians who were asked to name hospitals they consider tops in their specialty for difficult cases.

Hospitals in the four remaining specialties (ophthalmology, psychiatry, rehabilitation and rheumatology) were ranked solely on the basis of the annual physician surveys. That's because so few patients die in these specialties that mortality data, which carry heavy weight in the 12 other specialties, mean little.

To be considered for ranking in the 12 data-driven specialties, a hospital had to meet one of four criteria: It had to be a teaching hospital, be affiliated with a medical school, have at least 200 beds, or have at least 100 beds and offer at least four out of eight medical technologies that are key to high-quality care, such as a PET/CT scanner and certain precision radiation therapies. This year 2,259 hospitals met that test.

The hospitals next had to meet a volume requirement in each specialty – a minimum number of traditional fee-for-service Medicare inpatients from 2012 to 2014 who received certain procedures and treatment for specific conditions. The minimum number for cardiology and heart surgery, for example, was 1,333, of which 500 had to be surgical cases. The orthopedics minimum was 293, of which 269 had to be surgical. A hospital that fell short was still eligible in a specialty if it was nominated by at least 1 percent of the physicians responding to the 2014, 2015 and 2016 reputational surveys.

At the end of the process, 1,891 hospitals were candidates for ranking in at least one specialty. Each received a U.S. News score of 0 to 100 based on four elements: patient survival; patient safety; care-related factors such as nursing, volume, technology, and special accreditations and recognitions, and reputation. The 50 top performers in each specialty were ranked. Scores and data for the rest are available at usnews.com/best-hospitals. The four elements and their weights in brief:

Survival score (37.5 percent). Success at keeping patients alive was judged by comparing the number of Medicare inpatients with certain conditions who died within 30 days of admission in 2012, 2013 and 2014 with the number expected given the severity of their illness, the complexity of their care and factors such as advanced age, obesity and high blood pressure that increase risk. A score of 10 indicates the highest survival relative to other hospitals; 1 is the worst. Industry-standard software (3M Health Information Systems Medicare Severity Grouper) was used to adjust each patient's risk in calculating survival odds.

Patient safety score (5 percent). Patients are unnecessarily harmed at every hospital; this score reflects efforts to prevent the six kinds of harm listed in the box below.

Other care-related indicators (30 percent). Trauma center status, arthritis center certification, and availability of intensive care specialists are examples. The American Hospital Association's 2014 survey was the main source.

Reputation (27.5 percent). This part of a hospital's total score was drawn from the last three years of annual physician surveys. Specialists were asked to name up to five hospitals, setting aside location and cost, that they consider best in their area of expertise for patients with the most difficult medical problems. In the latest three-year period, responses were tallied from some 33,000 physicians.

The figures shown under "specialists recommending" in the ranking tables show the average percentages of specialists in 2014, 2015 and 2016 who named a particular hospital. An adjustment is made to keep a relatively small number of hospitals with high reputational scores from monopolizing the final rankings. Hospitals with low reputational scores but strong clinical numbers can and do outrank centers with higher reputations, as shown by the many ranked hospitals with low and even zero reputational scores.

In the four reputation-based specialties, a hospital had to be cited by at least 5 percent of responding physicians in the latest three years of U.S. News surveys to be ranked. That created lists of 12 hospitals in ophthalmology, psychiatry and rehabilitation and 15 in rheumatology.

We made changes for 2016-17, as we do every year based on expert input and the professional literature. After eliminating one element of the patient safety score, we cut the weight of that score in half and transferred the 5 points to survival. A transparency measure was added in cardiology and heart surgery to credit hospitals that report outcomes; it's weighted at 3 percent. Reputation in that specialty was lowered to 24.5 percent.

Monitor usnews.com over the year for new Best Hospitals content. Be sure to add your own fact-gathering to ours and consult with your doctor or other health professional. No hospital is best for every patient. ●

WHAT THE TERMS MEAN

FACT accreditation level: hospital meets Foundation for the Accreditation of Cellular Therapy standards as of March 1, 2016, for harvesting and transplanting stem cells from a patient's own bone marrow and tissue (level 1) and from a donor (level 2) to treat cancer.

Intensivists: at least one critical-care specialist manages patients in intensive care units.

NAEC epilepsy center: designated by the National Association of Epilepsy Centers as of March 1, 2016, as a regional or national referral facility (level 4) for staffing, technology and training in epilepsy care.

NCI cancer center: designated by the National Cancer Institute as of March 1, 2016, as a clinical or comprehensive cancer hospital.

NIA Alzheimer's center: designated by the National Institute on Aging as of March 1, 2016, as an Alzheimer's Disease Center, indicating high quality of research and clinical care.

Number of patients: number of fee-for-service Medicare inpatients in 2012, 2013 and 2014 who received certain high-level care as defined by U.S. News. In geriatrics, only patients age 75 and older are included.

Nurse Magnet status: certified by the American Nurses Credentialing Center as of April 1, 2016, for nursing excellence.

Nurse staffing score: relative balance of nonsupervisory registered nurses (inpatient and outpatient) to average daily number of all patients. Inpatient nurse staffing receives greater weight. Agency and temporary nurses are not counted.

Patient safety score: indicates ability to protect patients from six types of preventable harm: death from preventable postsurgical complications, collapsed lung during certain procedures, major postsurgical bleeding and bruising, postsurgical respiratory failure, surgical incisions that reopen, and injury during surgery.

Patient services score: number of services offered out of the number considered important to quality (such as genetic testing in cancer and an Alzheimer's center in geriatrics).

Rank: based on U.S. News score except in ophthalmology, psychiatry, rehabilitation and rheumatology, where specialist recommendations determine rank.

Specialists recommending: percentage of physicians responding to U.S. News surveys in 2014, 2015 and 2016 who named the hospital as among the best in their specialty for especially challenging cases and procedures, setting aside location and cost.

Survival score: reflects inpatient deaths in the specialty within 30 days of admission.

Technology score: reflects availability of technologies considered important to quality of care, such as PET/CT scanner in pulmonology and diagnostic radioisotope services in urology.

Transparency score: indicates whether hospital publicly reports heart outcomes through the American College of Cardiology and the Society of Thoracic Surgeons. Worth 3 percent of U.S. News score.

Trauma center: indicates certification as Level 1 or 2 trauma center, which can properly care for the most severe injuries.

U.S. News score: 0 to 100 summary of quality of hospital inpatient care. Survival is worth 37.5 percent, operational quality data such as nurse staffing and patient volume 30 percent, specialists' recommendations 27.5 percent (24.5 percent in cardiology and heart surgery), and patient safety 5 percent.

KEEPING SOFTWARE ALIVE IS NOT A SIGNIFICANT CONTRIBUTION TO MEDICINE.

CANCER

Rank	Hospital	U.S. News score	Survival score (10=best)	Patient safety score (5=best)	Number of patients	Nurse staffing score (higher is better)	Nurse Magnet status	NCI cancer center	FACT accredita- tion level (2=best)	Patient services score (8=best)	Specialists recom- mending
1	University of Texas MD Anderson Cancer Center, Houston	100.0	10	2	5,638	2.0	Yes	Yes	2	8	62.0%
2	Memorial Sloan Kettering Cancer Center, New York	97.9	10	4	3,843	2.0	Yes	Yes	2	8	61.1%
3	Mayo Clinic, Rochester, Minn.	91.0	10	5	3,206	2.7	Yes	Yes	2	8	26.3%
4	Dana-Farber/Brigham and Women's Cancer Center, Boston	80.9	9	5	2,984	2.4	No	Yes	2	8	33.5%
5	UCLA Medical Center, Los Angeles	75.2	10	4	1,646	3.1	Yes	Yes	2	8	6.8%
6	Moffitt Cancer Center and Research Institute, Tampa	75.0	10	1	2,105	1.2	Yes	Yes	2	8	4.0%
7	Seattle Cancer Care Alliance/U. of Washington Medical Center	74.9	10	3	1,046	2.1	Yes	Yes	2	8	10.8%
8	Cleveland Clinic	73.8	10	5	2,449	2.1	Yes	Yes	2	8	8.5%
9	Johns Hopkins Hospital, Baltimore	72.7	8	2	1,573	2.1	Yes	Yes	2	8	20.1%
10	UCSF Medical Center, San Francisco	71.8	9	5	1,315	2.7	Yes	Yes	2	8	8.0%
11	Massachusetts General Hospital, Boston	70.6	9	3	2,431	2.3	Yes	Yes	2	8	10.3%
12	Hospitals of the U. of Pennsylvania-Penn Presbyterian, Philadelphia	69.4	9	5	2,330	2.5	Yes	Yes	2	8	7.7%
13	Stanford Health Care-Stanford Hospital, Stanford, Calif.	69.0	9	5	1,260	2.4	Yes	Yes	2	8	8.0%
14	Northwestern Memorial Hospital, Chicago	68.6	10	4	1,722	1.6	Yes	Yes	2	8	1.6%
15	Barnes-Jewish Hospital/Washington University, St. Louis	68.5	9	3	3,043	2.2	Yes	Yes	2	8	4.8%
16	University of North Carolina Hospitals, Chapel Hill	67.0	10	2	1,365	1.8	Yes	Yes	2	8	2.5%
17	New York-Presbyterian U. Hospital of Columbia and Cornell, N.Y.	66.8	10	3	4,161	2.5	No	Yes	2	8	2.4%
18	USC Norris Cancer Hosp.-Keck Medical Cen. of USC, Los Angeles	66.7	10	1	877	3.8	No	Yes	2	8	1.1%
19	Wake Forest Baptist Medical Center, Winston-Salem, N.C.	66.4	10	2	2,030	1.6	Yes	Yes	2	8	1.4%
20	City of Hope, Duarte, Calif.	65.9	10	5	910	2.3	No	Yes	2	8	5.4%
21	University of Maryland Medical Center, Baltimore	65.5	10	1	1,071	2.9	Yes	Yes	2	8	1.1%
22	University of Colorado Hospital, Aurora	65.1	10	3	853	2.2	Yes	Yes	2	8	0.6%
23	UPMC Presbyterian Shadyside, Pittsburgh	64.9	9	1	3,422	1.9	Yes	Yes	2	8	2.9%
24	University of Michigan Hospitals and Health Centers, Ann Arbor	64.8	9	5	2,206	2.9	No	Yes	2	8	5.1%
25	University of Kansas Hospital, Kansas City	64.4	10	2	1,353	1.9	Yes	Yes	2	8	0.7%
26	Fox Chase Cancer Center, Philadelphia	64.3	9	2	1,187	2.1	Yes	Yes	2	8	3.5%
26	Mayo Clinic, Phoenix	64.3	10	5	995	3.2	No	Yes	2	8	2.0%
28	Seidman Cancer Center at UH Case Medical, Cleveland	63.6	9	2	1,525	2.3	Yes	Yes	2	8	3.0%
29	Mayo Clinic Jacksonville, Fla.	63.5	10	5	816	2.1	Yes	Yes	2	8	1.9%
29	Thomas Jefferson University Hospital, Philadelphia	63.5	9	4	1,770	2.2	Yes	Yes	2	8	1.6%
31	University of Virginia Medical Center, Charlottesville	62.9	10	4	1,128	2.1	Yes	Yes	2	7	0.4%
32	University of Chicago Medical Center	62.7	10	4	1,720	2.3	No	Yes	2	8	2.6%
33	NYU Langone Medical Center, New York	62.6	9	4	1,182	2.6	Yes	Yes	1	8	1.3%
34	University of Iowa Hospitals and Clinics, Iowa City	62.4	10	4	1,148	1.8	Yes	Yes	2	8	0.5%
35	UC San Diego Medical Center - UC San Diego Health, Calif.	62.3	9	5	868	1.8	Yes	Yes	2	8	1.5%
36	Oregon Health and Science University Hospital, Portland	61.6	10	2	1,126	2.1	Yes	Yes	2	8	0.5%
37	Ohio State University James Cancer Hospital, Columbus	61.5	9	2	2,671	2.1	Yes	Yes	2	8	2.8%
38	Mount Sinai Hospital, New York	61.4	9	4	1,953	2.0	Yes	Yes	2	8	1.5%
38	Rush University Medical Center, Chicago	61.4	10	4	1,530	2.2	Yes	No	2	8	1.1%
40	Duke University Hospital, Durham, N.C.	60.9	7	4	2,069	2.2	Yes	Yes	2	8	6.8%
40	University of California, Davis Medical Center, Sacramento	60.9	9	4	809	2.7	Yes	Yes	2	8	0.8%
42	Vanderbilt University Medical Center, Nashville	60.7	9	4	1,263	1.9	Yes	Yes	2	8	1.1%
43	University of Wisconsin Hospital and Clinics, Madison	60.6	9	2	1,259	1.9	Yes	Yes	2	8	0.5%
44	Houston Methodist Hospital	60.1	10	3	1,372	1.9	Yes	No	2	8	1.1%
44	University of Minnesota Medical Center, Fairview	60.1	10	1	987	2.1	No	Yes	2	8	0.3%
46	Emory University Hospital, Atlanta	58.7	8	5	1,474	2.0	Yes	Yes	2	8	2.6%
47	Huntsman Cancer Institute at the U. of Utah, Salt Lake City	58.5	10	4	860	2.4	No	Yes	2	8	0.5%
47	Medical University of South Carolina Medical Center, Charleston	58.5	9	3	1,001	2.1	Yes	Yes	2	8	0.2%
49	UF Health Shands Hospital, Gainesville, Fla.	57.9	9	3	1,381	2.0	Yes	No	2	8	0.9%
50	Yale-New Haven Hospital, New Haven, Conn.	57.5	8	1	2,272	1.8	Yes	Yes	2	8	2.5%

Terms are explained on Page 90.

More @ usnews.com/besthospitals

Top 10 in the nation.
10 years in a row.

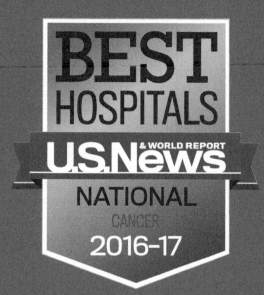

Here are 3 reasons why.

Fred Hutch · Seattle Children's · UW Medicine

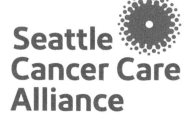

At Seattle Cancer Care Alliance, we bring together the leading research teams and cancer specialists of Fred Hutch, Seattle Children's and UW Medicine. It's one extraordinary group whose sole mission is the pursuit of better, longer, richer lives for our patients. And thanks to our collaboration and dedication we are one of the Top 10 Cancer Hospitals in the nation. Learn more about how working together is better at **SeattleCCA.org.**

CARDIOLOGY & HEART SURGERY

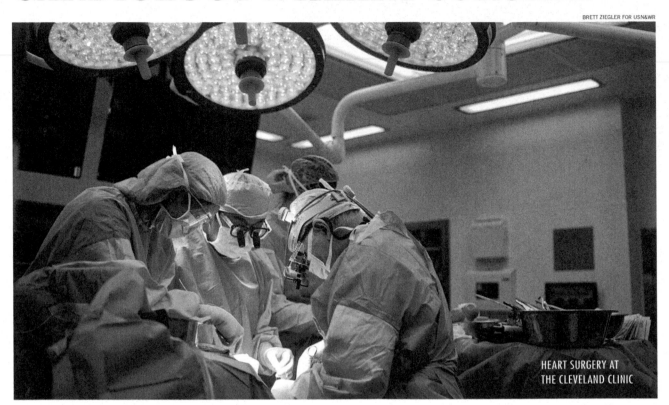

BRETT ZIEGLER FOR USN&WR

HEART SURGERY AT
THE CLEVELAND CLINIC

Rank	Hospital	U.S. News score	Survival score (10=best)	Patient safety score (5=best)	Trans- parency score (3=best)	Number of patients	Nurse staffing score (higher is better)	Nurse Magnet status	Technology score (6=best)	Patient services score (7=best)	Intensivists	Specialists recom- mending
1	Cleveland Clinic	100.0	10	5	3	13,183	2.1	Yes	6	7	Yes	52.8%
2	Mayo Clinic, Rochester, Minn.	96.7	10	5	2	9,946	2.7	Yes	6	7	Yes	47.6%
3	New York-Presbyterian U. Hospital of Columbia and Cornell, N.Y.	83.2	10	3	2	16,921	2.5	No	6	7	Yes	16.7%
4	Massachusetts General Hospital, Boston	78.2	9	3	3	7,510	2.3	Yes	6	7	Yes	18.6%
5	Duke University Hospital, Durham, N.C.	75.7	10	4	2	6,161	2.2	Yes	6	7	Yes	13.8%
6	Northwestern Memorial Hospital, Chicago	75.4	10	4	2	4,341	1.6	Yes	6	7	Yes	3.7%
7	Brigham and Women's Hospital, Boston	75.2	10	5	3	6,215	2.4	No	6	7	Yes	17.3%
8	Mount Sinai Hospital, New York	75.0	10	4	2	9,380	2.0	Yes	6	7	Yes	4.8%
9	Johns Hopkins Hospital, Baltimore	72.7	9	2	3	3,795	2.1	Yes	6	7	Yes	15.6%
10	Cedars-Sinai Medical Center, Los Angeles	72.5	9	3	2	6,857	2.6	Yes	6	7	Yes	6.3%
10	NYU Langone Medical Center, New York	72.5	10	4	3	4,220	2.6	Yes	5	7	Yes	2.7%
12	UCLA Medical Center, Los Angeles	70.4	9	4	3	4,028	3.1	Yes	6	7	Yes	3.3%
13	Hospitals of the U. of Pennsylvania-Penn Presbyterian, Philadelphia	69.6	9	5	0	9,398	2.5	Yes	6	7	Yes	8.3%
14	Barnes-Jewish Hospital/Washington University, St. Louis	69.0	10	3	2	6,784	2.2	Yes	6	7	Yes	3.8%
15	Stanford Health Care-Stanford Hospital, Stanford, Calif.	68.0	8	5	3	3,035	2.4	Yes	6	7	Yes	6.8%
16	Emory University Hospital, Atlanta	67.3	9	5	3	3,966	2.0	Yes	6	7	Yes	6.5%
16	St. Francis Hospital, Roslyn, N.Y.	67.3	10	2	2	9,309	1.9	Yes	5	7	Yes	1.1%
18	The Heart Hospital Baylor Plano, Texas	65.8	10	4	3	3,886	2.3	Yes	4	5	Yes	2.1%
19	UPMC Presbyterian Shadyside, Pittsburgh	65.3	9	1	3	10,381	1.9	Yes	6	7	Yes	1.9%
20	St. Luke's Hospital, Kansas City, Mo.	65.2	10	5	2	4,311	1.6	Yes	6	7	Yes	1.5%
21	Houston Methodist Hospital	65.0	9	3	2	6,473	1.9	Yes	6	7	Yes	3.6%
22	University of Michigan Hospitals and Health Centers, Ann Arbor	64.6	9	5	3	5,507	2.9	No	6	7	Yes	5.0%
23	Advocate Christ Medical Center, Oak Lawn, Ill.	64.2	9	4	3	6,920	2.4	Yes	5	7	Yes	0.6%
24	Sentara Norfolk General Hosp.-Sentara Heart Hosp., Norfolk, Va.	64.0	10	1	3	5,355	1.6	Yes	6	7	Yes	0.3%

(CONTINUED ON PAGE 96)

Terms are explained on Page 90.

▶ **More @ usnews.com/besthospitals**

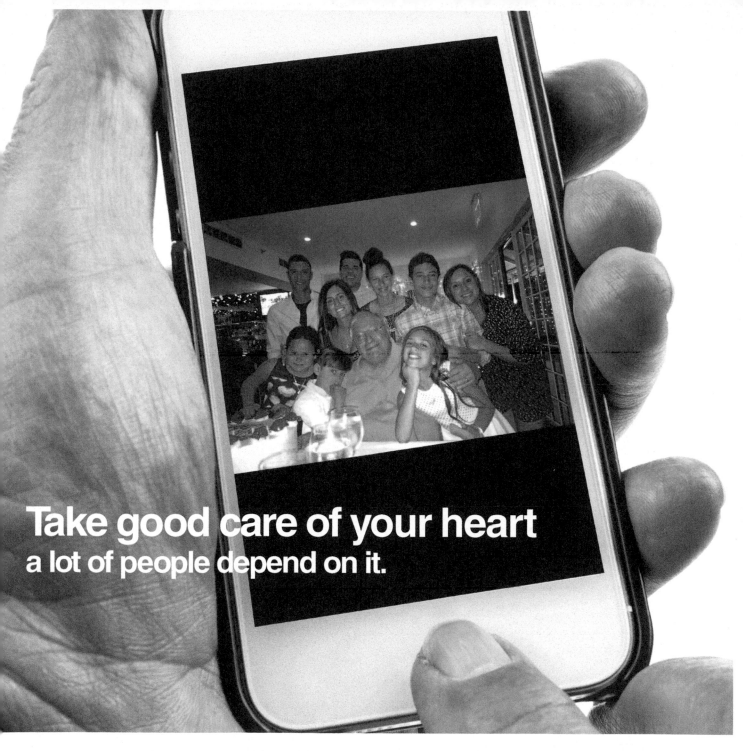

Take good care of your heart
a lot of people depend on it.

St. Francis is the only Long Island Hospital nationally ranked in Cardiology & Heart Surgery by *U.S. News & World Report* 10 years in a row.

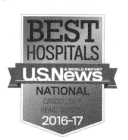

St. Francis Hospital, The Heart Center®
Catholic Health Services
At the heart of health

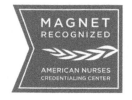
MAGNET RECOGNIZED
AMERICAN NURSES CREDENTIALING CENTER

Find us on Facebook at StFrancisHeartCenter

100 Port Washington Blvd., Roslyn, NY 11576   For a physician referral, call 1-888-HEARTNY.   www.stfrancisheartcenter.com

CARDIOLOGY & HEART SURGERY (CONTINUED)

Rank	Hospital	U.S. News score	Survival score (10=best)	Patient safety score (5=best)	Trans-parency score (3=best)	Number of patients	Nurse staffing score (higher is better)	Nurse Magnet status	Technology score (6=best)	Patient services score (7=best)	Intensivists	Specialists recom-mending
25	Beaumont Hospital-Royal Oak, Mich.	63.9	9	3	3	9,475	1.8	Yes	5	7	Yes	1.1%
26	Ohio State University Wexner Medical Center, Columbus	63.4	9	2	3	6,050	2.1	Yes	6	7	Yes	1.1%
27	Morristown Medical Center, Morristown, N.J.	63.1	9	4	3	7,428	1.9	Yes	5	7	Yes	0.2%
28	Scripps La Jolla Hospitals and Clinics, La Jolla, Calif.	62.6	9	4	2	5,030	2.9	Y/N*	5	7	Yes	1.9%
29	Vanderbilt University Medical Center, Nashville	62.4	9	4	2	4,785	1.9	Yes	6	7	Yes	2.2%
30	Tampa General Hospital	62.3	10	1	2	4,200	2.2	Yes	6	7	Yes	0.1%
31	Aurora St. Luke's Medical Center, Milwaukee	61.0	9	1	3	9,209	1.5	Yes	6	7	Yes	0.6%
31	Minneapolis Heart Institute at Abbott Northwestern Hospital	61.0	8	5	3	6,742	2.1	Yes	6	7	Yes	1.2%
31	UC San Diego Medical Center - UC San Diego Health, Calif.	61.0	9	5	2	2,215	1.8	Yes	6	6	Yes	0.7%
34	University of California, Davis Medical Center, Sacramento	60.4	9	4	2	2,319	2.7	Yes	5	7	Yes	0.1%
35	Lehigh Valley Hospital, Allentown, Pa.	60.2	8	4	3	7,518	1.8	Yes	5	7	Yes	0.3%
36	Oregon Health and Science University Hospital, Portland	60.1	10	2	3	2,402	2.1	Yes	6	7	Yes	0.2%
37	University of Alabama Hospital at Birmingham	60.0	9	4	2	4,401	1.8	Yes	6	6	Yes	0.8%
38	Texas Heart Institute at Baylor St. Luke's Medical Cen., Houston	59.9	8	1	0	6,301	1.8	Yes	5	6	Yes	10.5%
38	University of Kansas Hospital, Kansas City	59.9	10	2	0	3,651	1.9	Yes	5	7	Yes	0.2%
40	Mayo Clinic, Phoenix	59.6	10	5	2	2,246	3.2	No	6	7	Yes	1.7%
41	Fairview Hospital, Cleveland	59.1	10	5	2	3,398	1.7	Yes	4	7	Yes	0.0%
42	Hackensack University Medical Center, Hackensack, N.J.	58.8	8	4	2	5,693	2.4	Yes	5	7	Yes	0.1%
42	University of Colorado Hospital, Aurora	58.8	8	3	3	2,195	2.2	Yes	6	7	Yes	0.6%
44	IU Health Academic Health Center, Indianapolis	58.7	8	2	3	4,588	1.8	Yes	6	7	Yes	0.2%
45	Memorial Hermann-Texas Medical Center, Houston	58.4	9	5	0	3,451	2.2	Yes	6	7	Yes	0.7%
45	UCSF Medical Center, San Francisco	58.4	8	5	2	1,787	2.7	Yes	5	6	Yes	2.7%
45	University of Washington Medical Center, Seattle	58.4	10	3	2	1,923	2.1	Yes	6	7	Yes	1.2%
48	Kaiser Permanente San Francisco Medical Center	58.3	10	4	2	3,490	2.3	No	5	7	Yes	0.5%
48	Keck Medical Center of USC, Los Angeles†	58.3	10	1	2	1,558	3.8	No	6	7	Yes	1.0%
48	Munson Medical Center, Traverse City, Mich.	58.3	9	2	2	5,222	1.8	Yes	5	7	Yes	0.3%
48	Thomas Jefferson University Hospital, Philadelphia	58.3	8	4	2	4,197	2.2	Yes	6	7	Yes	0.6%

*Reflects more than one hospital's status. The secondary hospital lacks Nurse Magnet recognition.
†Due to a data processing error, this hospital was initially omitted from these rankings. Rankings for other hospitals have not been changed.

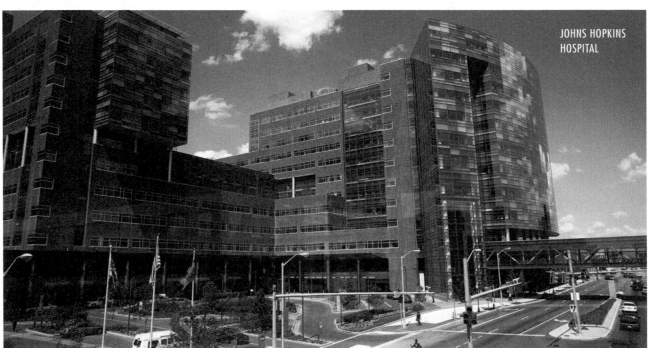

JOHNS HOPKINS HOSPITAL

BRETT ZIEGLER FOR USN&WR

▶ More @ usnews.com/besthospitals

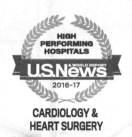

HOW FAR DO YOU GO TO SAVE A LIFE? 400 MILES IN THE MIDDLE OF THE NIGHT. OR WHATEVER IT TAKES.

We developed the world's first transvenous cardiac pacemaker, performed the world's first coronary bypass, and have world-renowned specialists taking on complex cases others can't handle. Like recently flying a young mom to Montefiore for lifesaving care. To learn more about this story, and how we're doing more in heart care, go to **doingmoremontefiore.org**

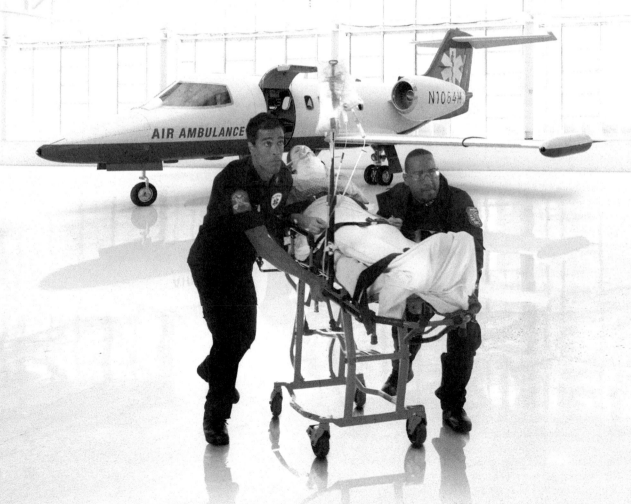

Westchester   Hudson Valley   Bronx

Montefiore
DOING MORE℠

DIABETES & ENDOCRINOLOGY

Rank	Hospital	U.S. News score	Survival score (10=best)	Patient safety score (5=best)	Number of patients	Nurse staffing score (higher is better)	Nurse Magnet status	Technology score (4=best)	Patient services score (8=best)	Intensivists	Specialists recom-mending
1	Mayo Clinic, Rochester, Minn.	100.0	9	5	551	2.7	Yes	4	8	Yes	54.7%
2	Massachusetts General Hospital, Boston	85.1	7	3	491	2.3	Yes	4	8	Yes	35.2%
3	Cleveland Clinic	83.9	8	5	699	2.1	Yes	4	8	Yes	22.5%
4	Johns Hopkins Hospital, Baltimore	80.8	8	2	308	2.1	Yes	4	8	Yes	25.3%
5	New York-Presbyterian U. Hospital of Columbia and Cornell, N.Y.	80.6	9	3	1,294	2.5	No	4	8	Yes	10.5%
6	UCSF Medical Center, San Francisco	78.6	9	5	261	2.7	Yes	4	8	Yes	9.1%
7	Stanford Health Care-Stanford Hospital, Stanford, Calif.	73.7	9	5	242	2.4	Yes	4	8	Yes	1.8%
8	Houston Methodist Hospital	71.5	9	3	472	1.9	Yes	4	8	Yes	2.6%
9	Hospitals of the U. of Pennsylvania-Penn Presbyterian, Philadelphia	70.6	7	5	527	2.5	Yes	4	8	Yes	7.0%
10	Beaumont Hospital-Royal Oak, Mich.	69.5	8	3	892	1.8	Yes	4	8	Yes	0.4%
11	Mount Sinai Hospital, New York	69.4	7	4	722	2.0	Yes	4	8	Yes	5.7%
11	Northwestern Memorial Hospital, Chicago	69.4	8	4	365	1.6	Yes	4	8	Yes	4.0%
13	Harper University Hospital, Detroit	67.9	10	3	217	1.6	No	4	8	Yes	0.1%
14	Cedars-Sinai Medical Center, Los Angeles	67.8	8	3	522	2.6	Yes	4	8	Yes	3.4%
14	University of Colorado Hospital, Aurora	67.8	8	3	269	2.2	Yes	4	8	Yes	2.6%
16	Yale-New Haven Hospital, New Haven, Conn.	67.5	7	1	829	1.8	Yes	4	8	Yes	7.2%
17	Brigham and Women's Hospital, Boston	67.2	7	5	395	2.4	No	4	8	Yes	10.9%
18	Christiana Care Christiana Hospital, Newark, Del.	66.9	8	4	787	2.0	Yes	4	8	Yes	0.1%
18	Duke University Hospital, Durham, N.C.	66.9	8	4	293	2.2	Yes	4	8	Yes	3.3%
20	NYU Langone Medical Center, New York	66.7	8	4	299	2.6	Yes	4	8	Yes	1.8%
20	Queen's Medical Center, Honolulu	66.7	9	3	348	1.8	Yes	4	8	Yes	0.0%
22	Montefiore Medical Center, New York	66.4	8	1	1,043	2.2	No	4	8	Yes	1.8%
23	University of North Carolina Hospitals, Chapel Hill	66.3	8	2	274	1.8	Yes	4	8	Yes	2.7%
24	Scripps La Jolla Hospitals and Clinics, La Jolla, Calif.	66.2	9	4	275	2.9	Y/N*	4	8	Yes	0.2%
24	Sentara Norfolk General Hospital, Norfolk, Va.	66.2	9	1	290	1.6	Yes	4	8	Yes	0.7%
26	Baylor St. Luke's Medical Center, Houston	66.1	9	1	323	1.8	Yes	4	7	Yes	2.1%
27	Tampa General Hospital	65.9	9	1	325	2.2	Yes	4	8	Yes	0.0%
27	UCLA Medical Center, Los Angeles	65.9	7	4	379	3.1	Yes	4	8	Yes	6.4%
29	Barnes-Jewish Hospital/Washington University, St. Louis	65.8	7	3	527	2.2	Yes	4	8	Yes	4.9%
30	University of Alabama Hospital at Birmingham	65.7	9	4	401	1.8	Yes	4	7	Yes	0.5%
31	Baylor University Medical Center, Dallas	65.3	8	4	537	1.7	Yes	4	8	Yes	1.1%
32	UPMC Presbyterian Shadyside, Pittsburgh	65.2	7	1	774	1.9	Yes	4	8	Yes	3.7%
33	University of Kansas Hospital, Kansas City	64.8	9	2	255	1.9	Yes	4	8	Yes	0.2%
34	Thomas Jefferson University Hospital, Philadelphia	64.7	8	4	529	2.2	Yes	4	8	Yes	0.9%
35	Oregon Health and Science University Hospital, Portland	64.5	8	2	186	2.1	Yes	4	8	Yes	3.0%
36	Ohio State University Wexner Medical Center, Columbus	64.4	8	2	458	2.1	Yes	4	8	Yes	1.5%
36	Wake Forest Baptist Medical Center, Winston-Salem, N.C.	64.4	8	2	365	1.6	Yes	4	8	Yes	0.7%
38	UR Medicine Strong Memorial Hospital, Rochester, N.Y.	64.3	8	2	364	1.7	Yes	4	8	Yes	0.1%
39	Huntington Hospital, Huntington, N.Y.	64.1	9	4	197	1.8	Yes	4	8	Yes	0.0%
40	Baystate Medical Center, Springfield, Mass.	63.7	8	3	421	1.5	Yes	4	8	Yes	0.0%
40	University of Maryland Medical Center, Baltimore	63.7	8	1	149	2.9	Yes	4	8	Yes	1.0%
42	Vanderbilt University Medical Center, Nashville	63.4	8	4	315	1.9	Yes	4	8	Yes	2.2%
43	Flagstaff Medical Center, Flagstaff, Ariz.	63.2	10	3	147	2.8	No	4	7	Yes	0.0%
44	MetroHealth Medical Center, Cleveland	63.1	10	1	133	1.0	Yes	4	8	Yes	0.0%
45	Beth Israel Deaconess Medical Center, Boston	63.0	8	2	363	1.7	No	4	8	Yes	4.5%
46	Bon Secours Memorial Regional Medical Cen., Mechanicsville, Va.	62.7	9	2	192	1.4	Yes	4	6	Yes	0.0%
46	Rush University Medical Center, Chicago	62.7	8	4	336	2.2	Yes	4	8	Yes	0.7%
48	MedStar Georgetown University Hospital, Washington, D.C.	62.3	9	1	116	1.4	Yes	4	8	Yes	1.1%
48	UF Health Shands Hospital, Gainesville, Fla.	62.3	8	3	288	2.0	Yes	4	8	Yes	0.2%
50	Clear Lake Regional Medical Center, Webster, Texas	62.2	9	4	364	1.8	No	4	6	Yes	0.0%
50	Emory University Hospital, Atlanta	62.2	7	5	318	2.0	Yes	4	8	Yes	2.8%
50	Mayo Clinic, Phoenix	62.2	9	5	188	3.2	No	4	8	Yes	0.5%
50	Tufts Medical Center, Boston	62.2	10	2	170	1.6	No	4	8	Yes	0.8%

*Reflects more than one hospital's status. The secondary hospital lacks Nurse Magnet recognition.

Terms are explained on Page 90.

▶ **More @ usnews.com/besthospitals**

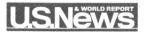

BEST HOSPITALS DASHBOARD

Rankings, tools and news for hospitals

ARE YOU IN HOSPITAL LEADERSHIP?

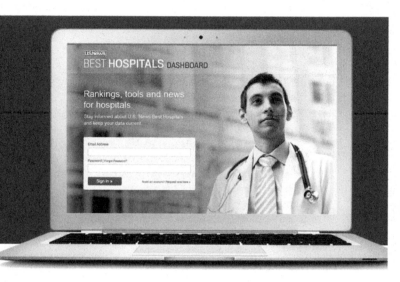

Update Hospital Information

Submit Photos

See Your Rankings Before Publication

Access PR Materials

Understand the Methodology

Contact Us

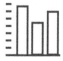

REQUEST A FREE ACCOUNT

hospitaldashboard.usnews.com

EAR, NOSE & THROAT

Rank	Hospital	U.S. News score	Survival score (10=best)	Patient safety score (5=best)	Number of patients	Nurse staffing score (higher is better)	Nurse Magnet status	Patient services score (8=best)	Trauma center	Intensivists	Specialists recom- mending
1	Massachusetts Eye and Ear Infirmary, Mass. General Hosp., Boston	100.0	10	3	395	2.3	N/Y*	8	Yes	Yes	27.2%
2	Mayo Clinic, Rochester, Minn.	96.5	10	5	299	2.7	Yes	8	Yes	Yes	15.0%
3	Johns Hopkins Hospital, Baltimore	95.7	9	2	157	2.1	Yes	8	Yes	Yes	34.1%
4	UCLA Medical Center, Los Angeles	88.7	10	4	304	3.1	Yes	8	Yes	Yes	6.5%
5	University of Iowa Hospitals and Clinics, Iowa City	88.1	9	4	151	1.8	Yes	8	Yes	Yes	17.7%
6	UPMC Presbyterian Shadyside, Pittsburgh	87.7	8	1	381	1.9	Yes	8	Yes	Yes	13.1%
7	Ohio State University Wexner Medical Center, Columbus	86.3	10	2	399	2.1	Yes	8	Yes	Yes	6.2%
8	University of Michigan Hospitals and Health Centers, Ann Arbor	86.1	8	5	322	2.9	No	8	Yes	Yes	14.6%
9	University of Texas MD Anderson Cancer Center, Houston	85.7	8	2	439	2.0	Yes	8	No	Yes	11.3%
10	Hospitals of the U. of Pennsylvania-Penn Presbyterian, Philadelphia	85.6	6	5	320	2.5	Yes	8	Yes	Yes	12.8%
11	UCSF Medical Center, San Francisco	85.0	10	5	140	2.7	Yes	8	Yes	Yes	7.4%
12	Cleveland Clinic	84.8	8	5	250	2.1	Yes	8	No	Yes	13.0%
13	Stanford Health Care-Stanford Hospital, Stanford, Calif.	83.4	7	5	216	2.4	Yes	8	Yes	Yes	10.2%
14	Medical University of South Carolina Medical Center, Charleston	81.9	9	3	196	2.1	Yes	8	Yes	Yes	6.4%
15	Barnes-Jewish Hospital/Washington University, St. Louis	80.9	7	3	269	2.2	Yes	8	Yes	Yes	8.0%
16	University of Washington Medical Center, Seattle	79.4	9	3	136	2.1	Yes	8	No	Yes	8.3%
17	University of North Carolina Hospitals, Chapel Hill	78.1	10	2	205	1.8	Yes	8	Yes	Yes	3.8%
18	Oregon Health and Science University Hospital, Portland	77.2	10	2	183	2.1	Yes	8	Yes	Yes	2.9%
18	Thomas Jefferson University Hospital, Philadelphia	77.2	8	4	319	2.2	Yes	8	Yes	Yes	1.9%
20	Mount Sinai Hospital, New York	77.1	6	4	299	2.0	Yes	8	Yes	Yes	5.7%
21	Memorial Sloan Kettering Cancer Center, New York	76.4	9	4	212	2.0	Yes	8	No	Yes	4.5%
22	University of Cincinnati Medical Center	75.7	10	1	221	1.8	No	8	Yes	Yes	5.4%
23	Vanderbilt University Medical Center, Nashville	75.0	3	4	264	1.9	Yes	8	Yes	Yes	11.5%
24	University of California, Davis Medical Center, Sacramento	74.9	9	4	111	2.7	Yes	8	Yes	Yes	1.9%
25	Rush University Medical Center, Chicago	74.4	10	4	99	2.2	Yes	8	Yes	Yes	1.0%
26	Baylor University Medical Center, Dallas	74.0	10	4	163	1.7	Yes	8	Yes	Yes	0.5%
27	Queen's Medical Center, Honolulu	73.6	10	3	86	1.8	Yes	8	Yes	Yes	0.0%
28	Mayo Clinic, Phoenix	73.5	10	5	182	3.2	No	8	No	Yes	1.4%
29	Mayo Clinic Jacksonville, Fla.	73.0	10	5	77	2.1	Yes	8	No	Yes	0.5%
29	University of Alabama Hospital at Birmingham	73.0	7	4	294	1.8	Yes	7	Yes	Yes	1.9%
31	University of Kansas Hospital, Kansas City	72.7	8	2	228	1.9	Yes	8	Yes	Yes	1.2%
32	Carolinas Medical Center, Charlotte, N.C.	72.6	10	3	154	1.7	Yes	8	Yes	Yes	0.0%
33	Yale-New Haven Hospital, New Haven, Conn.	72.4	8	1	335	1.8	Yes	8	Yes	Yes	0.6%
34	Cedars-Sinai Medical Center, Los Angeles	72.3	9	3	85	2.6	Yes	8	Yes	Yes	0.8%
35	University Hospitals Case Medical Center, Cleveland	71.4	6	2	261	2.3	Yes	8	Yes	Yes	2.9%
35	Wake Forest Baptist Medical Center, Winston-Salem, N.C.	71.4	8	2	277	1.6	Yes	8	Yes	Yes	0.7%
37	NYU Langone Medical Center, New York	70.9	8	4	60	2.6	Yes	8	Yes	Yes	2.5%
38	New York-Presbyterian U. Hospital of Columbia and Cornell, N.Y.	70.7	8	3	253	2.5	No	8	Yes	Yes	2.7%
39	Fox Chase Cancer Center, Philadelphia	70.5	10	2	83	2.1	Yes	8	No	Yes	0.1%
40	Porter Adventist Hospital, Denver	70.2	10	2	127	1.7	Yes	8	No	Yes	0.0%
41	University of California, Irvine Medical Center, Orange	70.0	8	2	102	2.6	Yes	7	Yes	Yes	1.2%
42	Ochsner Medical Center, New Orleans	69.9	8	3	136	1.9	Yes	8	Yes	Yes	0.5%
42	University of Chicago Medical Center	69.9	9	4	143	2.3	No	8	Yes	Yes	2.9%
44	Northwestern Memorial Hospital, Chicago	69.8	8	4	90	1.6	Yes	8	Yes	Yes	1.9%
45	University of Maryland Medical Center, Baltimore	69.5	8	1	197	2.9	Yes	8	Yes	Yes	0.6%
46	St. Vincent Hospital and Health Center, Indianapolis	69.4	9	3	162	1.6	Yes	8	Yes	Yes	0.0%
47	Hackensack University Medical Center, Hackensack, N.J.	69.3	8	4	99	2.4	Yes	8	Yes	Yes	0.0%
48	Froedtert Hosp. and the Medical College of Wisconsin, Milwaukee	69.2	7	4	111	1.8	Yes	8	Yes	Yes	1.6%
48	Penn State Milton S. Hershey Medical Center, Hershey	69.2	10	1	79	1.6	Yes	8	Yes	Yes	0.4%
50	Abington Memorial Hospital, Abington, Pa.	69.1	10	2	43	1.5	Yes	8	Yes	Yes	0.2%
50	University of Illinois Hospital, Chicago	69.1	10	3	36	1.7	No	8	No	Yes	1.3%

*Reflects more than one hospital's status. The specialized hospital lacks Nurse Magnet recognition.

Terms are explained on Page 90.

▶ **More @ usnews.com/besthospitals**

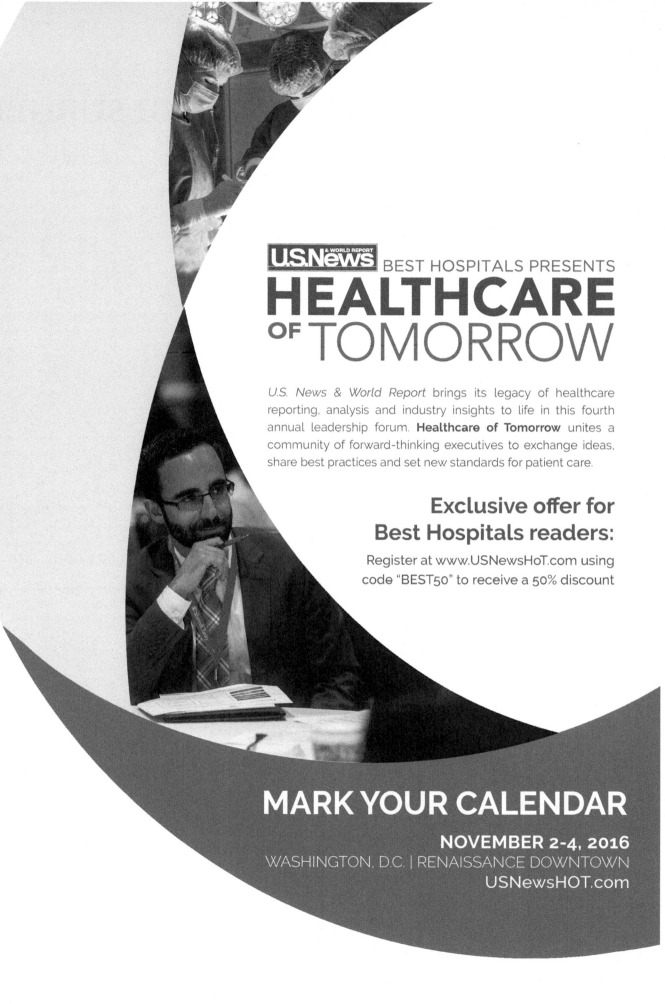

GASTROENTEROLOGY & GI SURGERY

Rank	Hospital	U.S. News score	Survival score (10=best)	Patient safety score (5=best)	Number of patients	Nurse staffing score (higher is better)	Nurse Magnet status	Technology score (7=best)	Patient services score (8=best)	Trauma center	Intensivists	Specialists recommending
1	Mayo Clinic, Rochester, Minn.	100.0	9	5	6,119	2.7	Yes	7	8	Yes	Yes	52.6%
2	Cleveland Clinic	89.1	10	5	5,392	2.1	Yes	7	8	No	Yes	36.0%
3	Johns Hopkins Hospital, Baltimore	77.1	7	2	2,645	2.1	Yes	7	8	Yes	Yes	23.5%
4	Massachusetts General Hospital, Boston	77.0	7	3	4,343	2.3	Yes	7	8	Yes	Yes	18.6%
5	UCLA Medical Center, Los Angeles	74.3	8	4	3,080	3.1	Yes	7	8	Yes	Yes	8.6%
6	UPMC Presbyterian Shadyside, Pittsburgh	73.6	8	1	6,898	1.9	Yes	7	8	Yes	Yes	9.2%
7	Mount Sinai Hospital, New York	72.7	7	4	5,040	2.0	Yes	7	8	Yes	Yes	11.8%
8	Mayo Clinic, Phoenix	72.4	10	5	2,011	3.2	No	7	8	No	Yes	4.2%
9	Cedars-Sinai Medical Center, Los Angeles	70.8	7	3	4,463	2.6	Yes	7	8	Yes	Yes	6.9%
10	Mayo Clinic Jacksonville, Fla.	70.5	10	5	1,935	2.1	Yes	7	8	No	Yes	3.8%
11	Houston Methodist Hospital	70.4	10	3	3,812	1.9	Yes	7	8	No	Yes	2.0%
12	Hospitals of the U. of Pennsylvania-Penn Presbyterian, Philadelphia	70.3	7	5	3,299	2.5	Yes	7	8	Yes	Yes	9.3%
13	NYU Langone Medical Center, New York	69.0	9	4	2,161	2.6	Yes	7	8	Yes	Yes	2.4%
14	New York-Presbyterian U. Hospital of Columbia and Cornell, N.Y.	68.9	8	3	7,389	2.5	No	7	8	Yes	Yes	5.7%
15	UCSF Medical Center, San Francisco	68.1	7	5	1,725	2.7	Yes	7	8	Yes	Yes	8.2%
16	Baylor University Medical Center, Dallas	68.0	8	4	3,462	1.7	Yes	7	8	Yes	Yes	3.4%
16	Northwestern Memorial Hospital, Chicago	68.0	8	4	2,702	1.6	Yes	7	8	Yes	Yes	5.7%
18	Beaumont Hospital-Royal Oak, Mich.	67.5	8	3	5,594	1.8	Yes	7	8	Yes	Yes	0.9%
19	St. Francis Hospital, Roslyn, N.Y.	66.5	10	2	2,243	1.9	Yes	6	8	Yes	Yes	0.1%
19	Thomas Jefferson University Hospital, Philadelphia	66.5	8	4	3,921	2.2	Yes	7	8	Yes	Yes	2.9%
21	Stanford Health Care-Stanford Hospital, Stanford, Calif.	66.4	7	5	2,389	2.4	Yes	7	8	Yes	Yes	3.5%
22	University of Colorado Hospital, Aurora	66.2	9	3	1,429	2.2	Yes	7	8	Yes	Yes	2.3%
23	University of Michigan Hospitals and Health Centers, Ann Arbor	66.1	8	5	3,572	2.9	No	7	8	Yes	Yes	6.5%
23	Yale-New Haven Hospital, New Haven, Conn.	66.1	8	1	5,514	1.8	Yes	7	8	Yes	Yes	2.6%
25	IU Health Academic Health Center, Indianapolis	65.9	8	2	3,864	1.8	Yes	7	8	Yes	Yes	3.0%
26	Tampa General Hospital	65.4	9	1	2,500	2.2	Yes	7	8	Yes	Yes	1.9%
27	Ochsner Medical Center, New Orleans	65.3	8	3	3,662	1.9	Yes	7	8	Yes	Yes	1.6%
27	University Hospitals Case Medical Center, Cleveland	65.3	8	2	2,670	2.3	Yes	7	8	Yes	Yes	2.3%
29	Barnes-Jewish Hospital/Washington University, St. Louis	64.7	6	3	4,533	2.2	Yes	7	8	Yes	Yes	4.6%
30	University of Wisconsin Hospital and Clinics, Madison	64.6	9	2	2,322	1.9	Yes	7	8	Yes	Yes	0.5%
31	University of Washington Medical Center, Seattle	64.4	9	3	1,264	2.1	Yes	7	8	No	Yes	2.4%
32	Fairview Hospital, Cleveland	64.2	9	5	1,738	1.7	Yes	6	8	Yes	Yes	0.0%
32	Sanford USD Medical Center, Sioux Falls, S.D.	64.2	9	2	2,051	2.6	Yes	6	8	Yes	Yes	0.0%
34	Hoag Memorial Hospital Presbyterian, Newport Beach, Calif.	64.0	10	3	2,922	2.2	Yes	6	8	No	Yes	0.0%
35	University of Kansas Hospital, Kansas City	63.9	9	2	2,056	1.9	Yes	7	8	Yes	Yes	0.6%
36	University of Chicago Medical Center	63.4	7	4	2,057	2.3	No	7	8	Yes	Yes	9.9%
37	Lancaster General Hospital, Lancaster, Pa.	63.3	8	4	3,175	1.7	Yes	6	8	Trauma	Yes	0.3%
38	Duke University Hospital, Durham, N.C.	63.2	6	4	2,863	2.2	Yes	7	8	Yes	Yes	5.4%
38	Lehigh Valley Hospital, Allentown, Pa.	63.2	8	4	3,914	1.8	Yes	6	8	Yes	Yes	0.1%
40	Memorial Hermann-Texas Medical Center, Houston	62.9	8	5	1,110	2.2	Yes	7	8	Yes	Yes	0.7%
41	University of North Carolina Hospitals, Chapel Hill	62.8	7	2	2,436	1.8	Yes	7	8	Yes	Yes	4.2%
42	Advocate Lutheran General Hospital, Park Ridge, Ill.	62.7	8	5	2,420	1.6	Yes	6	8	Yes	Yes	0.0%
42	Christ Hospital, Cincinnati	62.7	9	2	2,027	1.8	Yes	6	8	No	Yes	1.4%
44	Harper University Hospital, Detroit	62.5	10	3	1,050	1.6	No	6	8	Yes	Yes	0.0%
45	Aurora St. Luke's Medical Center, Milwaukee	62.4	9	1	3,869	1.5	Yes	6	8	No	Yes	0.2%
45	Brigham and Women's Hospital, Boston	62.4	7	5	3,635	2.4	No	6	8	Yes	Yes	5.0%
45	Christiana Care Christiana Hospital, Newark, Del.	62.4	7	4	4,981	2.0	Yes	6	8	Yes	Yes	0.1%
45	Scripps La Jolla Hospitals and Clinics, La Jolla, Calif.	62.4	8	4	2,404	2.9	Y/N*	7	8	Yes	Yes	0.6%
49	Cleveland Clinic Florida, Weston	61.7	10	4	1,247	1.9	No	5	8	No	Yes	4.0%
50	St. Luke's Hospital, Kansas City, Mo.	61.5	8	5	1,494	1.6	Yes	7	8	Yes	Yes	0.1%

*Reflects more than one hospital's status. The secondary hospital lacks Nurse Magnet recognition.

Terms are explained on Page 90.

▶ **More @ usnews.com/besthospitals**

GERIATRICS

Rank	Hospital	U.S. News score	Survival score (10=best)	Patient safety score (5=best)	Number of patients	Nurse staffing score (higher is better)	Nurse Magnet status	NIA Alzheimer's center	Patient services score (9=best)	Intensivists	Specialists recommending
1	Mayo Clinic, Rochester, Minn.	100.0	9	5	26,018	2.7	Yes	Yes	9	Yes	15.3%
2	UCLA Medical Center, Los Angeles	95.8	8	4	15,380	3.1	Yes	Yes	9	Yes	21.7%
3	Mount Sinai Hospital, New York	94.3	8	4	23,226	2.0	Yes	Yes	9	Yes	23.6%
4	Johns Hopkins Hospital, Baltimore	92.2	9	2	7,883	2.1	Yes	Yes	9	Yes	23.0%
5	NYU Langone Medical Center, New York	88.4	10	4	12,927	2.6	Yes	Yes	9	Yes	3.5%
6	Massachusetts General Hospital, Boston	87.5	8	3	20,279	2.3	Yes	Yes	9	Yes	12.6%
7	New York-Presbyterian U. Hospital of Columbia and Cornell, N.Y.	87.4	9	3	41,087	2.5	No	Yes	9	Yes	7.6%
8	Cleveland Clinic	86.7	10	5	20,573	2.1	Yes	No	9	Yes	10.8%
9	Northwestern Memorial Hospital, Chicago	82.5	10	4	11,232	1.6	Yes	Yes	9	Yes	1.8%
10	Yale-New Haven Hospital, New Haven, Conn.	81.2	7	1	30,759	1.8	Yes	Yes	9	Yes	6.9%
11	Rush University Medical Center, Chicago	80.8	10	4	8,625	2.2	Yes	Yes	9	Yes	1.8%
12	UPMC Presbyterian Shadyside, Pittsburgh	78.9	7	1	28,504	1.9	Yes	Yes	9	Yes	5.4%
13	University of Kansas Hospital, Kansas City	77.8	9	2	8,409	1.9	Yes	Yes	9	Yes	1.0%
14	Hospitals of the U. of Pennsylvania-Penn Presbyterian, Philadelphia	77.5	8	5	15,918	2.5	Yes	Yes	9	Yes	2.2%
15	UCSF Medical Center, San Francisco	76.6	7	5	6,827	2.7	Yes	Yes	9	Yes	7.0%
16	Mayo Clinic, Phoenix	76.0	9	5	8,464	3.2	No	Yes	9	Yes	0.6%
17	University of California, Davis Medical Center, Sacramento	75.4	9	4	6,568	2.7	Yes	Yes	9	Yes	0.2%
18	Barnes-Jewish Hospital/Washington University, St. Louis	75.1	8	3	15,997	2.2	Yes	Yes	9	Yes	1.0%
19	Houston Methodist Hospital	74.7	10	3	16,635	1.9	Yes	No	9	Yes	2.9%
20	University of Washington Medical Center, Seattle	73.9	9	3	3,676	2.1	Yes	Yes	8	Yes	1.5%
21	Keck Medical Center of USC, Los Angeles	73.6	10	1	3,748	3.8	No	Yes	9	Yes	2.0%
22	Stanford Health Care-Stanford Hospital, Stanford, Calif.	73.1	7	5	10,324	2.4	Yes	Yes	9	Yes	1.9%
23	IU Health Academic Health Center, Indianapolis	72.7	8	2	12,660	1.8	Yes	Yes	9	Yes	2.0%
24	Brigham and Women's Hospital, Boston	72.4	8	5	14,395	2.4	No	Yes	9	Yes	1.6%
24	Cedars-Sinai Medical Center, Los Angeles	72.4	8	3	21,822	2.6	Yes	No	8	Yes	3.4%
26	Beaumont Hospital-Royal Oak, Mich.	72.3	8	3	33,380	1.8	Yes	No	9	Yes	1.4%
27	Emory University Hospital at Wesley Woods, Atlanta	72.1	7	5	9,729	2.0	Yes	Yes	8	Yes	1.7%
28	UC San Diego Medical Center - UC San Diego Health, Calif.	72.0	8	5	6,415	1.8	Yes	Yes	9	Yes	1.3%
29	Mayo Clinic Jacksonville, Fla.	71.3	8	5	7,735	2.1	Yes	Yes	8	Yes	1.5%
30	University of Wisconsin Hospital and Clinics, Madison	70.3	7	2	8,337	1.9	Yes	Yes	9	Yes	2.0%
31	UT Southwestern Medical Center, Dallas	69.8	8	5	5,753	2.0	No	Yes	9	Yes	1.7%
32	Banner University Medical Center Phoenix	69.5	8	2	8,832	2.1	Yes	Yes	9	Yes	0.2%
33	UF Health Shands Hospital, Gainesville, Fla.	68.9	7	3	10,863	2.0	Yes	Yes	9	Yes	0.1%
34	St. Francis Hospital, Roslyn, N.Y.	68.2	9	2	14,870	1.9	Yes	No	8	Yes	0.1%
35	Duke University Hospital, Durham, N.C.	67.9	7	4	11,654	2.2	Yes	No	9	Yes	7.1%
36	University of Colorado Hospital, Aurora	67.7	9	3	5,445	2.2	Yes	No	9	Yes	1.4%
37	Aurora St. Luke's Medical Center, Milwaukee	66.7	9	1	23,950	1.5	Yes	No	8	Yes	0.3%
38	Oregon Health and Science University Hospital, Portland	66.6	7	2	5,683	2.1	Yes	Yes	9	Yes	0.0%
38	Thomas Jefferson University Hospital, Philadelphia	66.6	8	4	16,195	2.2	Yes	No	9	Yes	2.5%
40	Lehigh Valley Hospital, Allentown, Pa.	66.4	8	4	23,516	1.8	Yes	No	8	Yes	0.8%
41	Abbott Northwestern Hospital, Minneapolis	66.1	8	5	15,280	2.1	Yes	No	9	Yes	0.0%
41	Fairview Hospital, Cleveland	66.1	9	5	9,760	1.7	Yes	No	9	Yes	0.0%
41	University Hospitals Case Medical Center, Cleveland	66.1	8	2	11,685	2.3	Yes	No	9	Yes	2.3%
44	Ohio State University Wexner Medical Center, Columbus	65.6	9	2	13,396	2.1	Yes	No	9	Yes	0.8%
45	University of Kentucky Albert B. Chandler Hospital, Lexington	65.2	7	2	7,320	1.8	Yes	Yes	9	Yes	0.0%
46	Banner University Medical Center Tucson, Ariz.	65.1	7	2	6,353	1.6	Yes	Yes	7	Yes	0.3%
47	University of Michigan Hospitals and Health Centers, Ann Arbor	64.9	8	5	11,790	2.9	No	No	9	Yes	5.4%
48	Scripps La Jolla Hospitals and Clinics, La Jolla, Calif.	64.8	8	4	14,754	2.9	Y/N*	No	8	Yes	0.5%
49	Winthrop-University Hospital, Mineola, N.Y.	63.8	8	2	15,592	1.7	Yes	No	9	Yes	0.6%
50	Huntington Memorial Hospital, Pasadena, Calif.	63.7	7	4	11,487	2.5	Yes	No	9	Yes	0.5%

Terms are explained on Page 90.

*Reflects more than one hospital's status. The secondary hospital lacks Nurse Magnet recognition.

GYNECOLOGY

Rank	Hospital	U.S. News score	Survival score (10=best)	Patient safety score (5=best)	Number of patients	Nurse staffing score (higher is better)	Nurse Magnet status	Technology score (5=best)	Patient services score (9=best)	Intensivists	Specialists recom- mending
1	Mayo Clinic, Rochester, Minn.	100.0	10	5	463	2.7	Yes	5	9	Yes	15.3%
2	Memorial Sloan Kettering Cancer Center, New York	92.3	10	4	466	2.0	Yes	5	8	Yes	7.2%
3	Cleveland Clinic	91.0	9	5	255	2.1	Yes	5	9	Yes	13.9%
4	UCSF Medical Center, San Francisco	90.3	10	5	124	2.7	Yes	5	9	Yes	8.7%
5	Massachusetts General Hospital, Boston	88.5	10	3	326	2.3	Yes	5	9	Yes	6.9%
6	Brigham and Women's Hospital, Boston	88.3	10	5	346	2.4	No	5	9	Yes	11.7%
7	Johns Hopkins Hospital, Baltimore	87.4	10	2	123	2.1	Yes	5	9	Yes	11.5%
8	Stanford Health Care-Stanford Hospital, Stanford, Calif.	85.7	10	5	132	2.4	Yes	5	9	Yes	5.0%
9	University of Texas MD Anderson Cancer Center, Houston	85.2	9	2	321	2.0	Yes	5	9	Yes	9.0%
10	UCLA Medical Center, Los Angeles	84.7	10	4	136	3.1	Yes	5	9	Yes	4.9%
11	University of North Carolina Hospitals, Chapel Hill	82.6	10	2	254	1.8	Yes	5	9	Yes	5.4%
12	Magee-Womens Hospital of UPMC, Pittsburgh	81.8	9	1	500	1.4	No	5	9	Yes	9.2%
13	University of Wisconsin Hospital and Clinics, Madison	81.7	10	2	357	1.9	Yes	5	9	Yes	1.8%
14	University of Michigan Hospitals and Health Centers, Ann Arbor	81.4	10	5	202	2.9	No	5	9	Yes	2.2%
15	Cedars-Sinai Medical Center, Los Angeles	81.3	9	3	227	2.6	Yes	5	9	Yes	3.8%
16	Abbott Northwestern Hospital, Minneapolis	80.4	9	5	269	2.1	Yes	5	9	Yes	1.0%
16	University of Alabama Hospital at Birmingham	80.4	9	4	360	1.8	Yes	5	8	Yes	3.2%
18	Vanderbilt University Medical Center, Nashville	80.2	10	4	128	1.9	Yes	5	9	Yes	1.2%
19	St. Luke's Hospital, Kansas City, Mo.	80.0	10	5	209	1.6	Yes	5	8	Yes	0.7%
20	Barnes-Jewish Hospital/Washington University, St. Louis	79.7	8	3	428	2.2	Yes	5	9	Yes	2.3%
21	Rush University Medical Center, Chicago	79.5	9	4	334	2.2	Yes	5	9	Yes	0.3%
21	Scripps La Jolla Hospitals and Clinics, La Jolla, Calif.	79.5	10	4	132	2.9	Y/N*	5	8	Yes	1.0%
23	Duke University Hospital, Durham, N.C.	79.3	8	4	168	2.2	Yes	5	9	Yes	5.7%
23	Queen's Medical Center, Honolulu	79.3	10	3	146	1.8	Yes	5	8	Yes	0.0%
25	John Muir Medical Center, Walnut Creek, Calif.	79.2	10	2	178	2.5	Yes	5	9	Yes	0.9%
25	New York-Presbyterian U. Hospital of Columbia and Cornell, N.Y.	79.2	9	3	318	2.5	No	5	9	Yes	7.6%
27	Good Samaritan Hospital, Cincinnati	79.1	10	3	111	1.7	Yes	5	9	Yes	0.9%
28	Memorial Hermann-Texas Medical Center, Houston	78.5	10	5	55	2.2	Yes	5	8	Yes	0.4%
29	UF Health Shands Hospital, Gainesville, Fla.	78.4	10	3	165	2.0	Yes	5	9	Yes	0.8%
30	University Hospitals Case Medical Center, Cleveland	78.2	10	2	277	2.3	Yes	5	9	Yes	0.5%
31	Northwestern Memorial Hospital, Chicago	77.9	9	4	117	1.6	Yes	5	9	Yes	4.5%
32	University of Colorado Hospital, Aurora	77.8	10	3	180	2.2	Yes	5	9	Yes	0.3%
33	Advocate Christ Medical Center, Oak Lawn, Ill.	77.6	9	4	212	2.4	Yes	5	9	Yes	0.7%
34	Advocate Lutheran General Hospital, Park Ridge, Ill.	77.5	10	5	129	1.6	Yes	5	8	Yes	0.8%
35	Mayo Clinic Jacksonville, Fla.	77.1	9	5	143	2.1	Yes	5	8	Yes	2.1%
35	University Hospital, San Antonio	77.1	10	2	78	1.6	Yes	5	9	Yes	1.6%
35	Yale-New Haven Hospital, New Haven, Conn.	77.1	8	1	424	1.8	Yes	5	9	Yes	1.1%
38	University of Kansas Hospital, Kansas City	77.0	9	2	280	1.9	Yes	5	9	Yes	0.2%
39	Huntington Memorial Hospital, Pasadena, Calif.	76.9	10	4	153	2.5	Yes	4	9	Intensivists	0.7%
39	Medical University of South Carolina Medical Center, Charleston	76.9	9	3	235	2.1	Yes	5	9	Yes	0.7%
39	Sharp Memorial Hospital, San Diego	76.9	10	3	150	2.4	Yes	5	7	Yes	0.5%
39	University of California, Davis Medical Center, Sacramento	76.9	9	4	161	2.7	Yes	5	9	Yes	1.9%
43	University of Washington Medical Center, Seattle	76.2	9	3	230	2.1	Yes	5	9	Yes	1.5%
44	Christ Hospital, Cincinnati	76.0	10	2	104	1.8	Yes	5	8	Yes	1.5%
44	Medical City Dallas Hospital	76.0	10	1	167	2.0	Yes	4	8	Yes	0.4%
44	University of Texas Medical Branch Hospitals, Galveston	76.0	10	1	50	1.5	Yes	5	8	Yes	1.1%
47	Long Island Jewish Medical Center, New Hyde Park, N.Y.	75.9	10	2	187	1.6	Yes	5	9	Yes	0.4%
47	Providence Portland Medical Center, Portland, Ore.	75.9	10	3	122	1.6	Yes	4	7	Yes	0.0%
49	University of Iowa Hospitals and Clinics, Iowa City	75.8	8	4	224	1.8	Yes	5	9	Yes	3.7%
50	Banner Desert Medical Center, Mesa, Ariz.	75.7	10	4	84	2.1	No	5	9	Yes	0.0%
50	Baptist Medical Center, Jacksonville, Fla.	75.7	9	3	106	1.8	Yes	5	9	Yes	1.2%
50	West Penn Hospital, Pittsburgh	75.7	10	4	118	1.2	Yes	5	9	Yes	0.4%

*Reflects more than one hospital's status. The secondary hospital lacks Nurse Magnet recognition.   Terms are explained on Page 90.

▶ **More @ usnews.com/besthospitals**

NEPHROLOGY

Rank	Hospital	U.S. News score	Survival score (10=best)	Patient safety score (5=best)	Number of patients	Nurse staffing score (higher is better)	Nurse Magnet status	Technology score (7=best)	Patient services score (8=best)	Intensivists	Specialists recom-mending
1	Mayo Clinic, Rochester, Minn.	100.0	9	5	1,720	2.7	Yes	7	8	Yes	29.6%
2	Cleveland Clinic	96.6	10	5	2,086	2.1	Yes	7	8	Yes	26.8%
3	UCSF Medical Center, San Francisco	91.4	10	5	793	2.7	Yes	7	8	Yes	10.8%
4	New York-Presbyterian U. Hospital of Columbia and Cornell, N.Y.	90.6	9	3	3,286	2.5	No	7	8	Yes	21.0%
5	Johns Hopkins Hospital, Baltimore	89.3	9	2	969	2.1	Yes	7	8	Yes	19.7%
6	Massachusetts General Hospital, Boston	83.0	8	3	1,319	2.3	Yes	7	8	Yes	14.3%
7	UCLA Medical Center, Los Angeles	82.7	9	4	1,132	3.1	Yes	7	8	Yes	6.3%
8	Barnes-Jewish Hospital/Washington University, St. Louis	82.2	8	3	1,846	2.2	Yes	7	8	Yes	7.7%
8	Vanderbilt University Medical Center, Nashville	82.2	8	4	1,161	1.9	Yes	7	8	Yes	10.9%
10	University of California, Davis Medical Center, Sacramento	80.9	10	4	721	2.7	Yes	7	8	Yes	2.4%
11	Mount Sinai Hospital, New York	79.6	8	4	1,593	2.0	Yes	7	8	Yes	6.9%
11	UF Health Shands Hospital, Gainesville, Fla.	79.6	9	3	1,179	2.0	Yes	7	8	Yes	5.0%
13	Cedars-Sinai Medical Center, Los Angeles	79.5	9	3	1,422	2.6	Yes	7	8	Yes	3.6%
14	Northwestern Memorial Hospital, Chicago	79.1	10	4	1,172	1.6	Yes	7	8	Yes	2.4%
15	University of Colorado Hospital, Aurora	78.9	10	3	502	2.2	Yes	7	8	Yes	2.6%
16	IU Health Academic Health Center, Indianapolis	78.4	10	2	1,486	1.8	Yes	7	8	Yes	2.7%
17	Hospitals of the U. of Pennsylvania-Penn Presbyterian, Philadelphia	78.3	8	5	1,142	2.5	Yes	7	8	Yes	6.2%
18	Tampa General Hospital	78.0	10	1	1,128	2.2	Yes	7	8	Yes	0.9%
19	Rush University Medical Center, Chicago	77.4	8	4	741	2.2	Yes	7	8	Yes	4.9%
20	University of Alabama Hospital at Birmingham	76.7	9	4	1,065	1.8	Yes	7	7	Yes	3.8%
21	Brigham and Women's Hospital, Boston	76.6	6	5	960	2.4	No	7	8	Yes	16.6%
21	University of North Carolina Hospitals, Chapel Hill	76.6	9	2	936	1.8	Yes	7	8	Yes	4.8%
23	University of Michigan Hospitals and Health Centers, Ann Arbor	75.9	9	5	1,253	2.9	No	7	8	Yes	5.4%
24	UC San Diego Medical Center - UC San Diego Health, Calif.	75.6	10	5	504	1.8	Yes	7	8	Yes	1.0%
25	Ohio State University Wexner Medical Center, Columbus	75.5	9	2	1,419	2.1	Yes	7	8	Yes	2.5%
25	Wake Forest Baptist Medical Center, Winston-Salem, N.C.	75.5	8	2	1,795	1.6	Yes	7	8	Yes	3.9%
27	University of Washington Medical Center, Seattle	75.2	9	3	474	2.1	Yes	7	8	Yes	4.6%
28	Duke University Hospital, Durham, N.C.	75.1	7	4	979	2.2	Yes	7	8	Yes	5.4%
28	Mayo Clinic, Phoenix	75.1	10	5	745	3.2	No	7	8	Yes	1.7%
28	University of Wisconsin Hospital and Clinics, Madison	75.1	10	2	750	1.9	Yes	7	8	Yes	1.9%
31	Beaumont Hospital-Royal Oak, Mich.	74.6	9	3	2,087	1.8	Yes	7	8	Yes	0.4%
32	University Hospital, San Antonio	74.5	10	2	226	1.6	Yes	7	8	Yes	0.1%
33	UPMC Presbyterian Shadyside, Pittsburgh	74.4	8	1	2,201	1.9	Yes	7	8	Yes	3.0%
34	Yale-New Haven Hospital, New Haven, Conn.	74.3	6	1	2,322	1.8	Yes	7	8	Yes	8.1%
35	Banner University Medical Center Phoenix	73.7	9	2	668	2.1	Yes	7	8	Yes	0.7%
36	Stanford Health Care-Stanford Hospital, Stanford, Calif.	73.2	6	5	753	2.4	Yes	7	8	Yes	6.7%
37	Keck Medical Center of USC, Los Angeles†	73.0	10	1	886	3.8	No	7	8	Yes	0.8%
37	Oregon Health and Science University Hospital, Portland	72.9	9	2	503	2.1	Yes	7	8	Yes	1.0%
38	Houston Methodist Hospital	72.7	9	3	1,410	1.9	Yes	7	8	Yes	1.4%
39	Banner University Medical Center Tucson, Ariz.	72.2	10	2	457	1.6	Yes	7	7	Yes	0.7%
40	Queen's Medical Center, Honolulu	71.8	9	3	773	1.8	Yes	7	8	Yes	0.0%
41	University of Chicago Medical Center	71.7	9	4	824	2.3	No	7	8	Yes	1.5%
42	Christiana Care Christiana Hospital, Newark, Del.	71.6	8	4	1,985	2.0	Yes	7	8	Yes	0.1%
43	Medical University of South Carolina Medical Center, Charleston	71.0	8	3	803	2.1	Yes	7	8	Yes	1.0%
43	Memorial Hermann-Texas Medical Center, Houston	71.0	8	5	481	2.2	Yes	7	8	Yes	0.2%
45	Froedtert Hosp. and the Medical College of Wisconsin, Milwaukee	70.9	8	4	742	1.8	Yes	7	8	Yes	1.2%
46	University of Virginia Medical Center, Charlottesville	70.7	8	4	713	2.1	Yes	7	7	Yes	0.8%
46	Virginia Commonwealth University Medical Center, Richmond	70.7	9	3	492	2.2	Yes	7	7	Yes	0.2%
48	Loyola University Medical Center, Maywood, Ill.	70.5	8	4	843	1.6	Yes	7	8	Yes	0.4%
49	Thomas Jefferson University Hospital, Philadelphia	70.2	8	4	1,196	2.2	Yes	7	8	Yes	0.3%

Terms are explained on Page 90.   †Due to a data processing error, this hospital was initially misranked. Rankings for other hospitals have not been changed.

NEUROLOGY & NEUROSURGERY

Rank	Hospital	U.S. News score	Survival score (10=best)	Patient safety score (5=best)	Number of patients	Nurse staffing score (higher is better)	Nurse Magnet status	NAEC epilepsy center	Technology score (5=best)	Patient services score (9=best)	Intensivists	Specialists recommending
1	Mayo Clinic, Rochester, Minn.	100.0	8	5	4,160	2.7	Yes	Yes	5	9	Yes	35.7%
2	Johns Hopkins Hospital, Baltimore	92.2	8	2	2,087	2.1	Yes	Yes	5	9	Yes	32.9%
3	New York-Presbyterian U. Hospital of Columbia and Cornell, N.Y.	87.0	8	3	6,136	2.5	No	Yes	5	9	Yes	19.1%
4	Massachusetts General Hospital, Boston	86.2	6	3	4,375	2.3	Yes	Yes	5	9	Yes	27.4%
5	UCSF Medical Center, San Francisco	85.1	7	5	1,908	2.7	Yes	Yes	4	9	Yes	23.4%
6	Cleveland Clinic	84.2	9	5	3,738	2.1	Yes	Yes	5	9	Yes	19.9%
7	NYU Langone Medical Center, New York	82.3	9	4	1,536	2.6	Yes	Yes	5	9	Yes	6.0%
8	UCLA Medical Center, Los Angeles	79.8	7	4	2,571	3.1	Yes	Yes	5	9	Yes	10.5%
9	Northwestern Memorial Hospital, Chicago	77.2	9	4	1,942	1.6	Yes	Yes	5	9	Yes	2.5%
10	Barnes-Jewish Hospital/Washington University, St. Louis	77.1	7	3	3,950	2.2	Yes	Yes	5	9	Yes	8.0%
11	Brigham and Women's Hospital, Boston	76.3	7	5	2,976	2.4	No	Yes	5	9	Yes	9.6%
12	Mount Sinai Hospital, New York	75.7	8	4	2,723	2.0	Yes	Yes	5	9	Yes	4.5%
13	Rush University Medical Center, Chicago	74.8	9	4	2,311	2.2	Yes	Yes	5	9	Yes	3.4%
14	Hospitals of the U. of Pennsylvania-Penn Presbyterian, Philadelphia	74.2	6	5	2,479	2.5	Yes	Yes	5	9	Yes	8.4%
15	Emory University Hospital, Atlanta	72.4	7	5	2,677	2.0	Yes	Yes	5	9	Yes	5.2%
16	St. Joseph's Hospital and Medical Center, Phoenix	71.5	7	2	3,989	1.8	No	Yes	5	9	Yes	8.5%
17	Houston Methodist Hospital	70.0	9	3	3,307	1.9	Yes	Yes	5	9	Yes	2.5%
18	Cedars-Sinai Medical Center, Los Angeles	69.5	8	3	2,878	2.6	Yes	Yes	5	9	Yes	2.4%
19	Stanford Health Care-Stanford Hospital, Stanford, Calif.	68.7	6	5	1,786	2.4	Yes	Yes	5	9	Yes	4.8%
19	UPMC Presbyterian Shadyside, Pittsburgh	68.7	6	1	7,024	1.9	Yes	Yes	5	9	Yes	2.4%
21	UF Health Shands Hospital, Gainesville, Fla.	67.3	6	3	3,221	2.0	Yes	Yes	5	9	Yes	4.0%
22	University of Kansas Hospital, Kansas City	66.8	7	2	1,727	1.9	Yes	Yes	5	9	Yes	1.7%
23	Ochsner Medical Center, New Orleans	65.9	8	3	2,547	1.9	Yes	Yes	5	9	Yes	0.3%
24	Thomas Jefferson University Hospital, Philadelphia	65.6	7	4	4,332	2.2	Yes	Yes	5	9	Yes	2.6%
25	University of Alabama Hospital at Birmingham	65.5	7	4	3,147	1.8	Yes	Yes	5	8	Yes	2.7%
25	Yale-New Haven Hospital, New Haven, Conn.	65.5	6	1	4,005	1.8	Yes	Yes	5	9	Yes	2.3%
27	Harper University Hospital, Detroit	65.4	10	3	813	1.6	No	Yes	5	9	Yes	0.4%
28	Beaumont Hospital-Royal Oak, Mich.	65.1	8	3	4,502	1.8	Yes	Yes	5	9	Yes	0.1%
29	IU Health Academic Health Center, Indianapolis	65.0	7	2	3,045	1.8	Yes	Yes	5	9	Yes	1.4%
30	Ohio State University Wexner Medical Center, Columbus	64.7	8	2	2,930	2.1	Yes	Yes	5	9	Yes	1.2%
31	Mayo Clinic Jacksonville, Fla.	64.3	6	5	1,541	2.1	Yes	Yes	5	9	Yes	2.4%
32	University of Michigan Hospitals and Health Centers, Ann Arbor	63.1	7	5	2,095	2.9	No	Yes	5	9	Yes	5.1%
33	Duke University Hospital, Durham, N.C.	63.0	5	4	2,354	2.2	Yes	Yes	5	9	Yes	5.9%
34	UR Medicine Strong Memorial Hospital, Rochester, N.Y.	62.9	7	2	2,892	1.7	Yes	Yes	5	9	Yes	2.5%
34	University of California, Davis Medical Center, Sacramento	62.9	6	4	1,156	2.7	Yes	Yes	5	9	Yes	0.2%
36	Sinai Hospital of Baltimore	62.4	8	1	1,924	1.7	Yes	Yes	5	9	Yes	1.5%
37	UC San Diego Medical Center - UC San Diego Health, Calif.	61.9	6	5	1,221	1.8	Yes	Yes	5	9	Yes	0.6%
38	Baylor University Medical Center, Dallas	61.8	7	4	3,296	1.7	Yes	Yes	5	9	Yes	0.5%
38	MedStar Southern Maryland Hospital Center, Clinton, Md.	61.8	10	3	3,347	1.6	No	No	5	9	Yes	0.0%
40	University of Wisconsin Hospital and Clinics, Madison	61.7	6	2	2,005	1.9	Yes	Yes	5	9	Yes	1.5%
41	Memorial Hermann-Texas Medical Center, Houston	61.5	6	5	3,938	2.2	Yes	Yes	5	9	Yes	1.7%
42	UT Southwestern Medical Center, Dallas	61.0	8	5	1,384	2.0	No	No	5	9	Yes	1.8%
43	University of Colorado Hospital, Aurora	60.8	7	3	1,087	2.2	Yes	Yes	5	9	Yes	1.4%
43	Vanderbilt University Medical Center, Nashville	60.8	6	4	2,699	1.9	Yes	Yes	5	9	Yes	3.4%
45	Mayo Clinic, Phoenix	60.7	6	5	1,346	3.2	No	Yes	5	9	Yes	2.9%
46	Wake Forest Baptist Medical Center, Winston-Salem, N.C.	60.4	7	2	3,064	1.6	Yes	Yes	5	9	Yes	1.0%
47	Abbott Northwestern Hospital, Minneapolis	60.0	7	5	2,402	2.1	Yes	Yes	5	9	Yes	0.0%
47	Huntington Memorial Hospital, Pasadena, Calif.	60.0	7	4	1,552	2.5	Yes	Yes	5	9	Yes	0.1%
47	OhioHealth Riverside Hospital, Columbus	60.0	6	2	5,645	2.0	Yes	Yes	5	9	Yes	0.4%
47	University Hospitals Case Medical Center, Cleveland	60.0	7	2	2,898	2.3	Yes	Yes	5	9	Yes	1.0%
47	University of Iowa Hospitals and Clinics, Iowa City	60.0	7	4	3,056	1.8	Yes	Yes	5	9	Yes	1.4%

Terms are explained on Page 90.

▶ **More @ usnews.com/besthospitals**

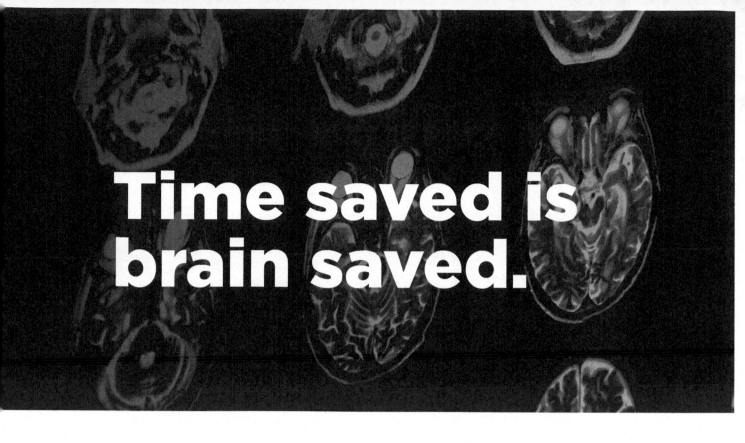

Time saved is brain saved.

To learn more, visit

ChiBrain.org

UI Health is proud to be a **Comprehensive Stroke Center**, providing the highest level of care to our patients **24/7**.

The Joint Commission

American Heart Association **American Stroke Association**

CERTIFICATION

Meets standards for
Comprehensive Stroke Center

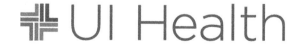

The University of Illinois Hospital & Health Sciences System
is part of the University of Illinois at Chicago

ORTHOPEDICS

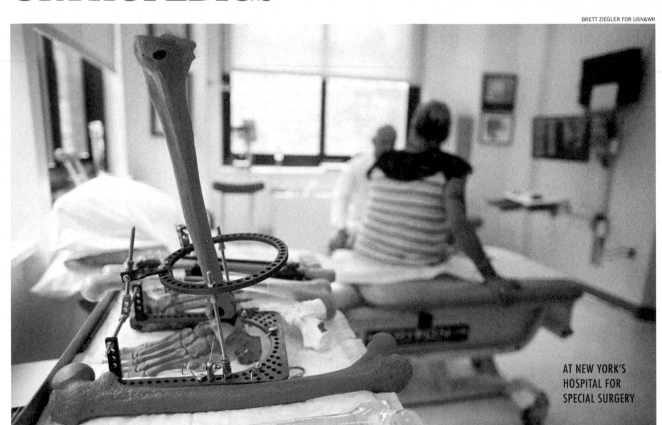

BRETT ZIEGLER FOR USN&WR

AT NEW YORK'S
HOSPITAL FOR
SPECIAL SURGERY

Rank	Hospital	U.S. News score	Survival score (10=best)	Patient safety score (5=best)	Number of patients	Nurse staffing score (higher is better)	Nurse Magnet status	Technology score (2=best)	Patient services score (7=best)	Intensivists	Specialists recom-mending
1	Hospital for Special Surgery, New York	100.0	10	5	9,954	3.2	Yes	2	7	Yes	36.7%
2	Mayo Clinic, Rochester, Minn.	86.9	9	5	6,587	2.7	Yes	2	7	Yes	32.1%
3	Cleveland Clinic	76.7	10	5	3,046	2.1	Yes	2	7	Yes	17.8%
4	Rush University Medical Center, Chicago	73.6	10	4	2,462	2.2	Yes	2	7	Yes	11.3%
5	Hospital for Joint Diseases, NYU Langone Medical Cen., New York	72.1	10	4	3,818	2.6	Yes	2	7	Yes	5.8%
6	Northwestern Memorial Hospital, Chicago	69.1	10	4	2,839	1.6	Yes	2	7	Yes	3.3%
7	Rothman Institute at Thomas Jefferson University Hosp. Philadelphia	68.9	9	4	4,186	2.2	Yes	2	7	Yes	6.6%
8	Massachusetts General Hospital, Boston	68.4	9	3	3,113	2.3	Yes	2	7	Yes	10.6%
9	Johns Hopkins Hospital, Baltimore	65.7	9	2	1,006	2.1	Yes	2	7	Yes	9.7%
10	UCSF Medical Center, San Francisco	65.3	10	5	1,973	2.7	Yes	2	7	Yes	2.8%
11	Cedars-Sinai Medical Center, Los Angeles	64.7	10	3	3,785	2.6	Yes	2	7	Yes	2.3%
11	UPMC Presbyterian Shadyside, Pittsburgh	64.7	9	1	5,032	1.9	Yes	2	7	Yes	6.8%
13	Barnes-Jewish Hospital/Washington University, St. Louis	64.6	8	3	3,149	2.2	Yes	2	7	Yes	6.8%
14	Abbott Northwestern Hospital, Minneapolis	63.6	10	5	4,118	2.1	Yes	2	7	Yes	0.9%
15	Duke University Hospital, Durham, N.C.	63.2	7	4	2,571	2.2	Yes	2	7	Yes	7.6%
16	University of Iowa Hospitals and Clinics, Iowa City	63.0	9	4	1,771	1.8	Yes	2	7	Yes	4.9%
17	Stanford Health Care-Stanford Hospital, Stanford, Calif.	62.9	9	5	2,870	2.4	Yes	2	7	Yes	1.9%
18	UCLA Medical Center, Los Angeles	62.6	8	4	1,941	3.1	Yes	2	7	Yes	3.7%
19	Patewood Memorial Hospital, Greenville, S.C.	62.5	10	5	683	4.8	No	2	7	Yes	0.1%
20	University of California, Davis Medical Center, Sacramento	62.3	9	4	1,266	2.7	Yes	2	7	Yes	2.1%
21	Hosp. of the U. of Pennsylvania-Penn Presbyterian, Philadelphia	62.2	9	5	1,864	2.5	Yes	2	7	Yes	2.9%
22	Keck Medical Center of USC, Los Angeles†	61.3	10	1	1,306	3.8	No	2	7	Yes	2.3%

†Due to a data processing error, this hospital's results were initially miscalculated. They are correct as shown. Rankings for other hospitals have not been changed.

Terms are explained on Page 90.

(CONTINUED ON PAGE 110)

▶ **More @ usnews.com/besthospitals**

#1 for Adult Orthopedics in the U.S.

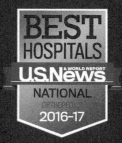

#2 for Rheumatology.

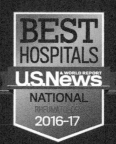

HSS has been among the top-ranked institutions for orthopedics and rheumatology in the U.S. for 25 consecutive years.

Our exclusive focus on musculoskeletal conditions, together with our industry-leading research, personalized care and specialization, delivers a level of excellence to patients unmatched in U.S. healthcare. www.hss.edu

HSS

HOSPITAL FOR **SPECIAL SURGERY**
WHERE THE WORLD COMES TO GET BACK IN THE GAME

ORTHOPEDICS (CONTINUED)

Rank	Hospital	U.S. News score	Survival score (10=best)	Patient safety score (5=best)	Number of patients	Nurse staffing score (higher is better)	Nurse Magnet status	Technology score (2=best)	Patient services score (7=best)	Intensivists	Specialists recom-mending
22	Beaumont Hospital-Royal Oak, Mich.	61.0	8	3	6,358	1.8	Yes	2	7	Yes	1.0%
23	Houston Methodist Hospital	60.9	9	3	3,401	1.9	Yes	2	7	Yes	2.3%
24	University Hospitals Case Medical Center, Cleveland	60.7	9	2	1,623	2.3	Yes	2	7	Yes	3.5%
25	Northwestern Medicine Central DuPage Hospital, Winfield, Ill.	60.1	10	4	2,644	1.9	Yes	2	6	Yes	0.1%
26	Brigham and Women's Hospital, Boston	59.8	8	5	2,380	2.4	No	2	7	Yes	6.7%
26	Emory University Hospital, Atlanta	59.8	10	5	2,140	2.0	Yes	2	6	Yes	0.8%
28	UC San Diego Medical Center - UC San Diego Health, Calif.	59.6	9	5	1,246	1.8	Yes	2	7	Yes	1.1%
29	University of Washington Medical Center, Seattle	59.1	10	3	755	2.1	Yes	1	7	Yes	3.4%
30	Mayo Clinic Jacksonville, Fla.	58.9	10	5	2,121	2.1	Yes	2	7	Yes	1.0%
32	Magee-Womens Hospital of UPMC, Pittsburgh	58.5	10	1	1,195	1.4	No	2	7	Yes	0.0%
32	St. Cloud Hospital, St. Cloud, Minn.	58.5	10	3	2,572	2.2	Yes	2	6	Yes	0.0%
34	Scripps La Jolla Hospitals and Clinics, La Jolla, Calif.	58.3	8	4	3,046	2.9	Y/N*	2	7	Yes	1.3%
35	University of Kansas Hospital, Kansas City	58.2	9	2	1,565	1.9	Yes	2	7	Yes	0.1%
36	Virginia Commonwealth University Medical Center, Richmond	58.1	10	3	1,277	2.2	Yes	2	6	Yes	0.7%
37	New England Baptist Hospital, Boston	57.7	10	5	3,904	2.0	No	2	5	Yes	1.5%
38	Morristown Medical Center, Morristown, N.J.	57.6	8	4	3,616	1.9	Yes	2	7	Yes	0.1%
39	Lehigh Valley Hospital, Allentown, Pa.	57.5	8	4	3,934	1.8	Yes	2	6	Yes	0.4%
40	University of California, Irvine Medical Center, Orange	56.9	10	2	657	2.6	Yes	2	6	Yes	0.1%
41	Good Samaritan Hospital, Cincinnati	56.7	9	3	2,252	1.7	Yes	2	7	Yes	0.0%
42	Mount Sinai Hospital, New York	56.6	8	4	2,494	2.0	Yes	2	7	Yes	0.4%
42	University of Colorado Hospital, Aurora	56.6	8	3	1,080	2.2	Yes	2	7	Yes	1.0%
44	Nebraska Orthopaedic Hospital, Omaha	56.5	10	5	1,043	3.0	No	2	4	No	0.6%
44	New York-Presbyterian U. Hospital of Columbia and Cornell, N.Y.	56.5	8	3	2,911	2.5	No	2	7	Yes	3.9%
46	Mayo Clinic, Phoenix	56.4	9	5	1,976	3.2	No	2	7	Yes	1.3%
47	IU Health Academic Health Center, Indianapolis	56.3	9	2	1,968	1.8	Yes	2	7	Yes	0.5%
47	Mercy Medical Center, Baltimore	56.3	10	4	2,122	1.4	Yes	2	6	Yes	0.0%
49	Hackensack University Medical Center, Hackensack, N.J.	56.2	8	4	2,396	2.4	Yes	2	7	Yes	0.1%
49	Pennsylvania Hospital, Philadelphia†	56.2	10	4	1,592	1.6	Yes	2	7	Yes	0.5%
50	University of Wisconsin Hospital and Clinics, Madison	55.9	9	2	1,670	1.9	Yes	2	7	Yes	0.7%

*Reflects more than one hospital's status. The secondary hospital lacks Nurse Magnet recognition.
†Due to a data processing error, this hospital's results were initially miscalculated. They are correct as shown. Rankings for other hospitals have not been changed.

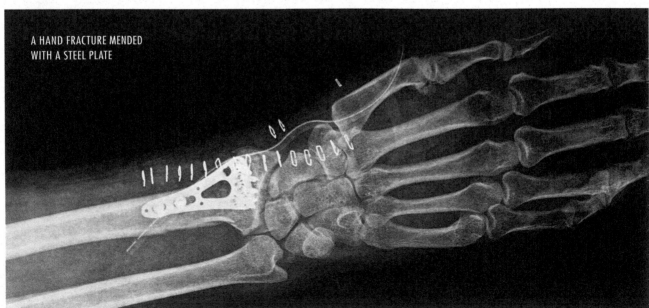

A HAND FRACTURE MENDED WITH A STEEL PLATE

DAVID PEDRE/GETTY IMAGES

▶ **More @ usnews.com/besthospitals**

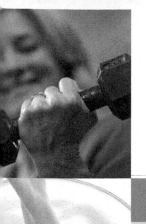

OUTSTANDING HOSPITALS DON'T SIMPLY TREAT FRAGILITY FRACTURES—
THEY PREVENT FRACTURES FROM RECURRING

THE BEST HOSPITALS AND PRACTICES OWN THE BONE.

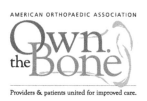

AMERICAN ORTHOPAEDIC ASSOCIATION

Own. the Bone

Providers & patients united for improved care.

The American Orthopaedic Association applauds the following institutions for their achievements and participation in the Own the Bone® quality improvement program:

STAR PERFORMERS | Institutions are recognized for at least 75% compliance on 5 of the 10 recommended measures over the last year.

Akron General Medical Center - Akron, OH

Anne Arundel Medical Group Orthopedics and Sports Medicine Specialists - Annapolis, MD

Beaumont Health - Royal Oak, MI

Berkshire Medical Center - Pittsfield, MA

Chippenham & Johnston Willis Hospitals/CJW Medical Center - Richmond, VA

^**Christiana Hospital** - Greenville, DE

^**CHRISTUS St. Vincent Regional Medical Center** - Santa Fe, NM

Coastal Fracture Prevention Center - Sebastian, FL

Colorado Spine Institute PLLC - Johnstown, CO

Concord Hospital - Concord, NH

Cooper Health System - Camden, NJ

Crystal Clinic Orthopaedic Center - Akron, OH

*****Doctors Hospital at Renaissance Health System** - Edinburg, TX

Doylestown Health - Doylestown, PA

*****ETMC First Physicians Orthopedic Institute** - Tyler, TX

Forsyth Medical Center - Winston Salem, NC

^**Greenville Hospital System University Medical Center** - Greenville, SC

*****Herrin Hospital** - Herrin, IL

Hoag Orthopedic Institute - Irvine, CA

^**Huntsville Hospital** - Huntsville, AL

Illinois Bone & Joint Institute, LLC - Morton Grove, IL

Jefferson Regional Medical Center - Pittsburgh, PA

Lafayette General Medical Center - Lafayette, LA

Lahey Hospital & Medical Center - Burlington, MA

Lakeshore Bone and Joint Institute - Chesterton, IN

MaineGeneral Medical Center - Augusta, ME

Medical Center Arlington - Arlington, TX

Memorial Hospital & Health Care Center - Jasper, IN

Mercy Regional Medical Center - Durango, CO

Michigan Neurosurgical Institute - Grand Blanc, MI

Mission Hospital - Asheville, NC

Nanticoke Memorial Hospital - Seaford, DE

NewYork-Presbyterian/Queens - Flushing, NY

Norton Health Care - Louisville, KY

NSLIJ-Lenox Hill Hospital - Manhasset, NY

NWIA Bone, Joint & Sports Surgeons - Spencer, IA

OhioHealth Grant Medical Center - Columbus, OH

^**Oklahoma Sports and Orthopedics Institute - Bone Health Clinic** - Norman, OK

Orthopaedic Associates of Michigan - Grand Rapids, MI

Orthopaedic Associates of Muskegon - Muskegon, MI

Palmetto Health - Columbia, SC

Paramount Care, Inc. - Maumee, OH

^**Park Nicollet Methodist Hospital** - Minneapolis, MN

Parkview Regional Medical Center - Fort Wayne, IN

Peninsula Regional Medical Center - Salisbury, MD

ProMedica Toledo Hospital - Toledo, OH

Regions Hospital/HealthPartners Orthopaedic and Sports Medicine - Minneapolis, MN

^**Roger Williams Medical Center** - Providence, RI

Sacred Heart Hospital - Pensacola - Pensacola, FL

^**Sanford Medical Center Fargo** - Fargo, ND

^**Shawnee Mission Health** - Shawnee Mission, KS

Southeast Georgia Health System - Brunswick, GA

St. Charles Health System - Bend, OR

St. Luke's University Hospital and Health Network - Bethlehem, PA

*****St. Peter's Hospital** - Helena, MT

*****St. Vincent's Medical Center** - Bridgeport, CT

Tahoe Forest Health System - Truckee, CA

Tallahassee Memorial HealthCare - Tallahassee, FL

Texas Health Arlington Memorial Hospital - Arlington, TX

*****The CORE Institute - Arizona** - Phoenix, AZ

The Medical Center of Aurora - Aurora, CO

The Methodist Hospitals Spine Care Center - Merrillville, IN

The Ohio State University Medical Center - Columbus, OH

^**The Queen's Medical Center** - Honolulu, HI

UF Health Orthopaedics and Sports Medicine Institute - Gainesville, FL

University Hospital - San Antonio, TX

University of Michigan Hospitals & Health Centers - Ann Arbor, MI

UW Medicine Northwest Hospital and Medical Center - Seattle, WA

*****VHS San Antonio Partners, LLC – Baptist Health System** - San Antonio, TX

Western Reserve Hospital - Cuyahoga Falls, OH

^**Wilmington Hospital** - Wilmington, DE

^**WVU Hospitals, Department of Orthopaedics** - Morgantown, WV

^First in State to enroll in Own the Bone®
*Also a Newly Enrolled Institution

NEWLY ENROLLED INSTITUTIONS

Own the Bone is a national post-fracture quality improvement initiative that provides institutions the tools to ensure fragility fracture patients receive the treatment to prevent future fractures.

Visit us: www.ownthebone.org

Baptist Medical Center - San Antonio, TX

Good Samaritan Hospital - Cincinnati, OH

Good Samaritan Hospital - San Jose - San Jose, CA

JPS Health Network - Fort Worth, TX

LewisGale Medical Center - Salem, VA

Marshfield Clinic - Marshfield, WI

Medical University of South Carolina - Charleston, SC

NewYork-Presbyterian/Hudson Valley Hospital - Cortlandt Manor, NY

North Central Baptist Hospital - San Antonio, TX

Northwestern Medicine Central DuPage Hospital - Winfield, IL

Northwestern Medicine Delnor Hospital - Geneva, IL

OhioHealth-Osteoporosis Clinic - Columbus, OH

Our Lady of Lourdes Memorial Hospital, Inc - Binghamton, NY

Randolph Hospital - Asheboro, NC

Sacred Heart Hospital on the Emerald Coast - Miramar Beach/Destin, FL

Sonoran Orthopaedic Trauma Surgeons - Phoenix, AZ

St. Mary's Medical Center - Evansville, IN

The Johns Hopkins Hospital - Baltimore, MD

Twin Cities Orthopedics - Golden Valley, MN

OU Medical Center - Oklahoma City, OK

VCU HealthSystem - Richmond, VA

Waterbury Hospital - Middlebury, CT

PULMONOLOGY

Rank	Hospital	U.S. News score	Survival score (10=best)	Patient safety score (5=best)	Number of patients	Nurse staffing score (higher is better)	Nurse Magnet status	Technology score (6=best)	Patient services score (8=best)	Intensivists	Specialists recommending
1	Mayo Clinic, Rochester, Minn.	100.0	9	5	6,470	2.7	Yes	6	8	Yes	34.1%
2	National Jewish Health, Denver-U. of Colorado Hospital, Aurora	94.4	9	3	2,168	2.2	N/Y*	6	8	Yes	50.3%
3	Cleveland Clinic	87.8	8	5	4,803	2.1	Yes	6	8	Yes	25.8%
4	Massachusetts General Hospital, Boston	82.4	8	3	5,380	2.3	Yes	6	8	Yes	12.5%
5	Duke University Hospital, Durham, N.C.	77.3	6	4	4,390	2.2	Yes	6	8	Yes	12.2%
5	Hospitals of the U. of Pennsylvania-Penn Presbyterian, Philadelphia	77.3	6	5	4,880	2.5	Yes	6	8	Yes	11.5%
7	UPMC Presbyterian Shadyside, Pittsburgh	76.8	6	1	7,608	1.9	Yes	6	8	Yes	11.5%
8	New York-Presbyterian U. Hospital of Columbia and Cornell, N.Y.	76.1	7	3	10,274	2.5	No	6	8	Yes	8.5%
9	UCLA Medical Center, Los Angeles	76.0	7	4	4,860	3.1	Yes	6	8	Yes	4.6%
10	Barnes-Jewish Hospital/Washington University, St. Louis	75.7	7	3	4,429	2.2	Yes	6	8	Yes	9.2%
11	UC San Diego Medical Center - UC San Diego Health, Calif.	75.2	7	5	2,244	1.8	Yes	6	8	Yes	7.9%
12	Yale-New Haven Hospital, New Haven, Conn.	74.2	8	1	9,988	1.8	Yes	5	8	Yes	2.4%
13	Johns Hopkins Hospital, Baltimore	73.9	5	2	2,104	2.1	Yes	6	8	Yes	19.2%
14	NYU Langone Medical Center, New York	73.7	9	4	2,946	2.6	Yes	5	8	Yes	2.1%
15	Brigham and Women's Hospital, Boston	73.3	7	5	4,501	2.4	No	6	8	Yes	7.7%
16	University of Michigan Hospitals and Health Centers, Ann Arbor	73.2	7	5	3,606	2.9	No	6	8	Yes	8.5%
17	Houston Methodist Hospital	72.9	9	3	4,625	1.9	Yes	6	8	Yes	1.4%
17	Northwestern Memorial Hospital, Chicago	72.9	9	4	3,235	1.6	Yes	5	8	Yes	2.2%
19	UCSF Medical Center, San Francisco	72.6	5	5	2,193	2.7	Yes	6	8	Yes	12.0%
20	University of California, Davis Medical Center, Sacramento	72.1	9	4	2,757	2.7	Yes	5	8	Yes	0.3%
21	Banner Estrella Medical Center, Phoenix	71.8	10	4	2,448	2.1	Yes	5	8	Yes	0.0%
22	Beaumont Hospital-Royal Oak, Mich.	71.7	8	3	8,667	1.8	Yes	5	8	Yes	0.1%
23	IU Health Academic Health Center, Indianapolis	71.5	8	2	4,790	1.8	Yes	6	8	Yes	0.4%
23	Miami Valley Hospital, Dayton, Ohio	71.5	9	2	5,860	2.1	Yes	5	8	Yes	0.0%
25	UF Health Shands Hospital, Gainesville, Fla.	71.4	8	3	3,599	2.0	Yes	6	8	Yes	2.4%
26	Fairview Hospital, Cleveland	71.3	9	5	3,077	1.7	Yes	5	8	Yes	0.0%
27	University of North Carolina Hospitals, Chapel Hill	70.7	8	2	2,854	1.8	Yes	6	8	Yes	3.2%
28	University of Kansas Hospital, Kansas City	70.5	9	2	2,972	1.9	Yes	5	8	Yes	0.9%
29	University of Alabama Hospital at Birmingham	70.4	8	4	4,280	1.8	Yes	6	7	Yes	1.6%
30	Mayo Clinic, Phoenix	70.3	10	5	2,899	3.2	No	5	8	Yes	1.2%
31	University of Washington Medical Center, Seattle	69.7	7	3	1,311	2.1	Yes	6	8	Yes	8.0%
32	Scripps La Jolla Hospitals and Clinics, La Jolla, Calif.	69.6	9	4	4,028	2.9	Y/N*	5	8	Yes	0.1%
33	Ohio State University Wexner Medical Center, Columbus	69.3	8	2	4,685	2.1	Yes	6	8	Yes	0.6%
33	University of Wisconsin Hospital and Clinics, Madison	69.3	8	2	2,643	1.9	Yes	6	8	Yes	1.5%
35	Loyola University Medical Center, Maywood, Ill.	69.1	8	4	2,351	1.6	Yes	6	8	Yes	0.9%
36	Cedars-Sinai Medical Center, Los Angeles	69.0	6	3	5,977	2.6	Nurse	6	8	Yes	1.8%
36	Lehigh Valley Hospital, Allentown, Pa.	69.0	8	4	5,852	1.8	Magnet	5	8	Yes	0.2%
38	St. Luke's Hospital, Kansas City, Mo.	68.7	9	5	2,433	1.6	Yes	5	8	Yes	0.0%
39	Spectrum Hlth. Butterworth-Blodgett Campuses, Grand Rapids, Mich.	68.4	7	2	7,973	1.7	Yes	6	8	Yes	0.1%
39	University of Tennessee Medical Center, Knoxville	68.4	9	3	4,626	1.5	Yes	5	8	Yes	0.3%
41	Lancaster General Hospital, Lancaster, Pa.	68.3	8	4	5,387	1.7	Yes	5	8	Yes	0.0%
42	Cleveland Clinic Akron General Medical Center, Ohio	68.1	9	2	4,606	1.2	Yes	5	8	Yes	0.0%
42	Froedtert Hosp. and the Medical College of Wisconsin, Milwaukee	68.1	7	4	3,177	1.8	Yes	6	8	Yes	0.4%
42	Vanderbilt University Medical Center, Nashville	68.1	7	4	3,113	1.9	Yes	6	8	Yes	3.8%
45	Christiana Care Christiana Hospital, Newark, Del.	68.0	7	4	7,659	2.0	Yes	5	8	Yes	0.1%
45	Mount Sinai Hospital, New York	68.0	6	4	6,391	2.0	Yes	6	8	Yes	2.9%
45	St. Luke's Regional Medical Center, Boise, Idaho	68.0	9	3	4,171	2.5	Yes	5	6	Yes	0.0%
48	Tampa General Hospital	67.9	8	1	2,837	2.2	Yes	6	8	Yes	1.1%
49	Mayo Clinic Jacksonville, Fla.	67.8	8	5	2,514	2.1	Yes	6	8	Yes	1.3%
49	Reading Hospital and Medical Center, West Reading, Pa.	67.8	9	2	7,140	1.7	No	5	7	Yes	1.3%

*Reflects more than one hospital's status. The specialized or secondary hospital lacks Nurse Magnet recognition.

Terms are explained on Page 90.

▶ **More @ usnews.com/besthospitals**

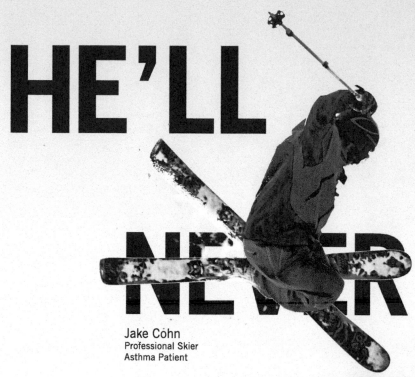

HE'LL NEVER FLY.

Jake Cohn
Professional Skier
Asthma Patient

AT THE NATION'S LEADING RESPIRATORY HOSPITAL, WE NEVER SAY NEVER.

Jake Cohn was born with severe asthma and spent much of his childhood in the hospital. For a while, it looked like he'd never lead a normal life. But then he came to **National Jewish Health in Denver.**

Thanks to our cutting-edge technology, groundbreaking research and expert care, Jake's spending his days on the slopes as a professional skier, instead of in a hospital bed. See more of Jake's story and many others at njhealth.org/patients. **To learn more or to make an appointment, call 1.800.621.0505 or visit njhealth.org.**

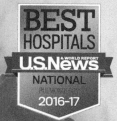

BEST HOSPITALS
U.S.News & WORLD REPORT
NATIONAL
PULMONOLOGY
2016-17

National Jewish
Health®

Science Transforming Life®

UROLOGY

Rank	Hospital	U.S. News score	Survival score (10=best)	Patient safety score (5=best)	Number of patients	Nurse staffing score (higher is better)	Nurse Magnet status	Technology score (6=best)	Patient services score (9=best)	Intensivists	Specialists recommending
1	Mayo Clinic, Rochester, Minn.	100.0	10	5	970	2.7	Yes	6	9	Yes	25.0%
2	Cleveland Clinic	99.2	9	5	818	2.1	Yes	6	9	Yes	48.9%
3	UCLA Medical Center, Los Angeles	89.2	8	4	532	3.1	Yes	6	9	Yes	17.7%
4	Johns Hopkins Hospital, Baltimore	87.8	6	2	488	2.1	Yes	6	9	Yes	38.9%
5	Memorial Sloan Kettering Cancer Center, New York	87.7	10	4	834	2.0	Yes	6	8	Yes	14.0%
6	New York-Presbyterian U. Hospital of Columbia and Cornell, N.Y.	83.7	9	3	1,311	2.5	No	6	9	Yes	10.0%
7	UCSF Medical Center, San Francisco	82.1	7	5	440	2.7	Yes	6	9	Yes	13.2%
8	Vanderbilt University Medical Center, Nashville	81.9	8	4	601	1.9	Yes	6	9	Yes	13.5%
9	Duke University Hospital, Durham, N.C.	80.9	7	4	437	2.2	Yes	6	9	Yes	13.8%
10	NYU Langone Medical Center, New York	80.4	9	4	308	2.6	Yes	6	9	Yes	7.1%
11	Northwestern Memorial Hospital, Chicago	79.9	10	4	352	1.6	Yes	6	9	Yes	4.7%
12	University of Michigan Hospitals and Health Centers, Ann Arbor	79.2	9	5	719	2.9	No	6	9	Yes	7.2%
13	Stanford Health Care-Stanford Hospital, Stanford, Calif.	76.3	8	5	373	2.4	Yes	6	9	Yes	4.1%
14	Barnes-Jewish Hospital/Washington University, St. Louis	76.0	8	3	625	2.2	Yes	6	9	Yes	5.8%
15	Hospitals of the U. of Pennsylvania-Penn Presbyterian, Philadelphia	75.3	8	5	552	2.5	Yes	6	9	Yes	2.6%
15	Keck Medical Center of USC, Los Angeles†	75.3	8	1	662	3.8	No	6	9	Yes	8.4%
16	University of North Carolina Hospitals, Chapel Hill	75.0	10	2	484	1.8	Yes	6	9	Yes	1.5%
17	University of Kansas Hospital, Kansas City	73.8	9	2	437	1.9	Yes	6	9	Yes	2.5%
18	Tampa General Hospital	73.5	10	1	474	2.2	Yes	6	9	Yes	0.7%
19	UPMC Presbyterian Shadyside, Pittsburgh	73.4	8	1	772	1.9	Yes	6	9	Yes	2.6%
20	University of California, Davis Medical Center, Sacramento	73.3	9	4	313	2.7	Yes	6	9	Yes	1.1%
21	University of Wisconsin Hospital and Clinics, Madison	73.1	10	2	401	1.9	Yes	6	9	Yes	1.1%
22	Beaumont Hospital-Royal Oak, Mich.	73.0	8	3	679	1.8	Yes	6	9	Yes	1.5%
22	Thomas Jefferson University Hospital, Philadelphia	73.0	8	4	474	2.2	Yes	6	9	Yes	1.8%
24	Oregon Health and Science University Hospital, Portland	72.9	10	2	250	2.1	Yes	6	9	Yes	1.1%
25	Cedars-Sinai Medical Center, Los Angeles	72.6	8	3	668	2.6	Yes	6	9	Yes	1.2%
26	Massachusetts General Hospital, Boston	72.5	6	3	556	2.3	Yes	6	9	Yes	5.5%
28	Brigham and Women's Hospital, Boston	72.3	7	5	428	2.4	No	6	9	Yes	6.3%
29	Mercy Health Hospital, Janesville, Wis.	72.2	10	1	71	1.7	Yes	5	9	Yes	0.0%
29	Mount Sinai Hospital, New York	72.2	7	4	613	2.0	Yes	6	9	Yes	2.8%
29	Yale-New Haven Hospital, New Haven, Conn.	72.2	8	1	747	1.8	Yes	6	9	Yes	1.8%
32	Houston Methodist Hospital	71.8	9	3	477	1.9	Yes	6	8	Yes	3.7%
33	University of Maryland Medical Center, Baltimore	71.6	10	1	292	2.9	Yes	6	9	Yes	0.2%
34	University of Iowa Hospitals and Clinics, Iowa City	71.4	8	4	300	1.8	Yes	6	9	Yes	2.5%
35	IU Health Academic Health Center, Indianapolis	71.2	7	2	674	1.8	Yes	6	9	Yes	3.7%
36	UT Southwestern Medical Center, Dallas	71.1	10	5	466	2.0	No	6	9	Yes	3.7%
36	University of Texas MD Anderson Cancer Center, Houston	71.1	5	2	680	2.0	Yes	6	9	Yes	9.7%
38	Rush University Medical Center, Chicago	70.1	9	4	315	2.2	Yes	6	9	Yes	0.1%
39	University Hospitals Case Medical Center, Cleveland	69.8	9	2	323	2.3	Yes	6	9	Yes	0.5%
40	City of Hope, Duarte, Calif.	69.7	10	5	336	2.3	No	6	8	Yes	0.8%
40	Memorial Hermann-Texas Medical Center, Houston	69.7	9	5	134	2.2	Yes	6	8	Yes	1.4%
42	UF Health Shands Hospital, Gainesville, Fla.	69.6	8	3	444	2.0	Yes	6	9	Yes	0.6%
43	Queen's Medical Center, Honolulu	69.5	9	3	339	1.8	Yes	6	8	Yes	0.0%
43	University of Virginia Medical Center, Charlottesville	69.5	8	4	251	2.1	Yes	6	8	Yes	1.8%
45	Medical University of South Carolina Medical Center, Charleston	69.3	8	3	276	2.1	Yes	6	9	Yes	0.5%
46	Sanford USD Medical Center, Sioux Falls, S.D.	69.2	9	2	199	2.6	Yes	6	9	Yes	0.0%
46	University of Cincinnati Medical Center	69.2	10	1	128	1.8	No	6	9	Yes	1.2%
48	Moffitt Cancer Center and Research Institute, Tampa	69.1	10	1	344	1.2	Yes	6	9	Yes	1.5%
49	Froedtert Hosp. and the Medical College of Wisconsin, Milwaukee	69.0	8	4	402	1.8	Yes	6	9	Yes	1.0%
49	Hackensack University Medical Center, Hackensack, N.J.	69.0	7	4	484	2.4	Yes	6	9	Yes	0.9%
49	UC San Diego Medical Center - UC San Diego Health, Calif.	69.0	8	5	234	1.8	Yes	6	9	Yes	0.7%
49	University of Alabama Hospital at Birmingham	69.0	8	4	308	1.8	Yes	6	8	Yes	0.7%
49	University of Washington Medical Center, Seattle	69.0	7	3	291	2.1	Yes	6	9	Yes	4.8%

†Due to a data processing error, this hospital was initially misranked. Rankings for other hospitals have not been changed.

Terms are explained on Page 90.

▶ **More @ usnews.com/besthospitals**

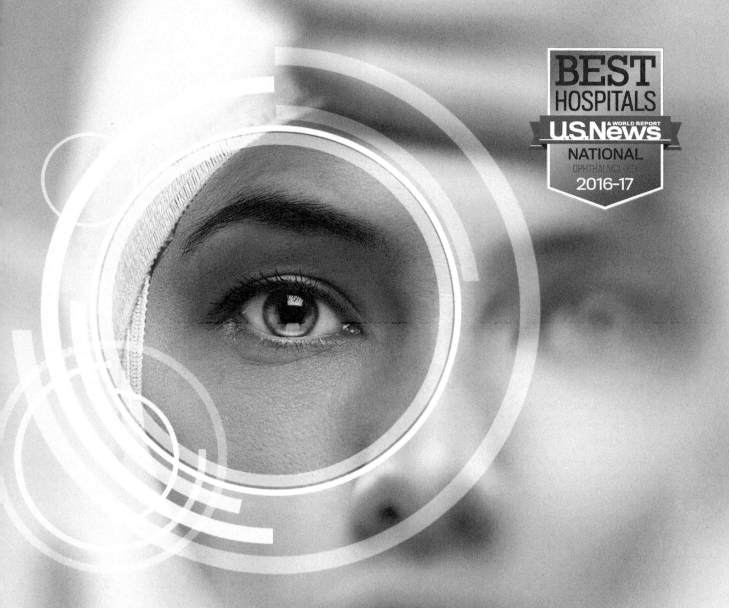

THESE HOSPITALS ARE AMONG THE BEST in their specialty for particularly challenging patients, in the view of at least 5 percent of specialists who responded to the latest three years of U.S. News physician surveys.

OPHTHALMOLOGY

Rank	Hospital	Specialists recommending
1	Bascom Palmer Eye Institute-Anne Bates Leach Eye Hosp., Miami	62.8%
2	Wills Eye Hospital, Thomas Jefferson U. Hospital, Philadelphia	51.8%
3	Wilmer Eye Institute, Johns Hopkins Hospital, Baltimore	50.1%
4	Massachusetts Eye and Ear Infirmary, Mass. General Hosp., Boston	33.2%
5	Stein and Doheny Eye Institutes, UCLA Medical Cen., Los Angeles	26.8%
6	Duke University Hospital, Durham, N.C.	13.5%
7	University of Iowa Hospitals and Clinics, Iowa City	11.7%
8	Cleveland Clinic	8.8%
9	W.K. Kellogg Eye Center, University of Michigan, Ann Arbor	8.3%
10	New York Eye and Ear Infirmary, N.Y.	6.7%
11	USC Eye Institute-Keck Medical Center of USC, Los Angeles	6.3%
12	UCSF Medical Center, San Francisco	5.3%

PSYCHIATRY

Rank	Hospital	Specialists recommending
1	Massachusetts General Hospital, Boston	22.7%
2	McLean Hospital, Belmont, Mass.	22.6%
3	New York-Presbyterian U. Hosp. of Columbia and Cornell, N.Y.	20.4%
4	Johns Hopkins Hospital, Baltimore	19.4%
5	Menninger Clinic, Houston	17.5%
6	Sheppard and Enoch Pratt Hospital, Baltimore	14.0%
7	Resnick Neuropsychiatric Hospital at UCLA, Los Angeles	13.6%
8	Mayo Clinic, Rochester, Minn.	8.8%
9	Austen Riggs Center, Stockbridge, Mass.	8.2%
10	Yale-New Haven Hospital, New Haven, Conn.	7.1%
11	UPMC Presbyterian Shadyside, Pittsburgh	6.3%
12	UCSF Medical Center, San Francisco	5.2%

REHABILITATION

Rank	Hospital	Specialists recommending
1	Rehabilitation Institute of Chicago	47.3%
2	TIRR Memorial Hermann, Houston	26.1%
3	Kessler Institute for Rehabilitation, West Orange, N.J.	22.0%
4	University of Washington Medical Center, Seattle	21.4%
5	Spaulding Rehabilitation Hosp. Mass. General Hosp, Boston	19.5%
6	Mayo Clinic, Rochester, Minn.	18.6%
7	Craig Hospital, Englewood, Colo.	15.0%
8	Shepherd Center, Atlanta	11.6%
9	Rusk Rehabilitation at NYU Langone Medical Center, New York	9.4%
10	MossRehab, Elkins Park, Pa.	8.9%
11	UPMC Presbyterian Shadyside, Pittsburgh	7.7%
12	New York-Presbyterian U. Hosp. of Columbia and Cornell, N.Y.	5.9%

RHEUMATOLOGY

Rank	Hospital	Specialists recommending
1	Johns Hopkins Hospital, Baltimore	45.4%
2	Hospital for Special Surgery, New York-Presbyterian University Hospital of Columbia and Cornell, N.Y	40.9%
3	Cleveland Clinic	39.8%
4	Mayo Clinic, Rochester, Minn.	36.4%
5	Brigham and Women's Hospital, Boston	23.3%
6	UCLA Medical Center, Los Angeles	20.1%
7	Massachusetts General Hospital, Boston	16.5%
8	Hospital for Joint Diseases, NYU Langone Medical Cen., New York	15.8%
9	UPMC Presbyterian Shadyside, Pittsburgh	12.8%
10	UCSF Medical Center, San Francisco	12.5%
11	University of Alabama Hospital at Birmingham	9.1%
12	Stanford Health Care-Stanford Hospital, Stanford, Calif.	7.6%
13	Duke University Hospital, Durham, N.C.	7.5%
14	University of Michigan Hospitals and Health Centers, Ann Arbor	6.0%
15	Northwestern Memorial Hospital, Chicago	5.9%

▶ More @ usnews.com/besthospitals

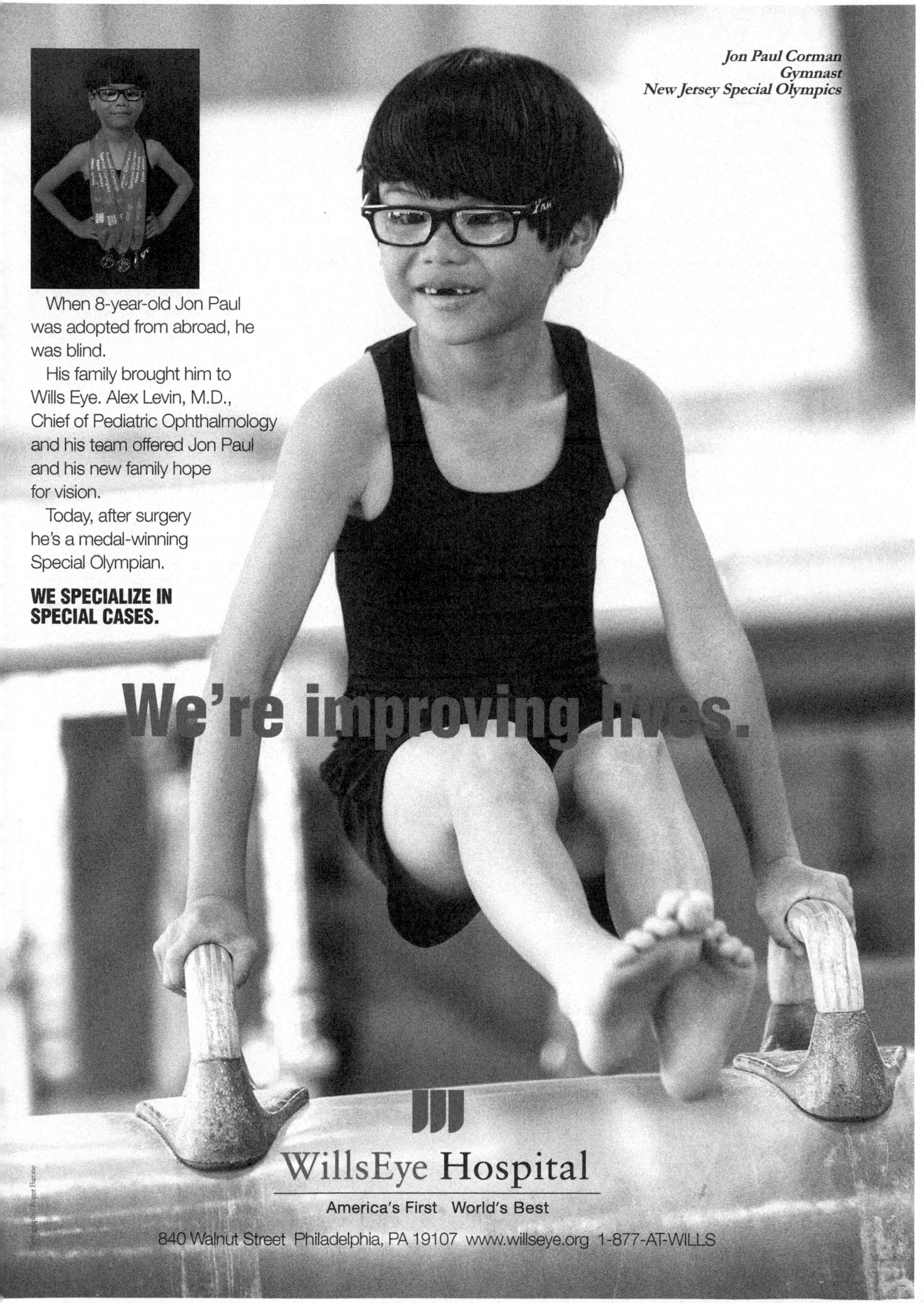

Jon Paul Corman
Gymnast
New Jersey Special Olympics

When 8-year-old Jon Paul was adopted from abroad, he was blind.

His family brought him to Wills Eye. Alex Levin, M.D., Chief of Pediatric Ophthalmology and his team offered Jon Paul and his new family hope for vision.

Today, after surgery he's a medal-winning Special Olympian.

WE SPECIALIZE IN SPECIAL CASES.

We're improving lives.

WillsEye Hospital

America's First   World's Best

840 Walnut Street Philadelphia, PA 19107 www.willseye.org 1-877-AT-WILLS

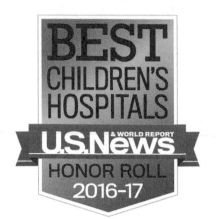

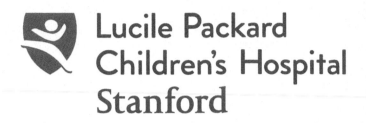

Top-ranked children's hospital in Northern California

We're honored to be the only children's hospital in Northern California, and one of just 11 nationwide, to be named on the 2016-17 U.S. News Best Children's Hospitals Honor Roll.

Ranked in all ten pediatric specialties

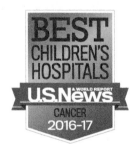 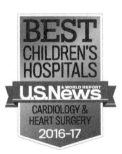 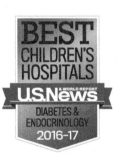 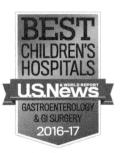 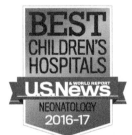

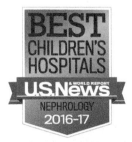 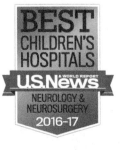 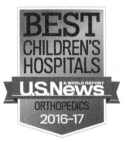 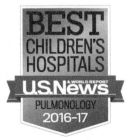 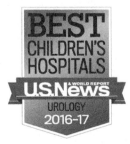

stanfordchildrens.org

Stanford | MEDICINE

CHILDREN'S HEALTH

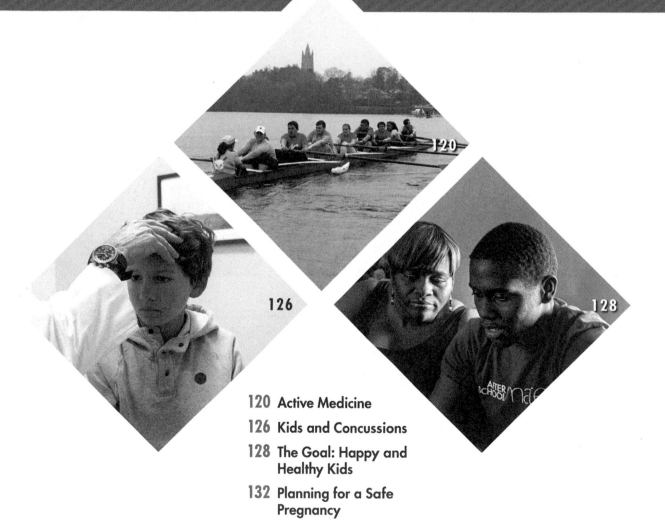

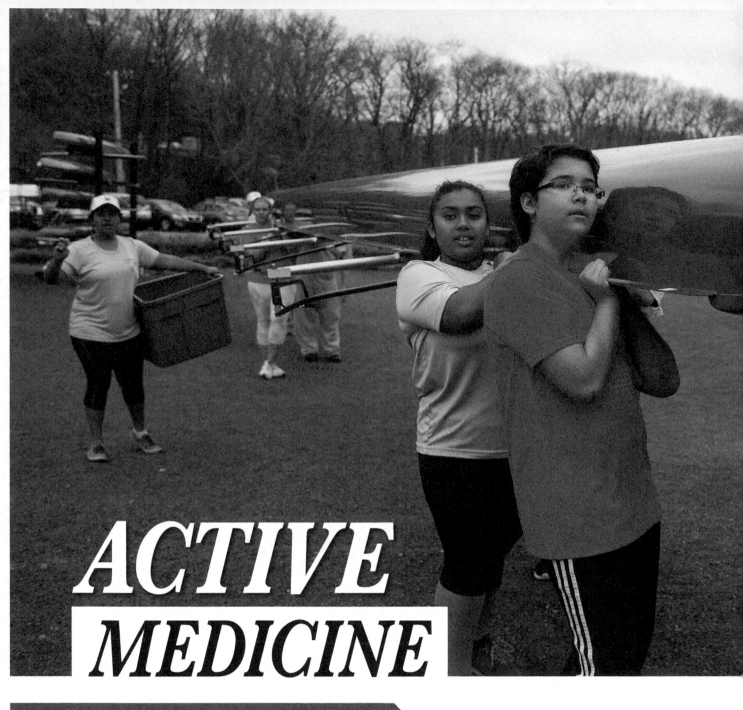

ACTIVE MEDICINE

born at 10 pounds and 13 ounces, Gigi Eisenstein of Philadelphia had been a robust baby. But when her weight was still outpacing her height at her 6-year check-up, the pediatrician referred her parents to Children's Hospital of Philadelphia. There, in consultations every six weeks or so including a medical evaluation and dietary, behavioral and fitness counseling, the family has learned ways to prepare healthier meals together and squeeze more physical activity into their day. Now Gigi and her sister and parents sub baked zucchini sticks for French fries, eat seconds of vegetables only, and walk the dog each night as

a family. Gigi, 10, has seen her body mass index drop from 24 to 21. (Nineteen is ideal.) "I used to be the snack mom – I always had something for the girls to eat," says Sarah Eisenstein, Gigi's mom. "Now I tell them 'I know you're hungry, but you'll be OK until we get home and make lunch.'"

It may seem surprising that families are getting this sort of hands-on help from a children's hospital. But in recent years many of these institutions have launched comprehensive weight management programs like the one at CHOP – and it's help that is sorely needed. Childhood obesity rates have nearly tripled since 1980; overall, nearly 18 percent of children and teens are now in that zone, putting them at risk for high blood pressure, high cholesterol, heart disease, diabetes, sleep apnea and other respiratory problems, and fatty liver disease. "We live in a toxic environment where the easy choices are overwhelmingly bad choices," says

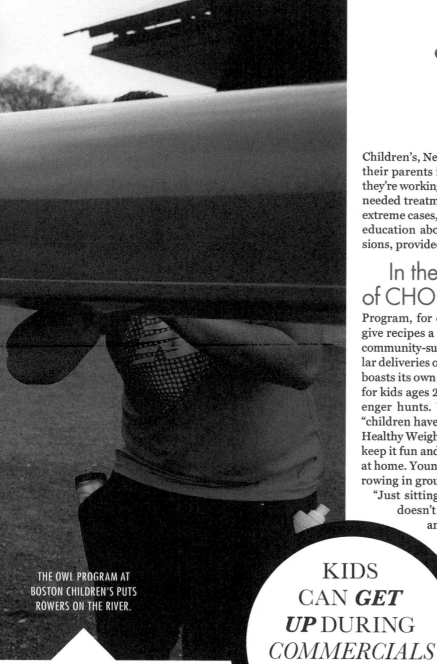

THE OWL PROGRAM AT BOSTON CHILDREN'S PUTS ROWERS ON THE RIVER.

Children's, Nemours and other centers bring children and their parents in regularly over the weeks or months that they're working toward a goal weight for evaluation and any needed treatment. This could include bariatric surgery in extreme cases, plus nutritional and behavioral counseling, education about physical fitness, and even exercise sessions, provided by a team of experts.

In the sparkling mock kitchen of CHOP's Healthy Weight

Program, for example, families learn to read labels and give recipes a healthier spin. They can also take part in a community-supported agriculture program, receiving regular deliveries of locally grown fruits and vegetables. CHOP boasts its own gym, too, and provides active programming for kids ages 2-19, everything from dance parties to scavenger hunts. When parents and siblings are included, "children have a lot more fun," says Amanda Holdridge, a Healthy Weight pediatric nurse practitioner. "The goal is to keep it fun and light" and to inspire families to get moving at home. Youngsters in the OWL program can work out by rowing in groups on the Charles River.

"Just sitting in a room and telling kids to lose weight doesn't work," says Madhu Mathur, a pediatrician and obesity medicine physician in Stamford, Connecticut, who developed and formerly directed the Kids' Fitness and Nutrition Services clinic at Stamford Hospital. "We needed something more." Participants in KIDS' FANS come in weekly over 12 weeks for nutrition guidance and an exercise session and adopt a new mantra: Eat fruits and vegetables, limit screen time, and get moving.

Besides the intensive weight-management services for patients, many hospitals offer guidance and resources to the community at large. Boston Children's has created a 10-week "OWL on the Road" curriculum, guided by a dietitian and a psychologist, that it provides free at several inner-city community health centers. Nemours offers guidance and resources about obesity prevention and treatment to local doctors. "Most pediatricians have not been trained to tackle childhood obesity," Hassink says.

Children's Hospitals and Clinics of Minnesota, partnering with other community organizations, offers its city's Latino residents the Vida Sana program, featuring instruction on healthy living (and dance classes). The Children's Hospital of Pittsburgh works with pediatrics practices, schools, and the Pittsburgh Parks Conservancy to get the word out. Texas Children's Hospital runs a two-week residential camp for kids ages 10-14 who are struggling

KIDS CAN *GET UP* DURING *COMMERCIALS* FOR JUMPING JACKS.

David Ludwig, an endocrinologist and director of the Optimal Weight for Life, or OWL, program at Boston Children's Hospital, the country's oldest weight management clinic for children and adolescents. "The consequences are grim."

Nemours/Alfred I. duPont Hospital for Children in Wilmington, Delaware, is another pioneer. As early as the late 1980s, Nemours pediatrician Sandra Hassink, who became president of the American Academy of Pediatrics upon retiring and now directs the AAP Institute for Healthy Childhood Weight, became alarmed when she began seeing a growing number of kids with serious weight problems. She assembled a team that included a nutritionist, psychologist, exercise physiologist and nurses to help young patients get healthier. The multidisciplinary model has caught on. The comprehensive programs at CHOP, Boston

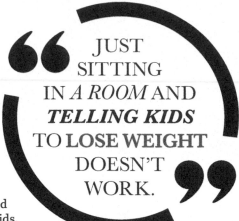

with their weight, plus a Saturday wellness program designed to teach children and teens about active living and nutrition. Besides running a summer camp and offering cooking classes, Children's Hospital Colorado provides bikes and safety training to local kids.

Some institutions are broadcasting their message statewide. The Barbara Bush Children's Hospital of Maine Medical Center in Portland has launched a Let's Go! campaign that forges connections with schools, child care sites, after-school programs, and doctors' offices to teach healthy living habits to hundreds of thousands of children. The campaign uses an easy-to-remember meme to put kids on a healthy track: 5-2-1-0, for five or more servings of fruits and vegetables; two hours or less of screen time; at least one hour

of exercise; and zero sugary beverages a day. Students take a five-minute active "brain break" each hour, and in some places sit at their desks on large inflatable balls so they can balance (or fidget) while they learn. They grow vegetables that are served in the school cafeteria. ("If you label carrots 'X-ray vision carrots,' kids will eat more of them," notes pediatrician Tory Rogers, the program's director.) Radio ads and posters displayed in schools and in doctors' offices reinforce the healthy message.

Crucially, schools, recreation centers, and after-school programs pledge not to use food as rewards for good performance and to nix the hundreds of calories of pizza, cupcakes and candy typically served up at every birthday party and soccer practice. The latest data

WHAT PARENTS CAN DO

Further tips on how to safeguard children from gaining too much weight – or help them lose it:

● **Set the stage at birth.** Excess weight gain during pregnancy can result in a bigger baby and increase the risk of weight struggles. Ask your doctor what is appropriate based on your pre-pregnancy weight. After birth, "breastfeeding and delaying solid foods for six months have a protective effect," says Sandra Hassink, director of the American Academy of Pediatrics Institute for Healthy Childhood Weight. You can help babies develop a taste for healthy fare by introducing fruits and vegetables early on.

● **Establish boundaries for screen time.** Sit down with

older children and a weekly calendar. If the TV shows they want to watch add up to more than two hours a day, ask what they are willing to give up. "Letting children negotiate is more apt to be successful than just turning the TV off," says Joanne Ikeda, co-founder of the University of California–Berkeley Center for Weight and Health. While they're watching favorite shows, have them get up during commercial breaks and do jumping jacks or silly dances. "In an hour of TV, that's 20 minutes of exercise," says Kristi King, a senior dietitian at Texas Children's Hospital in Houston.

● **Think outside the activity box.** Children, particularly young children, do not need

special classes or sports to get the exercise they need. You might, for instance, turn on some music and dance. Ikeda recommends getting active with inexpensive dollar-store toys: punch balls, gliders constructed of balsawood to throw around, balloons, a bottle of bubbles.

● **Promote eating habits that last a lifetime.** It's best to avoid putting kids on a diet. "It's risky because it can stunt their growth in height," says Ikeda. And restricting certain foods can lead kids to crave them more than ever. Encourage eating breakfast, even if it's just a spoonful of peanut butter on a banana. When kids skip a morning meal they tend to binge later. –*B.H.*

Our best ranking ever.
High fives all around.

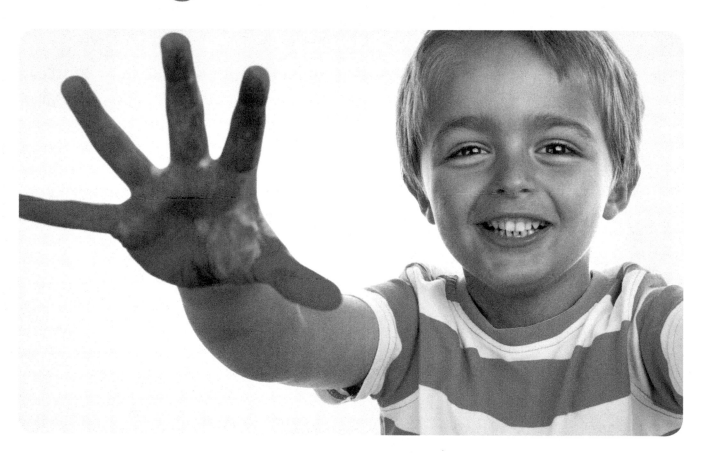

BEST CHILDREN'S HOSPITALS
U.S.News & WORLD REPORT
HONOR ROLL 2016-17

U.S. News & World Report **ranked Seattle Children's as the #5 children's hospital in the nation.** It's our highest ranking ever, and we couldn't have done it without the unwavering support of our dedicated clinicians, tireless research team, generous donors and, of course, the patients and families we treat every day. Thanks to everyone in the community for supporting Seattle Children's—and for making our continued success possible. To learn more, visit **seattlechildrens.org/usnews**.

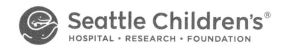

Seattle Children's®
HOSPITAL · RESEARCH · FOUNDATION

Hope. Care. Cure.™

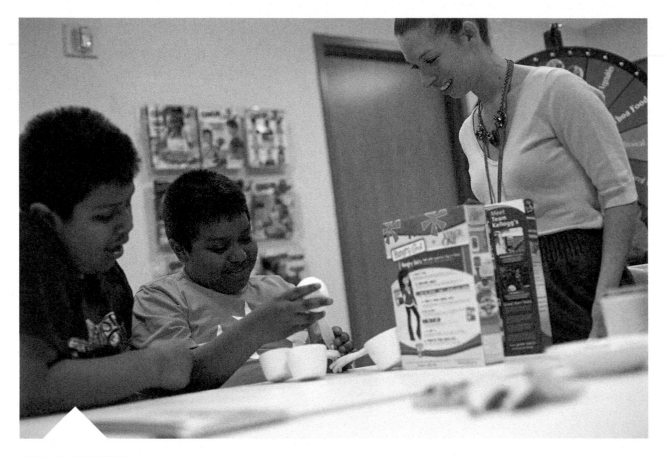

LUIS AND ALEXANDER DOMINGUEZ LEARN ABOUT PORTION SIZES IN CHOP'S TEACHING KITCHEN.

show obesity rates in the state are leveling off. The program has also made forays into New Hampshire.

Georgia hopes to duplicate that success with its statewide Strong4Life initiative, which was launched by Children's Healthcare of Atlanta in 2010. Like other efforts, the program uses multiple channels – pediatric practices, schools, and community partnerships – to spark change in families whose children are overweight. Instead of overwhelming them with onerous food and exercise rules, the Strong4Life idea is to make one small change at a time. Says Stephanie Walsh, the program's medical director of child wellness: "Our message is you don't have to get there tomorrow. If your goal is to eliminate soda, it might take six months to make the change. If you do it slowly, and patients have the experience of succeeding, you get buy-in."

So far, the program has trained 3,000 health care providers and 1,200 school nutrition staff across the state and racked up 2 million visits to its website, Strong4Life.com.

A cornerstone of most weight management programs is making lifestyle change a family affair (box, Page 122). "The child gets more support when parents are modeling healthy behaviors and the rules apply to everybody in the home," says Ludwig.

And just as curious toddlers need the safety of a baby-proofed house, a child struggling with weight issues needs the home to be made nutritionally safe, a place "where all choices are healthy, so parents don't have to micromanage a child's behavior all day long," Hassink says. Experts endorse eating together as a family, and on as regular as possible a schedule to minimize grazing. And it's important to keep in mind that children are still growing and may still grow into their weight.

Finally, Rogers says, parents should remember that change is tough and the process is ongoing; there will undoubtedly be setbacks. It's an outlook that easily applies to reversing the childhood obesity epidemic itself. "It took 30 years to get into this predicament," she says. "Turning it around won't happen overnight." ●

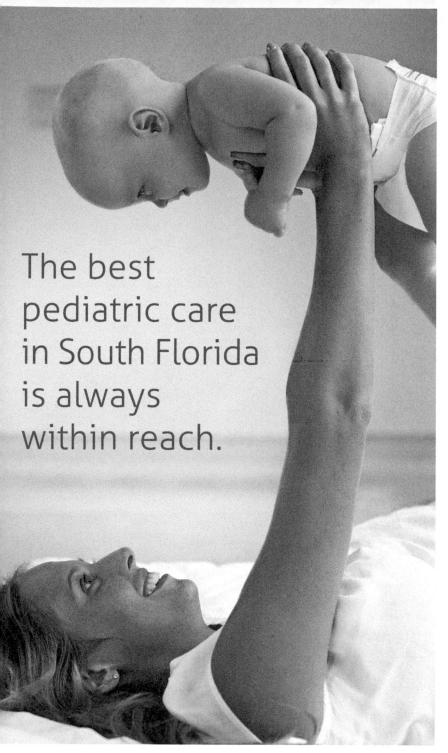

The best
pediatric care
in South Florida
is always
within reach.

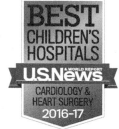

BEST CHILDREN'S HOSPITALS
U.S.News & WORLD REPORT
CARDIOLOGY & HEART SURGERY
2016-17

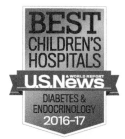

BEST CHILDREN'S HOSPITALS
U.S.News & WORLD REPORT
DIABETES & ENDOCRINOLOGY
2016-17

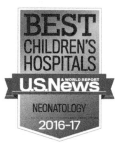

BEST CHILDREN'S HOSPITALS
U.S.News & WORLD REPORT
GASTROENTEROLOGY & GI SURGERY
2016-17

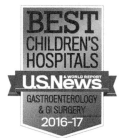

BEST CHILDREN'S HOSPITALS
U.S.News & WORLD REPORT
NEONATOLOGY
2016-17

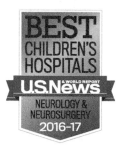

BEST CHILDREN'S HOSPITALS
U.S.News & WORLD REPORT
NEUROLOGY & NEUROSURGERY
2016-17

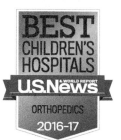

BEST CHILDREN'S HOSPITALS
U.S.News & WORLD REPORT
ORTHOPEDICS
2016-17

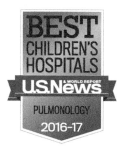

BEST CHILDREN'S HOSPITALS
U.S.News & WORLD REPORT
PULMONOLOGY
2016-17

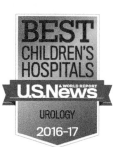

BEST CHILDREN'S HOSPITALS
U.S.News & WORLD REPORT
UROLOGY
2016-17

Once again, Nicklaus Children's Hospital has more programs ranked in *U.S.News & World Report's* 2016-17 pediatric rankings than any other hospital in South Florida. In addition, **our neurology and neurosurgery program is ranked in the top 15 nationally.** That means, you have world-class pediatric care right here in our own backyard. And through our network of outpatient and urgent care centers, chances are, we are only a few blocks away. It's great to be a leader, but even better to lead with compassion, innovation and extraordinary care. We thank our doctors, nurses, support staff, volunteers and donors for helping us achieve another year of excellence in care.

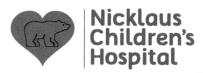

Nicklaus Children's Hospital

MIAMI CHILDREN'S HEALTH SYSTEM

For Health. For Life.

Nicklaus Children's Hospital | 3100 SW 62 Avenue, Miami, FL 33155 | 305-666-6511 | **nicklauschildrens.org**

Nicklaus Children's is proud to have more programs included within
U.S.News & World Report's 2016-17 "Best Children's Hospitals" rankings than any other hospital in South Florida.

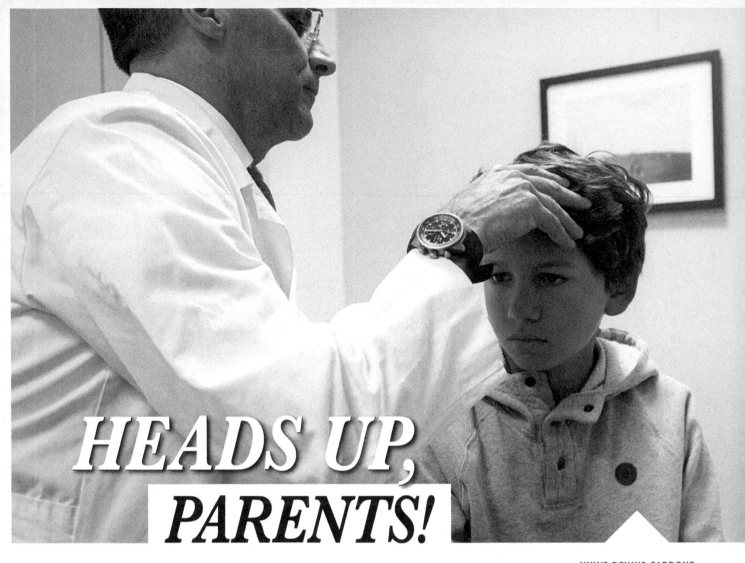

HEADS UP, PARENTS!

Here's what you need to know to safeguard your young athlete from concussion

BY ELIZABETH GARDNER

When Erick Goble of Glen Ellyn, Illinois, then 8, whacked the back of his head on the ice during a hockey game, he complained of a headache and was benched for the rest of the game. Afterward he claimed he was fine, and he played in another game the next day. But his headache persisted, so his worried parents whisked him to the pediatrician, who diagnosed a mild concussion. The doctor's orders included staying home from school for a day and laying off all intellectual activity, including homework, electronics, TV and reading, for a week. Erick also sat out gym, recess and hockey practice.

All seems well two years later, and Erick now plays competitive travel hockey. However, Rita Colorito, his mom, says that as the kids become bigger and more aggressive, she's taking all head bumps much more seriously. Indeed, concern about the long-term effects of concussion is rampant these days in the wake of revelations that pro football players have suffered permanent brain damage from the abuse they took during their playing years. And it's increasingly clear that the risk of worrisome head injury is not limited to the most serious athletes. The Centers for Disease Control and Prevention says that more than 170,000 children and teenagers go to the emergency room every year for sports-related brain injuries – and that's a small fraction of the kids who hit their heads during practices and games.

While most kids recover from concussions within a few weeks, a few struggle with the aftereffects for months or years. They can include headache, dizziness, fatigue, irritability, anxiety, and problems with concentration and memory. To lower the risk, Practice Like Pros, an anti-concussion group endorsed by several NFL coaches, advocates only flag football for younger players, and very limited full-contact practices in high school. The U.S. Soccer Federation changed its rules late last year to prohibit "heading" the ball by players 10 and under, and to reduce headers in practice for players between ages 11 and 13. Early this year, the coaches of the Ivy League voted to eliminate full-contact hitting from regular season football practices, and also to explore ways to reduce hits to the head in hockey, soccer and lacrosse.

IT'S EASY TO SEE THE DANGER OF CONCUSSION (caused by a blow to or violent shaking of the head that causes the brain to bounce around or twist in the skull) in football and soccer, where head impacts have long been part of the game. But any sport, from swimming to cheerleading, can pose some risk. "Being a flyer in cheer is more dangerous than playing football," says Robert Cantu, a clinical professor of neurology and neurosurgery at Boston University School of Medicine and co-founder of BU's Chronic Traumatic Encephalopathy Center. There doesn't even have to be a blow to the head: A youngster can give his brain a severe jolt just by slamming into a goal post with his chest and shoulder.

WITH NEW URGENCY to understand the cumulative effects, scientists are studying sports-related head impacts on several fronts. "We don't know a lot of the answers, and we're learning on the go," says Dennis Cardone, co-director of the Concussion Center at NYU Langone Medical Center in New York. He says the unanswered questions are many: for example, whether there's a maximum number of concussions that is "safe," and to what extent "subclinical" hits – impacts that fall short of concussion – may cause permanent damage. Sensors in the helmets of football players reveal hundreds of hits in people who have never been diagnosed with a concussion, Cardone says. "If you add it all up over a lifetime," he says, these players might be at "a big risk for long-term consequences."

The National Collegiate Athletic Association and the Department of Defense have begun enrolling thousands of college athletes for a three-year study of concussion and its aftereffects. The National Institutes of Health is underwriting a two-year study of 400 adult amateur soccer players who have been playing since their youth. While results are not yet available, an earlier pilot study by the same researchers found brain abnormalities and cognitive problems in amateur soccer players who frequently headed the ball, even when they had no history of concussion.

"It's remarkable how common it is for players to have concussive symptoms related to heading that they don't recognize or acknowledge as concussion," says Michael Lipton, a neuroradiologist at the Albert Einstein College of Medicine in New York and lead investigator of the NIH study. "Things like disorientation, dizziness, balance problems and nausea are

DANGER SIGNS

According to the CDC, symptoms of concussion break down as follows:

Parents or coaches may observe that a child:
- Appears dazed or stunned
- Forgets an instruction or is confused by it
- Moves clumsily
- Answers questions slowly
- Loses consciousness (even briefly)
- Shows mood, behavior or personality changes
- Can't recall events prior to or after a hit or fall

The player may report or exhibit:
- Headache or pressure in head
- Nausea or vomiting
- Balance problems or dizziness, or double or blurry vision
- Being bothered by light or noise
- Feeling sluggish, hazy, foggy or groggy
- Confusion, or concentration or memory problems
- Just not "feeling right," or "feeling down"

What requires an immediate ER visit:
- One pupil being larger than the other
- Drowsiness or inability to wake up
- A headache that gets worse and does not go away
- Slurred speech, weakness, numbness, or decreased coordination
- Repeated vomiting or nausea, convulsions or seizures
- Unusual behavior, increased confusion, restlessness, or agitation
- Loss of consciousness

not at all rare in people who just keep playing."

Colorito says the cumulative effects of lots of small concussions concern her just as much as the danger of one big one. Erick, now 11, can't wait until he turns 12 and is allowed to "check," or actively disrupt the opponent's possession of the puck. "Some kids drop the sport when checking starts, but Erick's looking forward to it," Colorito says. Because checking increases the risk of injury, his league's governing organization requires players to complete a checking clinic to learn safe techniques. Erick's coaches take a seminar every fall on concussion assessment, and Colorito says they benched Erick recently when he was knocked down and then failed a quick short-term memory test. "He remembered the words they asked him to repeat an hour later, but the coach still kept him out, which we appreciated."

BESIDES TRYING TO MAKE SURE THEIR KIDS play for enlightened coaches and keeping an eagle eye on injured players (box), what should parents know in order to keep their children safe?

First, while most kids survive a first concussion unscathed, the second one could be another story. "Long-term problems related to head injury in general are due to or exacerbated by multiple injuries," says Lipton.

When children do get injured, it's important to assess them carefully before sending them back into the game. "'Second impact' is a real phenomenon, when a football player takes a big hit, is concussed, sort of recovers, and then doesn't get up when he's tackled," says Yvonne Lui, chief of neuroradiology at Langone, whose research has shown changes in the brain up to a year after a concussion. "Those players can develop dramatic and life-threatening brain edema."

Second, some people are more vulnerable to serious aftereffects, especially those with conditions like depression, anxiety, attention deficit hyperactivity disorder, migraines, or learning disabilities. "If you have a brain challenge and then put a brain injury on top of it, the underlying challenge can become much worse," says Cantu. He recommends that parents of kids with any type of neuropsychological issue steer them away from activities associated with head injuries.

And finally, bear in mind that "the worst take-home message" is that you should avoid sports out of fear of concussion, Cardone says. "We should still be promoting sports and physical activity." ●

THE GOAL:
HEALTHY &
HAPPY KIDS

As hospitals focus on prevention and population health, many are
giving mental and emotional well-being greater attention

BY LINDA MARSA

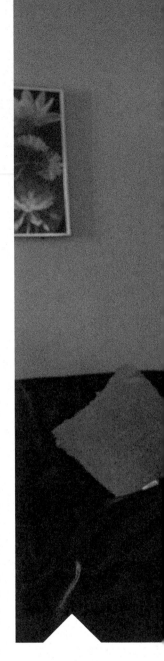

CHRISTOPHER BERRY
(WITH HIS MOM) SAYS
HE STILL SOMETIMES
TAPS THE CURB
PROGRAM'S HELPFUL
TECHNIQUES.

Christopher Berry, then 13, just wasn't his normal talkative self. The Chicago teenager was quiet and withdrawn and would hide out in his room. "This wasn't like him, and I knew it," says his mom, LaToya. When she shared her concerns with the pediatrician, he turned not to medication but to an innovative prevention program developed by doctors at a local children's hospital. The goal: to teach youngsters coping strategies to help them avoid tumbling into depression.

Called CURB, for Chicago Urban Resiliency Building, the three-month program at Children's Hospital University of Illinois uses a combination of counseling and weekly web-based lessons based on proven interventions to arm children and teens with resiliency and social skills. They hear stories about how other kids their age have overcome adversity and learn how to banish the blues by focusing on ways to change the common negative thoughts that make youngsters feel down ("I'm a loser!" "No one likes me!"). Christopher was taught, for example, to stop, freeze and think more realistically when he was on the verge of falling into a vortex of such thoughts and to look at his problems with some distance so he could see possible solutions.

"This helped me evaluate my problems and provided an outlet for me to express feelings that I didn't want to tell people directly," says Christopher, now 17 and a senior in high school. "Every once in a while I still use the techniques."

CURB is one of a rapidly growing number of hospital-based initiatives designed to catch and treat mental health issues in children and adolescents before they take root or worsen. Benjamin Van Voorhees, who helped develop this program and is interim chairman of the department of pediatrics at UI College of Medicine and physician-in-chief at Children's Hospital University of Illinois, considers it a "behavioral vaccine" intended to inoculate adolescents from mental illness. Depressive episodes often hit between the ages of 13 and 17, when they can create neural pathways in still-developing brains that can trigger recurrences over a lifetime. "The goal is to identify people in the incipient stages," says Van Voorhees. "These coping skills can reprogram the brain and hopefully abort the development of full-blown depression."

Other efforts range from devising more effective screening tools that can be used by primary care doctors to initiatives that quickly connect children to mental health professionals located in the same office or who are available remotely. Still, experts say, medicine is scrambling. "There's an incredible shortage of resources," notes Giovanni Piedimonte, chair of the Pediatric Institute at the Cleveland Clinic, because so few mental health professionals treat children, and insurance companies only spottily reimburse pediatricians for screening and evaluations. But "this is not just an infection that can be easily treated," he says. "This is a lifelong sentence that affects the whole family. This is now a true public health crisis."

Indeed, much of the impetus to take mental health very seriously (in adult patients as well as children) springs from the recognition, in

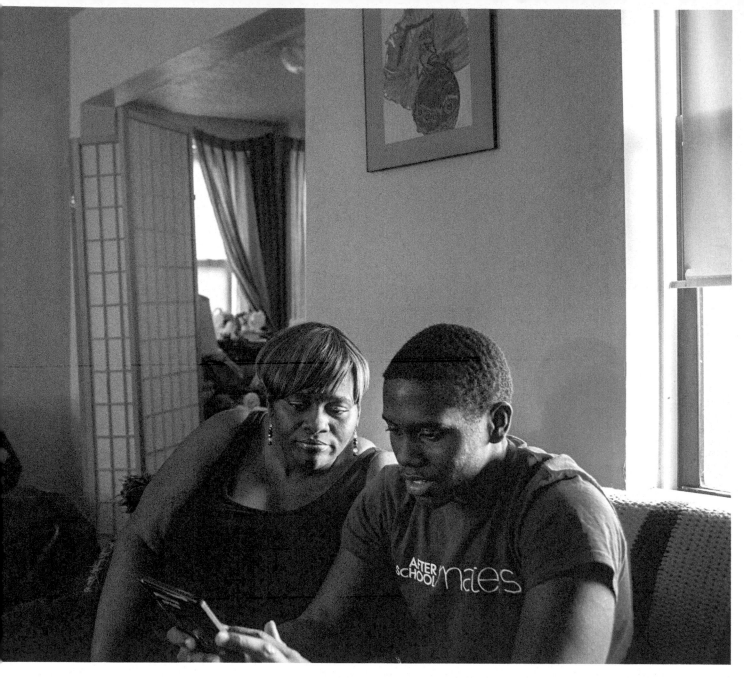

an age of population health, that depression and other ills play a huge role in physical well-being – in the lifestyle choices people make and how carefully they comply with doctors' orders, for example. And more than 17 million children, or as many as 1 in 5, have a challenge such as attention deficit hyperactivity disorder, autism, anxiety, substance abuse, behavior problems, an eating disorder, and depression. "When you look at the prevalence of these problems, they're very common in young children," says Carol Weitzman, director of the developmental-behavioral pediatrics program at Yale University. In fact, mental illness is the most common affliction of childhood, surpassing the number of kids with cancer, diabetes and AIDS combined.

YET STUDIES CONSISTENTLY SHOW that behavioral and emotional problems in children and adolescents have not been reliably detected or treated. Busy pediatricians rarely have enough time to diagnose mental health ills, nor do they typically have the expertise. And even when issues are detected, the shortage of child psychiatrists and psychologists translates to lengthy waiting lists. Fewer than half of those with serious mental health issues are identified, and of those, fewer than 1 in 8 receive treatment, according to the American Academy of Pediatrics. A 2015 report by the nonprofit Child Mind Institute

found that up to 80 percent of kids with anxiety disorders, about 60 percent of children with depression, and 40 percent of kids with ADHD do not get treatment.

The AAP has recommended early screening in primary care settings for even infants as young as 9 months if they're not hitting their developmental milestones or if they exhibit signs of autism. School-age children and adolescents should also be regularly screened, starting at age 5 (at their routine doctor's visits), and teenagers should also be screened for substance abuse. "Screening is an opportunity to start a conversation with the family and remove the stigma and talk honestly about these issues," says Weitzman. Parents and doctors should be on the lookout for troubling behaviors such as excessive crying, prolonged tantrums, or clinginess in young children, and problems with attention or mood, or poor performance in school.

The consequences of failing to intervene can be devastating. Suicide is the third leading cause of death among 10- to 24-year-olds; and half of children who suffer from depression will be plagued by it as an adult. Kids with undiagnosed psychological disorders are more likely to do poorly academically or drop out and have substance abuse issues, which can irrevocably alter the course of their lives.

THE HOSPITAL AND HEALTH system efforts aim to do a much better job. One approach is to integrate mental health screening into primary care, training pediatricians and family doctors to handle straightforward services. "Studies have shown that clinicians are more willing to manage problems and to prescribe medication" when they feel supported, Weitzman says.

Thanks to a program launched in the last year by Children's National Health System and MedStar Georgetown University Hospital, for instance, parents who take their kids to a pediatrician in Washington, D.C., now have a much easier time getting the proper diagnosis and treatment of a mental health issue. The two hospitals recently created DC MAP (for Mental Health Access in Pediatrics), an outreach program that provides any pediatrician in the city who wants to enroll with the screening tools and training to spot kids at risk during well-child visits. Expert help is just a phone call away. Doctors can talk over their questions with child psychiatrists, psychologists and social workers on staff at the hospitals.

The DC MAP team sets up face-to-face sessions with kids as needed and helps families get referrals, says Lee Beers, director of the program, which now serves providers taking care of more than half the children in the city. The number of kids receiving mental health screening has jumped from less than 10 percent to nearly 85 percent in participating practices over the past year, and children and teenagers are being routed to the appropriate professionals. The program is catching youngsters "before they end up in the ER," says Beers.

The Washington initiative is modeled on the Massachusetts Child Psychiatry Access Program, which launched more than a decade ago and has evolved into a national access program with projects now in 27 states, including California, Connecticut, New York, New Jersey, Louisiana, Pennsylvania and Georgia.

Some pioneering health systems, including Montefiore Medical Center in New York and Intermountain Healthcare in Utah, are putting behavioral health services themselves into the primary care setting, so that patients of all ages are regularly screened and can get treatment in the same location. As part of its effort, Carolinas HealthCare System, which has 39 hospitals in North Carolina, South Carolina and Georgia, launched a pilot program a year ago at two pediatric practices in suburban Charlotte to make behavioral health a component of basic care. During routine screenings, a parent or pediatrician worried about a child's mental health is immediately connected, over the phone or via video, with a mental health professional, who will assess the patient and provide treatment recommendations. Children in rural areas can do sessions with a psychologist via video.

Similarly, Texas Children's Hospital in Houston is testing a team approach to care, relying on "medical homes" that integrate mental health services on-site. "This is designed as an integrated one-stop shop, with pharmacy, dentistry, pediatrics and behavioral health all in the same place," says Angelo Giardino, senior vice president and chief quality officer at Texas Children's. "By introducing behavioral health professionals as part of the team, it sends the right message to families that health has many dimensions and this is just part of being healthy." A child who is identified as anxious or at risk of depression, say, is immediately introduced to the team's psychologist. Generally, only about 9 percent of kids in the system's health plan access mental health services; in these medical homes that figure is about 20 percent.

THE ACCESSIBILITY THAT characterizes such integrated care can be key to getting help that can be life-changing, as one Cleveland-area mom found out a number of years ago when her young son became disruptive and aggressive in kindergarten. When he got to second grade and began hiding under a table or desk, the family's pediatrician, who practiced at one of Cleveland Clinic Children's 53 locations, referred him to a staff psychiatrist. The diagnosis was unexpected: The boy wasn't dealing with oppositional defiant disorder or intermittent explosive disorder, even though his behavior suggested one of those, but rather he had severe anxiety that prompted him to lash out when confronted with challenging situations.

"This really helped us understand where he was coming from," says his mom, who prefers that he not be identified. Now 15 and entering high school in the fall, he still sees a Cleveland Clinic psychologist and psychiatrist regularly at the local center and has learned how to change his thought patterns so as not to worry so much.

The good news, says Lisa Cullins, a child psychiatrist at Children's National Hospital, is that programs like these "are the wave of the future." When mental health issues are identified and treated early, she says, a child's life trajectory can dramatically change. ●

KIDS SHOULD BE *SCREENED* REGULARLY STARTING AT *AGE 5.*

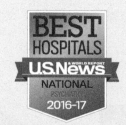

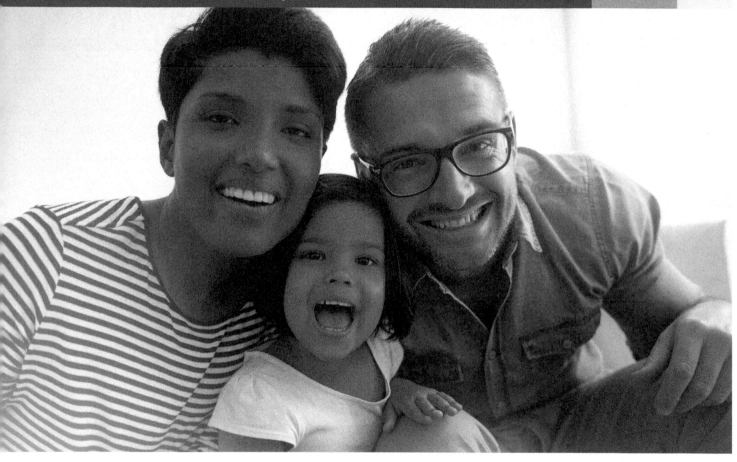

Proud to be Ranked Among the Nation's
Top Ten Psychiatric Hospitals for 2016-2017
by *U.S. News & World Report*

Sheppard Pratt Health System is dedicated to improving quality of life through mental health, special education, and substance use services for children, adolescents, and adults. Our patient-centered treatment approach, combined with our legacy of clinical excellence, sets us apart from other health systems on both a local and national level.

We are focused solely on mental health treatment, healing, and recovery, and provide our patients with the specialized care they need in a supportive and compassionate environment.

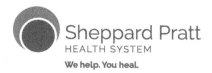

410.938.3000 • sheppardpratt.org
Nearly 40 locations throughout Maryland

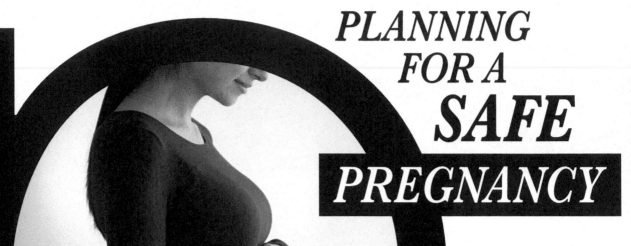

PLANNING FOR A *SAFE* PREGNANCY

Even women contemplating conceiving have plenty to think about these days

BY STACEY COLINO

W hether you're planning to get pregnant or already are, the headlines about the Zika virus and the government's new zero-alcohol recommendation may have you wondering about how best to keep your baby (and yourself) safe. Beyond the basics – taking prenatal vitamins, managing stress and limiting caffeine – what do you need to do these days to have the healthiest possible pregnancy?

The ideal way to avoid exposing a developing baby to potential harm would be for the pregnancy to be planned, says Jeffrey Ecker, chief of obstetrics and gynecology at Massachusetts General Hospital. But since half of pregnancies aren't, it's best to take certain steps if conceiving is even a possibility:

DEFEND AGAINST ZIKA. With the discovery of Zika-carrying mosquitoes in southern Florida this summer and the expectation that they could arrive in force in parts of the U.S., it's smart to stay alert for updates from the Centers for Disease Control and Prevention. Besides microcephaly (a smaller than expected head due to abnormal brain development), the virus has been linked with other brain defects in the babies of mothers infected during pregnancy, and with miscarriage. You'll want to both avoid exposure to the infected bugs and be aware that Zika can be transmitted during sex with an infected man. Several drugmakers are working on developing a vaccine, but it'll be a few years before one is available.

The CDC advises women who are pregnant or contemplating pregnancy to avoid traveling to areas with Zika. (Updated notices of hotspots can be found at wwwnc.cdc.gov/travel.) In fact, "both the woman and her partner should avoid travel to Zika endemic areas," says Neil Silverman, a spokesperson for the American College of Obstetricians and Gynecologists and a professor of obstetrics and gynecology at the UCLA School of Medicine.

If a man has traveled to a place where Zika is present, condoms should be used for eight weeks after his return even if he doesn't develop the telltale symptoms: fever, rash, joint pain, conjunctivitis. If he does, condoms should be used for six months. If you live in or must travel to an infected area, wear long sleeves and pants and use insect repellents that contain the chemicals DEET (20 percent concentration) or picaridin, Silverman says. Women who are infected when not pregnant will likely develop an immunity that will protect future pregnancies, the CDC says.

GO ALCOHOL-FREE. Having a cocktail or glass of wine per week was once thought to pose little risk. Those days are gone. Earlier this year, the CDC called for a zero-tolerance policy during pregnancy, recommending that even women trying to conceive not partake. The reason: It has become clear that many children – perhaps 1 in 20 – are affected by fetal alcohol spectrum disorders that create issues from low birth weight and heart ailments to intellectual disabilities and attention and behavioral problems. Plus some research suggests alcohol can increase the risk of miscarriage, stillbirth or premature birth.

While "there's no need to panic if you find out you're pregnant and you already had three glasses of wine," says Ecker, "what the CDC is saying is: We can't define a lower limit that is safe."

GET A FLU VACCINATION. The medical guidelines advise anyone 6 months old or older to get a vaccination, but half of pregnant women don't bother. "This is an ongoing source of frustration for those of us on the front lines of the vaccination effort," says Silverman. The shot is "absolutely safe" for mother and baby, he says, and pregnant women who get the flu are at increased risk of pneumonia and death. And a new Australian study found that the vaccine is associated with a 51 percent lower risk of stillbirth.

KEEP MOVING. Because pregnancy is a significant contributor to obesity in women, ACOG issued guidelines last December calling for at least 20 to 30 minutes of moderate-intensity aerobic exercise per day, plus moderate strength training two or three times per week. Besides assisting with weight control, the regimen should reduce the risk of gestational diabetes.

"In the past we said: Pregnancy is not a good time to change lifestyle. But it's the best time for behavior modification," says Raul Artal, professor

and chairman emeritus of obstetrics/gynecology and women's health at Saint Louis University and lead author of the guidelines. "Women have more access to medical care and supervision" than they do at any other time in their lives.

Of course, it's important to get the green light from your obstetrician. Assuming you do, walking, jogging, swimming, stationary cycling, modified yoga, low-impact aerobics and cardio machines are good choices.

EAT GOOD FISH. Both ACOG and the Food and Drug Administration recommend that women eat 8 to 12 ounces of fish each week to give their developing babies much-needed omega-3 fatty acids. But certain fish contain unsafe levels of mercury, a neurotoxin known to be harmful to developing brains. Now a 2016 study from the Environmental Working Group has ratcheted up this concern: After testing hair samples of 254 women of childbearing age who reported eating that much fish (or

WOMEN SHOULD *EAT* 8 *TO* 12 OUNCES OF *FISH* EACH WEEK.

more) per week, researchers found that nearly 30 percent had higher than safe levels of mercury; almost 60 percent exceeded what some experts deem to be a protective upper limit.

So what's an expectant mother to do? "You can get a win-win benefit from eating the right fish – wild salmon, sardines and rainbow trout, which are high in omega-3s and low in

mercury," says Tracey Woodruff, a professor in the department of obstetrics and gynecology and director of the Program on Reproductive Health and the Environment at the University of California–San Francisco. Steer clear of large predatory fish such as swordfish, tilefish, shark and king mackerel, which tend to have the highest mercury concentrations. You can also increase your intake of omega-3 fatty acids by eating walnuts, flaxseed, chia seeds, or boiled or roasted soybeans.

THINK TWICE ABOUT ANTIDEPRESSANTS. A couple of studies have suggested that pregnancy might be a reason to think about suspending or postponing antidepressant use. Researchers at the University of Montreal examined the records of more than 145,000 births and found that expectant mothers who took selective serotonin reuptake inhibitors during the second and/or third trimester had a twofold higher risk of giving birth to a child with an autism spectrum disorder, though the risk measured was still small. It rose from just under 1 percent in the general population to 2.17 percent. Meanwhile, a 2013 JAMA Psychiatry review of the research found an increased risk of preterm delivery and lower birth weight.

On the other hand, depression is very common during pregnancy and can be debilitating, says senior study author Anick Bérard, a professor of perinatal epidemiology at the University of Montreal. So a talk with your doctor is in order.

For mild to moderate depression, psychotherapy plus an exercise program might be sufficient. For moderate to severe depression, or when other approaches haven't worked, medication in combination with psychotherapy may be appropriate, says Elizabeth Fitelson, an assistant professor of psychiatry at Columbia University Medical Center.

"You're weighing risk against risk, because untreated maternal depression affects kids' emotional and cognitive development," she says. And it can take a real toll on family relationships. ●

To every top ranked hospital in the nation
well done.

We're all here for a reason. We're here because we know that at the end of the day, epilepsy doesn't care about rankings and congenital heart defects aren't impressed by individual accomplishments. We're here because we all know that **the only real enemy is disease itself.** We're here because our mutual collaboration helps us treat kids the best way we collectively know how. We're here because our shared knowledge keeps **pushing the boundaries of what's possible** for patient care.

So let's keep a good thing going. We'll continue to lead the way with breakthroughs in innovation, quality improvement and learning networks so that together, we can be the industry that chooses collaboration over competition.

Let's dedicate ourselves to changing the outcome together for every parent, child and future.

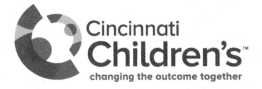

CHAPTER

BEST CHILDREN'S HOSPITALS

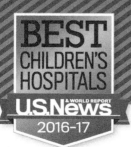

BEST CHILDREN'S HOSPITALS
U.S.News & WORLD REPORT
2016-17

BEST CHILDREN'S HOSPITALS

THE HONOR ROLL

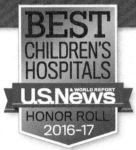

BEST CHILDREN'S HOSPITALS
U.S.News & WORLD REPORT
HONOR ROLL
2016-17

THE 11 HOSPITALS ON THIS YEAR'S ELITE PEDIATRIC LIST had to rank in the top 10 percent of all evaluated centers in at least three specialties. Position on the Honor Roll was determined by points; hospitals received two points per specialty for ranking in the top 5 percent and one point for ranking in the next 5 percent. Ties are ordered alphabetically.

1 **Boston Children's Hospital**
20 points in 10 specialties

2 **Children's Hospital of Philadelphia**
19 points in 10 specialties

3 **Cincinnati Children's Hospital Medical Center**
15 points in 8 specialties

4 **Texas Children's Hospital**
Houston
12 points in 7 specialties

5 **Seattle Children's Hospital**
6 points in 5 specialties

6 **Ann and Robert H. Lurie Children's Hospital of Chicago**
5 points in 4 specialties

7* **Children's Hospital Los Angeles**
4 points in 4 specialties

7* **Children's Hospital of Pittsburgh of UPMC**
4 points in 4 specialties

9 **Children's Hospital Colorado**
Aurora
4 points in 3 specialties

10* **Lucile Packard Children's Hospital at Stanford**
Palo Alto, Calif.
3 points in 3 specialties

10* **Nationwide Children's Hospital**
Columbus, Ohio
3 points in 3 specialties

*Denotes tie

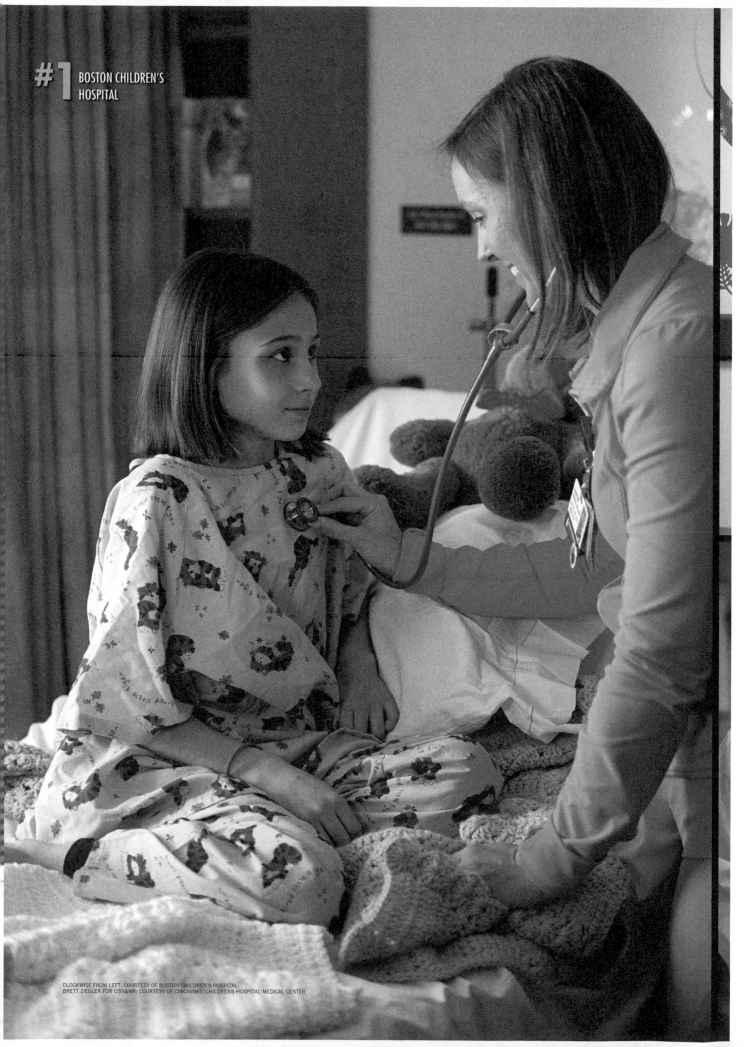

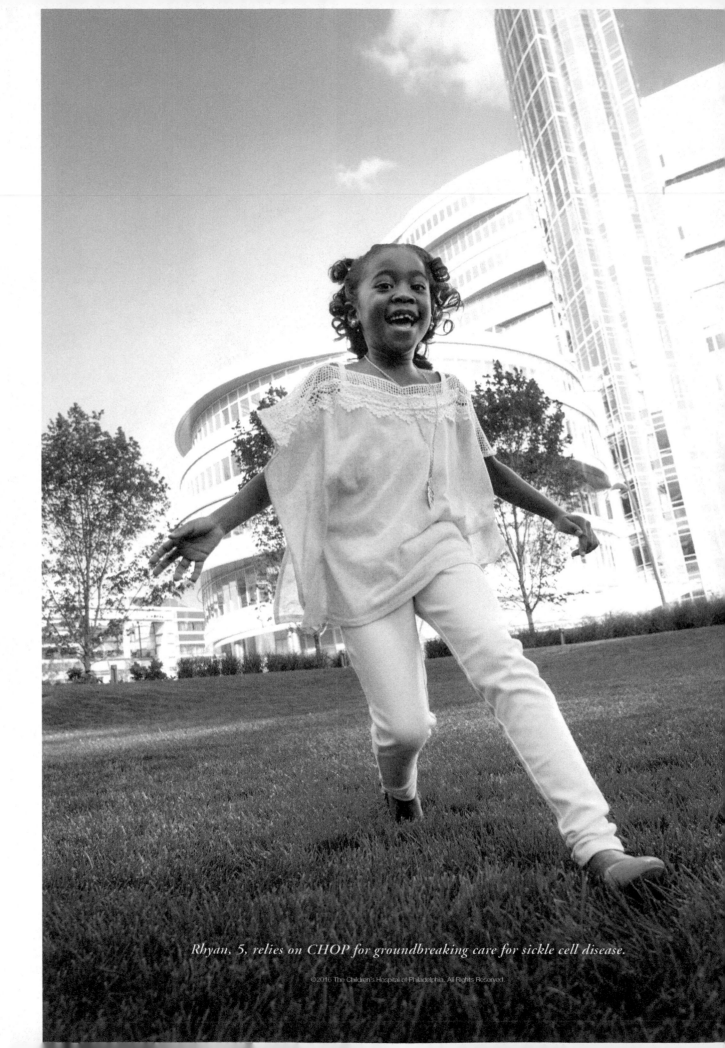

Rhyan, 5, relies on CHOP for groundbreaking care for sickle cell disease.

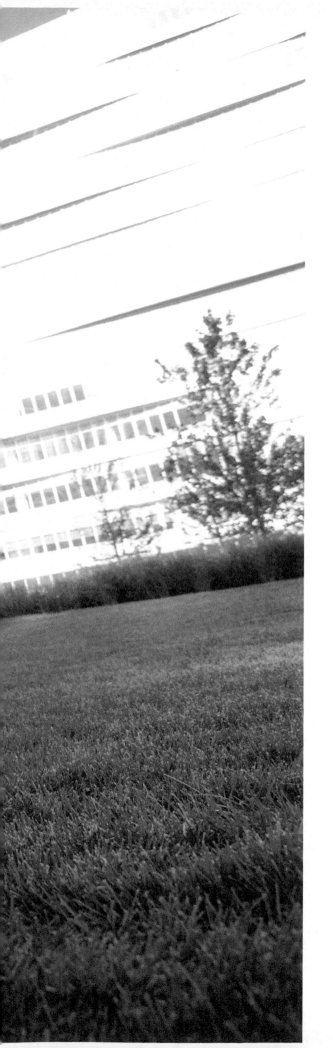

They're not our breakthroughs.
They're Rhyan's.

All children who come to Children's Hospital
of Philadelphia — and many who don't — benefit
from the discoveries and
advances that have been the
essence of who we are for
more than 160 years. It's our
work. It's their future.

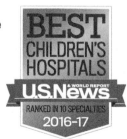

chop.edu/breakthroughs

CH The Children's Hospital
of Philadelphia®

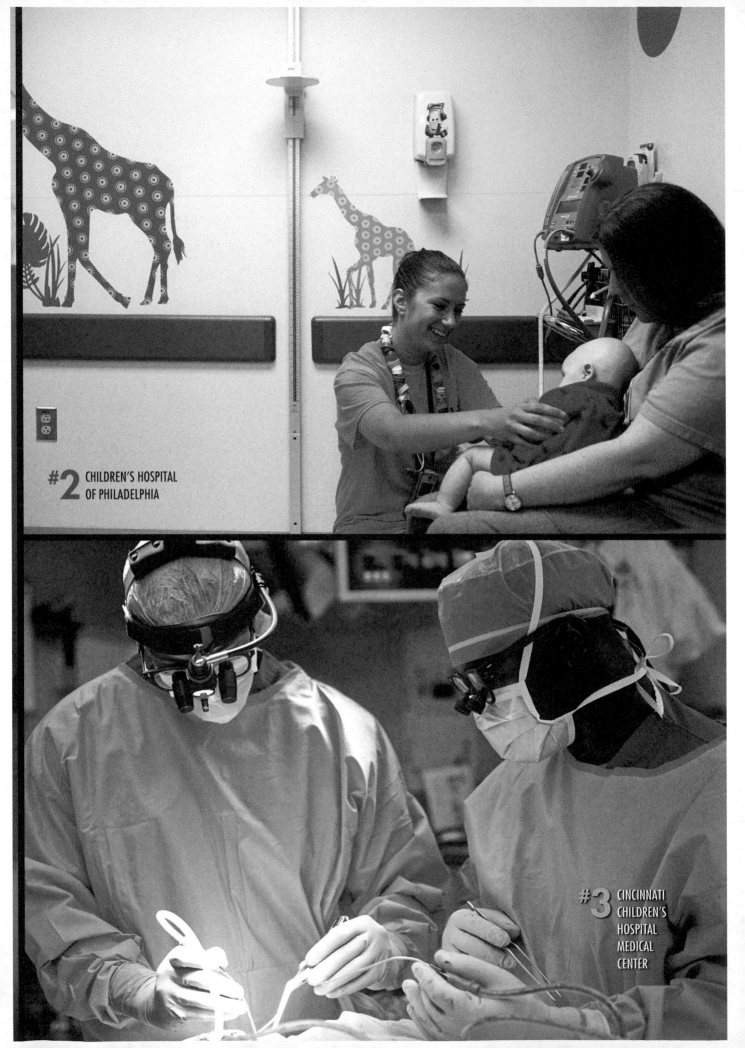

#2 CHILDREN'S HOSPITAL
OF PHILADELPHIA

#3 CINCINNATI
CHILDREN'S
HOSPITAL
MEDICAL
CENTER

BEHIND THE RANKINGS

How we identified 78 outstanding hospitals in 10 specialties

BY AVERY COMAROW

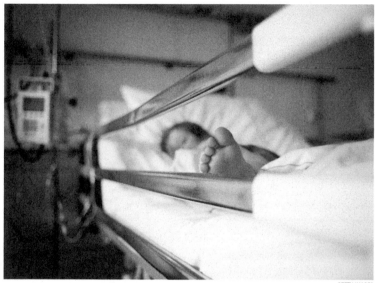

GETTY IMAGES

W here to take a newborn with a major heart defect, or find ongoing care for a child with failing kidneys or lung-clogging cystic fibrosis? A local hospital's pediatric department might see lots of kids, but few community hospitals have the skills to treat the sickest children. Even in the compact universe of fewer than 200 children's hospitals, some are better than others. U.S. News created the Best Children's Hospitals rankings to help parents find the ones that are the best for their child.

The 2016-17 rankings highlight top children's centers in 10 specialties: cancer, cardiology and heart surgery, diabetes and endocrinology, gastroenterology and GI surgery, neonatology, nephrology, neurology and neurosurgery, orthopedics, pulmonology and urology. This year, 78 hospitals ranked in at least one specialty, and the 2016-17 Honor Roll recognizes 11 standouts that scored at or near the top in at least three. Many ranked hospitals are stand-alone centers. Most of the rest are large multispecialty pediatric departments very much like hospitals within the walls of their parent institutions.

Putting children's hospitals under the microscope is much more challenging than evaluating adult care, as U.S. News does in Best Hospitals for high-risk patients in 16 specialties (page 84). Which data to collect, or even agreement on standards for how to interpret it, are a constant source of debate. Nor is there a pediatric version of the federal Medicare database that U.S. News draws on for the adult rankings.

Almost all of the medical data used in these rankings is therefore obtained by asking hospitals to complete a lengthy online survey. This year, 106 of the 183 hospitals surveyed by U.S. News provided enough data to be evaluated in at least one specialty. Most surveyed hospitals are members of the Children's Hospital Association; a few are specialty centers or non-CHA hospitals that were previously ranked or were recommended by trusted sources.

This year's survey was updated with the help of more than 100 medical directors, clinical specialists and other pediatric experts who served on 10 U.S. News specialty task forces. RTI International, a North Carolina-based research and consulting firm, ran the survey and analyzed the findings.

Whether and how high an institution was ranked depended on its clinical outcomes (such as survival and surgical complications), delivery of care (how well it orchestrates the many steps involved in treating patients and keeping them safe), and resources (such as staffing and technology). Complete details on the methodology are available at usnews.com/aboutchildrens.

Each of the three elements was worth one-third of a hospital's overall score. Here are the basics:

Clinical outcomes. These reveal a hospital's success at keeping kids alive after their treatment or surgery, protecting them from infections and complications, and improving their quality of life.

Delivery of care. How well a hospital handles day-to-day care was determined in part by compliance with accepted "best practices," such as having a full-time infection preventionist and holding regular conferences to discuss unexpected deaths and complications. U.S. News also surveys pediatric specialists annually, asking them to name up to 10 hospitals they consider best for children with serious or difficult medical problems in their area of expertise, ignoring location and cost. Results from the latest three surveys made up 15 percent of a hospital's total score. More than 25 percent of the surveyed physicians responded in 2016.

Resources. Surgical volume, nurse-patient ratio and the existence of clinics and programs for specific conditions such as asthma are a few of more than 30 measures and hundreds of submeasures that were evaluated in the rankings. ●

WHAT THE TERMS MEAN

USED ACROSS MULTIPLE SPECIALTIES

Best practices: examples include documenting a high percentage of outpatients' blood sugar results (diabetes & endocrinology); conducting simulator training for chest tube placement (neonatology); conducting hip exams with ultrasound specialists (orthopedics).
ICU infection prevention score: ability to prevent central-line bloodstream infections and urinary tract infections in intensive care units.
Nurse Magnet status: hospital recognized as meeting American Nurses Credentialing Center standards for excellence.
Nurse-patient ratio: balance of full-time registered nurses to inpatients.
Overall infection prevention score: ability to prevent infections through measures such as hand hygiene and vaccination.
Patient volume score: relative number of patients in past year with specified disorders.
Procedure volume score: relative number of tests and nonsurgical procedures in past one, two or three years depending on specialty, such as implanting radioactive seeds in a cancerous thyroid (diabetes & endocrinology) and using an endoscope for diagnosis (gastroenterology). Surgical procedures are included in orthopedics.
Specialists recommending: percentage of physician specialists responding to surveys in 2014, 2015 and 2016 and naming hospital among best for very challenging patients.
Surgery volume score: relative number of patients who had specified surgical procedures in past year.

Surgical complications prevention score: ability to prevent surgery-related complications and readmissions within 30 days (neurology & neurosurgery, orthopedics, urology).
U.S. News score: 0 to 100; summary of overall specialty performance.
NA: not applicable.
NR: not reported.

USED IN ONE SPECIALTY

CANCER
Bone marrow transplant survival score: survival of stem cell recipients at 100 days.
Five-year survival score: survival five years after treatment for acute lymphoblastic leukemia, acute myeloid leukemia, and neuroblastoma.
Palliative care score: how well program meets specified training and staffing standards for children with terminal or life-limiting conditions, and number of cancer patients referred to program.

CARDIOLOGY & HEART SURGERY
Catheter procedure volume score: relative number of specified catheter-based procedures in past year, such as inserting stents and treating heart rhythm problems.
Complex surgery survival score: survival following moderately complex to very difficult heart surgery in past four years.
Norwood/hybrid surgery survival score: survival at three years after having either of two surgeries to reconstruct the heart.

DIABETES & ENDOCRINOLOGY
Diabetes management score: ability to prevent serious problems in children with Type 1 diabetes and to keep blood sugar levels in check.
Hypothyroid management score: relative proportions of children treated for underactive thyroid who test normal and of infants who begin treatment by three weeks of age.

GASTROENTEROLOGY & GI SURGERY
Liver transplant survival score: relative survival one year after liver transplant.
Nonsurgical procedure volume score: relative number of tests and noninvasive procedures.
Selected treatments success score: shown, for example, by high remission rates for inflammatory bowel disease and few complications from endoscopic procedures.

NEONATOLOGY
Breast milk score: relative percentage of infants discharged from neonatal ICU receiving at least some nutrition from breast milk.
NICU infection prevention score: see ICU infection prevention score, above.
Readmissions prevention score: ability to minimize unplanned readmissions to NICU within 30 days after discharge.

NEPHROLOGY
Biopsy complications prevention score: ability to minimize complications after kidney biopsy.
Dialysis infection prevention score: ability to minimize dialysis-related infection.
Dialysis management score: relative proportion of dialysis patients in past two years who tested normal.
Kidney transplant survival score: based on patient survival and functioning kidney at one and three years.

NEUROLOGY & NEUROSURGERY
Clinic patient volume score: relative number of clinic patients in past year with specified disorders or procedures.
Epilepsy management score: ability to treat children with epilepsy.
Surgical survival score: survival at 30 days after complex surgery and procedures, such as those involving brain tumors, epilepsy and head trauma.

ORTHOPEDICS
Fracture repair score: ability to treat complex leg and forearm fractures efficiently.

PULMONOLOGY
Asthma inpatient score: ability to minimize asthmatic children's asthma-related deaths, length of stay, and readmissions.
Cystic fibrosis management score: ability to improve lung function and nutritional status.
Lung transplant survival score: reflects number of transplants in past two years, one-year survival, and recognition by United Network for Organ Sharing.

UROLOGY
Minimally invasive volume score: relative number of patients in past year who had specified nonsurgical procedures.
Testicular torsion care score: ability to perform prompt emergency surgery to correct twisted spermatic cord.
Urinary-tract infection prevention score: ability to minimize infections from urinary catheters.

WHERE THE MIRACLES ARE.

Because you give, our member hospitals are the best of the best.

Akron Children's Hospital, Akron, OH

Ann & Robert H. Lurie Children's Hospital of Chicago, Chicago, IL

Arkansas Children's Hospital, Little Rock, AR

Arnold Palmer Medical Center, Orlando, FL

Boston Children's Hospital, Boston, MA

Children's Healthcare of Atlanta, Atlanta, GA

Children's Health Children's Medical Center, Dallas, TX

Children's Hospital Colorado, Aurora, CO

Children's Hospital Los Angeles, Los Angeles, CA

Children's Hospital & Medical Center, Omaha, NE

Children's Hospital of Illinois, Peoria, IL

Children's Hospital of Pittsburgh of UPMC, Pittsburgh, PA

Children's Hospital of Wisconsin, Milwaukee, WI

Children's National Health System, Washington, DC

Children's of Alabama, Birmingham, AL

CHOC Children's, Orange, CA

Cincinnati Children's Hospital Medical Center, Cincinnati, OH

Cohen Children's Medical Center of New York, New Hyde Park, NY

Cook Children's Medical Center, Fort Worth, TX

Dell Children's Medical Center of Central Texas, Austin, TX

Duke Children's, Durham, NC

Helen DeVos Children's Hospital, Grand Rapids, MI

Johns Hopkins All Children's Hospital, St. Petersburg, FL

Johns Hopkins Children's Center, Baltimore, MD

Kosair Children's Hospital, Louisville, KY

Le Bonheur Children's Hospital, Memphis, TN

Levine Children's Hospital, Charlotte, NC

Maria Fareri Children's Hospital, Valhalla, NY

Medical University of South Carolina Shawn Jenkins Children's Hospital, Charleston, SC

Monroe Carell Jr. Children's Hospital at Vanderbilt, Nashville, TN

Nationwide Children's Hospital, Columbus, OH

Nicklaus Children's Hospital, Miami, FL

OHSU Doernbecher Children's Hospital, Portland, OR

Penn State Hershey Children's Hospital, Hershey, PA

Phoenix Children's Hospital, Phoenix, AZ

Primary Children's Hospital, Salt Lake City, UT

Rady Children's Hospital-San Diego, San Diego, CA

Riley Hospital for Children, Indianapolis, IN

Seattle Children's Hospital, Seattle, WA

SSM Health Cardinal Glennon Children's Hospital, St. Louis, MO

St. Louis Children's Hospital, St. Louis, MO

Texas Children's Hospital, Houston, TX

The Children's Hospital of Philadelphia, Philadelphia, PA

UC Davis Children's Hospital, Sacramento, CA

UCSF Benioff Children's Hospitals, Oakland, CA

UF Health Shands Children's Hospital, Gainesville, FL

University Hospitals Rainbow Babies & Children's Hospital, Cleveland, OH

University of Iowa Children's Hospital, Iowa City, IA

University of Virginia Children's Hospital, Charlottesville, VA

Valley Children's Hospital, Madera, CA

Wolfson Children's Hospital, Jacksonville, FL

It's no coincidence every hospital on the Best Children's Hospitals Honor Roll is one of ours. Children's Miracle Network Hospitals® are able to provide best-in-class care thanks to local donations.

CMNHospitals.org

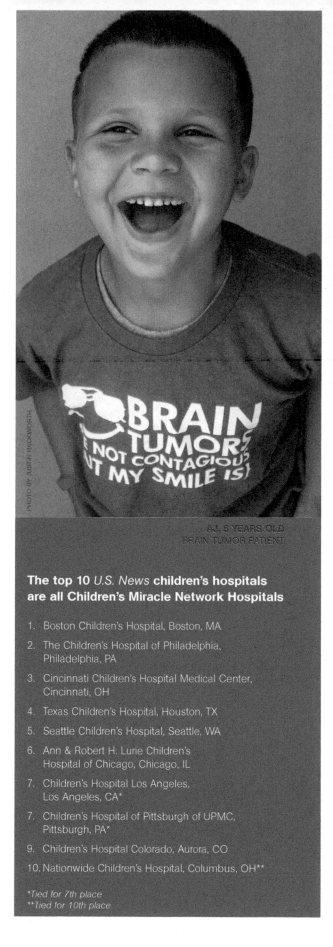

AJ, 5 YEARS OLD
BRAIN TUMOR PATIENT

The top 10 *U.S. News* children's hospitals are all Children's Miracle Network Hospitals

1. Boston Children's Hospital, Boston, MA

2. The Children's Hospital of Philadelphia, Philadelphia, PA

3. Cincinnati Children's Hospital Medical Center, Cincinnati, OH

4. Texas Children's Hospital, Houston, TX

5. Seattle Children's Hospital, Seattle, WA

6. Ann & Robert H. Lurie Children's Hospital of Chicago, Chicago, IL

7. Children's Hospital Los Angeles, Los Angeles, CA*

7. Children's Hospital of Pittsburgh of UPMC, Pittsburgh, PA*

9. Children's Hospital Colorado, Aurora, CO

10. Nationwide Children's Hospital, Columbus, OH**

*Tied for 7th place
**Tied for 10th place

Children's
Miracle Network
Hospitals'

Give Today
to your children's hospital

CANCER

Rank	Hospital	U.S. News score	Five-year survival score (12=best)	Bone marrow transplant survival score (6=best)	Overall infection prevention score (28=best)	ICU infection prevention score (20=best)	Patient volume score (9=best)	Nurse-patient ratio (higher is better)	Nurse Magnet status	Palliative care score (8=best)	Specialists recommending
1	Dana-Farber/Boston Children's Cancer and Blood Disorders Center	100.0	11	5	24	12	9	3.9	Yes	8	70.8%
2	Texas Children's Hospital, Houston	99.4	10	5	27	15	9	3.3	Yes	8	49.5%
3	Children's Hospital of Philadelphia	98.0	11	6	27	9	9	3.2	Yes	8	77.9%
4	St. Jude Children's Research Hospital, Memphis	93.4	10	4	23	16	9	4.6	Yes	8	58.3%
5	Johns Hopkins Children's Center, Baltimore	91.5	12	6	22	13	7	3.1	Yes	8	21.1%
6	Seattle Children's Hospital	90.1	10	6	27	12	9	2.9	Yes	8	43.2%
7	Children's Hospital Los Angeles	90.0	11	6	26	12	9	3.7	Yes	8	34.8%
8	Nationwide Children's Hospital, Columbus, Ohio	89.6	11	6	25	15	8	3.0	Yes	8	14.8%
9	Children's Hospital Colorado, Aurora	85.6	11	4	25	11	9	3.6	Yes	7	28.1%
10	Children's Healthcare of Atlanta	84.9	11	5	27	12	9	4.2	No	8	23.5%
11	Ann and Robert H. Lurie Children's Hospital of Chicago	84.7	10	4	25	15	9	3.5	Yes	8	19.9%
12	Cincinnati Children's Hospital Medical Center	83.9	10	2	25	12	9	3.1	Yes	8	62.0%
13	Children's National Medical Center, Washington, D.C.	81.9	9	4	27	14	9	3.1	Yes	8	16.4%
14	Memorial Sloan-Kettering Cancer Center, New York	79.5	11	3	23	16	4	3.6	Yes	8	21.8%
15	Children's Medical Center Dallas	77.4	11	3	28	15	9	3.0	Yes	7	9.6%
16	UCSF Benioff Children's Hospitals, San Francisco and Oakland	76.5	10	4	25	11	7	3.0	Yes	8	14.8%
17	Rainbow Babies and Children's Hospital, Cleveland	75.9	9	4	25	18	7	3.1	Yes	8	4.2%
18	Monroe Carell Jr. Children's Hospital at Vanderbilt, Nashville	75.6	11	4	23	15	8	3.4	Yes	8	3.0%
19	Rady Children's Hospital, San Diego	75.4	10	6	28	14	8	3.1	No	8	1.6%
20	Primary Children's Hospital, Salt Lake City	71.8	11	6	25	11	6	3.9	No	8	4.0%
21	Lucile Packard Children's Hospital at Stanford, Palo Alto, Calif.	70.8	8	4	27	14	8	3.5	No	8	9.1%
22	UF Health Shands Children's Hospital, Gainesville, Fla.	70.3	10	6	25	13	6	2.6	Yes	8	1.2%
23	St. Louis Children's Hospital-Washington University	70.0	8	5	26	13	4	3.4	Yes	8	8.8%
24	Phoenix Children's Hospital	69.4	11	4	23	14	8	3.3	No	8	3.2%
25	Duke Children's Hospital and Health Center, Durham, N.C.	69.0	9	5	26	11	5	3.0	Yes	8	8.6%
26	Mattel Children's Hospital UCLA, Los Angeles	68.7	5	6	23	15	5	3.8	Yes	8	3.3%
27	University of Iowa Children's Hospital, Iowa City	66.4	11	5	24	12	6	2.9	Yes	8	0.9%
28	North Carolina Children's Hospital at UNC, Chapel Hill	66.3	11	4	28	13	6	3.8	Yes	7	0.6%
29	Children's Hospital of Pittsburgh of UPMC	65.8	8	4	27	11	8	3.3	Yes	8	5.8%
30	Children's Mercy Kansas City, Mo.	65.7	9	4	26	9	7	4.2	Yes	6	5.9%
31	Mayo Clinic Children's Center, Rochester, Minn.	64.2	9	6	23	5	6	3.6	Yes	8	1.7%
31	NY-Presby. Morgan Stanley-Komansky Children's Hosp., N.Y.	64.2	10	4	28	12	7	2.9	No	8	3.3%
33	Children's Hospital of Wisconsin, Milwaukee	63.9	9	2	24	14	6	4.2	Yes	8	2.6%
34	Riley Hospital for Children at IU Health, Indianapolis	63.8	11	4	23	10	4	3.1	Yes	8	3.8%
35	Yale-New Haven Children's Hospital, New Haven, Conn.	63.7	11	6	22	6	5	2.4	Yes	7	0.3%
36	American Family Children's Hospital, Madison, Wis.	63.4	11	4	19	14	3	4.6	Yes	5	1.3%
37	Medical Univ. of South Carolina Children's Hosp., Charleston	61.8	9	4	26	16	3	2.7	Yes	8	1.1%
38	Penn State Children's Hospital, Hershey, Pa.	61.3	9	5	21	12	5	2.6	Yes	8	1.1%
39	Cleveland Clinic Children's Hospital	61.2	8	5	18	13	3	3.2	Yes	8	0.2%
40	Cook Children's Medical Center, Fort Worth	60.7	10	4	20	12	8	3.4	Yes	8	2.0%
40	University of Michigan C.S. Mott Children's Hospital, Ann Arbor	60.7	10	4	20	12	3	3.6	No	8	4.2%
42	Spectrum Hlth. Helen DeVos Children's Hosp., Grand Rapids, Mich.	60.6	11	4	24	12	6	2.6	Yes	6	0.8%
43	Steven & Alexandra Cohen Children's Hosp., New Hyde Park, N.Y.	60.5	9	3	27	16	8	3.3	No	8	1.2%
44	Doernbecher Children's Hospital, Portland, Ore.	60.4	10	4	24	14	6	3.4	Yes	7	1.8%
45	CHOC Children's Hospital, Orange, Calif.	60.2	9	3	25	14	7	2.9	Yes	8	1.2%
46	Akron Children's Hospital, Ohio	59.4	11	4	26	11	3	3.2	Yes	8	0.7%
47	Nemours Alfred I. duPont Hosp. for Children, Wilmington, Del.	58.8	10	2	22	12	3	3.8	Yes	8	0.5%
48	Medical City Children's Hospital, Dallas	58.6	10	4	25	15	4	2.2	Yes	7	0.1%
49	SSM Health Cardinal Glennon Children's Hospital, St. Louis	57.0	11	6	23	10	3	2.9	No	8	0.6%
50	Johns Hopkins All Children's Hospital, St. Petersburg, Fla.	56.4	7	5	23	12	8	3.3	No	7	0.5%

Terms are explained on Page 142.

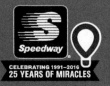

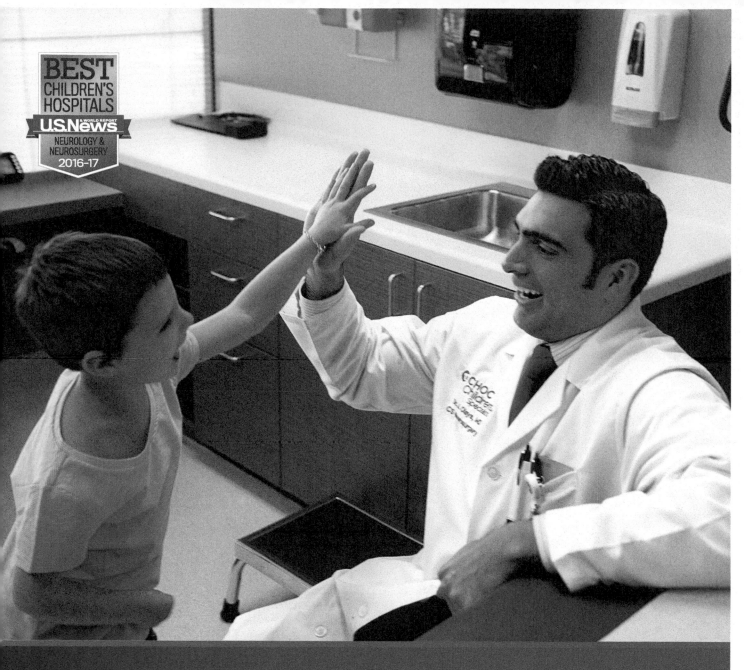

HOW DO YOU HEAL A CHILD'S BRAIN?
BY USING THE BEST OF OURS.

An epileptic seizure is one of the most frightening events a child and family can endure. At the CHOC
Children's Neuroscience Institute we offer state-of-the-art Epilepsy Monitoring Units in Orange and Mission
Viejo, allowing our pediatric epileptologists to gather valuable data that helps determine where a child's
seizures originate and how they spread in the brain. With this valuable information they can determine the
best course of treatment for each patient — ranging from minimally invasive surgery and clinical trials, to
alternative treatments. Recognized as one of the top 40 centers by *U.S. News & World Report* for neurology
and neurosurgery, CHOC offers the only specialists in Orange County with training in both child neurology
and clinical neurophysiology. **To learn more, visit choc.org/neuroscience**

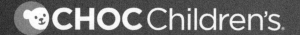

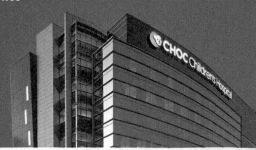

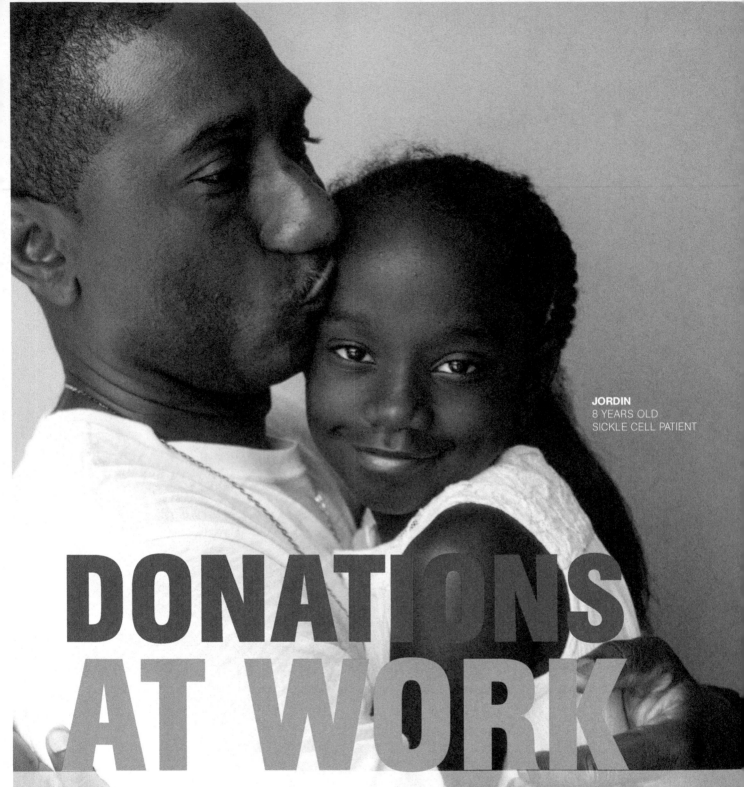

JORDIN
8 YEARS OLD
SICKLE CELL PATIENT

DONATIONS AT WORK

Jordin lives with sickle cell disease. To manage her pain and other complications caused by the red blood cell disorder, she frequently visits her children's hospital.

While waiting for a cure, this 8-year-old is doing all she can to fight, for her own health and for other sick and injured kids. **This year, Jordin is sharing her story across the United States, as a Champion for Children's Miracle Network Hospitals**. She is one of 52 kids — representing each state, Washington, D.C., and Puerto Rico — advocating for local donations to children's hospitals. Medicaid and insurance programs do not cover the full cost of caring for kids. Children's hospitals rely on local donations to fund critical

treatments, equipment and charitable care for more than 10 million kids each year.

At Jordin's hospital, donations purchase the 20 (or more) daily heat packs that help increase Jordin's blood circulation and provide comfort during a pain crisis. Donations also fund a bladder scanner that doctors use to monitor Jordin's organs.

As an aspiring doctor, Jordin is already helping kids. She and her family raised $42,000 for her children's hospital to purchase a machine that allows doctors to monitor blood disorders faster and more efficiently.

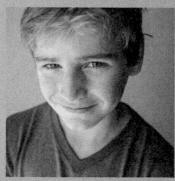

CHRISTOPHER
11 YEARS OLD
KIDNEY DISEASE PATIENT

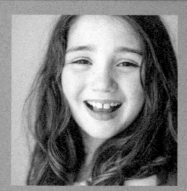

MORGAN
7 YEARS OLD
LEUKEMIA PATIENT

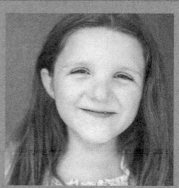

ELISE
6 YEARS OLD
JACOBSEN SYNDROME PATIENT

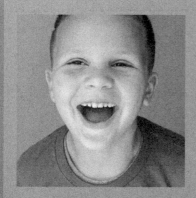

ANDREW
5 YEARS OLD
BRAIN TUMOR PATIENT

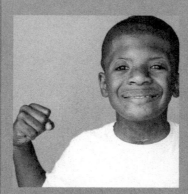

VICTOR
8 YEARS OLD
PIERRE ROBIN SYNDROME PATIENT

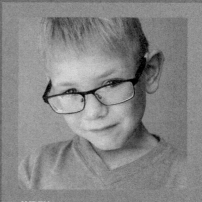

AYDEN
7 YEARS OLD
EXTREME PREMATURITY PATIENT

PHOTOS BY JUSTIN HACKWORTH

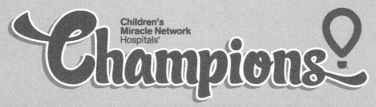

Children's Miracle Network Hospitals' **Champions**

The Children's Miracle Network Hospitals Champions program is possible thanks to these generous partners:

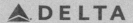
Give Today
to your children's hospital

Find your state's Champion and learn why children's hospitals need community support at *CMNHospitals.org.*

CARDIOLOGY & HEART SURGERY

Rank	Hospital	U.S. News score	Complex surgery survival score (24=best)	Norwood/ hybrid surgery survival score (12=best)	Overall infection prevention score (33=best)	ICU infection prevention score (10=best)	Surgery volume score (12=best)	Catheter procedure volume score (33=best)	Nurse-patient ratio (higher is better)	Nurse Magnet status	Specialists recom-mending
1	Boston Children's Hospital	100.0	22	10	30	6	12	33	3.9	Yes	85.7%
2	Texas Children's Hospital, Houston	98.3	22	11	32	7	10	31	3.3	Yes	64.2%
3	Children's Hospital of Philadelphia	87.9	18	9	33	3	11	28	3.2	Yes	80.4%
4	Children's Healthcare of Atlanta	85.1	19	9	33	6	10	32	4.2	No	36.8%
5	Lucile Packard Children's Hospital at Stanford, Palo Alto, Calif.	82.4	20	8	32	6	11	27	3.5	No	52.7%
6	Children's Hospital of Wisconsin, Milwaukee	81.9	17	12	29	8	9	14	4.2	Yes	25.3%
7	University of Michigan C.S. Mott Children's Hospital, Ann Arbor	81.7	17	10	26	6	11	23	3.6	No	52.0%
8	Cincinnati Children's Hospital Medical Center	81.3	21	9	31	6	8	22	3.1	Yes	36.0%
9	Nationwide Children's Hospital, Columbus, Ohio	79.3	19	10	31	7	8	27	3.0	Yes	26.3%
10	Children's Hospital Los Angeles	78.8	15	11	33	6	10	26	3.7	Yes	22.9%
11	Ann and Robert H. Lurie Children's Hospital of Chicago	77.6	23	9	31	7	6	16	3.5	Yes	13.3%
12	Children's Medical Center Dallas	77.5	22	12	33	7	8	24	3.0	Yes	3.6%
13	NY-Presby. Morgan Stanley-Komansky Children's Hosp., N.Y.	76.5	20	11	33	4	10	19	2.9	No	20.7%
14	Children's Hospital of Pittsburgh of UPMC	76.3	20	12	32	5	6	17	3.3	Yes	11.2%
15	Children's Hospital Colorado, Aurora	73.4	21	10	30	3	8	25	3.6	Yes	11.0%
16	Primary Children's Hospital, Salt Lake City	71.8	24	10	33	3	9	23	3.9	No	6.5%
17	Children's National Medical Center, Washington, D.C.	71.3	21	12	33	6	7	23	3.1	Yes	11.9%
18	Seattle Children's Hospital	71.0	18	7	33	6	8	20	2.9	Yes	9.6%
19	Monroe Carell Jr. Children's Hospital at Vanderbilt, Nashville	70.4	18	10	29	7	9	28	3.4	Yes	3.8%
20	MUSC Children's Heart Program of South Carolina, Charleston	70.3	19	10	31	8	7	20	2.7	Yes	10.9%
21	St. Louis Children's Hospital-Washington University	67.2	16	9	30	7	6	26	3.4	Yes	7.9%
22	Duke Children's Hospital and Health Center, Durham, N.C.	67.1	21	11	31	7	6	17	3.0	Yes	3.1%
23	Cleveland Clinic Children's Hospital	65.5	18	12	25	9	4	12	3.2	Yes	3.6%
24	UF Health Shands Children's Hospital, Gainesville, Fla.	64.3	22	11	30	7	5	10	2.6	Yes	1.6%
25	Mattel Children's Hospital UCLA, Los Angeles	64.0	17	7	29	5	5	28	3.8	Yes	6.0%
26	Phoenix Children's Hospital	62.4	21	10	29	6	8	27	3.3	No	3.0%
27	Mayo Clinic Children's Center, Rochester, Minn.	62.1	19	11	29	1	6	20	3.6	Yes	9.1%
28	Johns Hopkins Children's Center, Baltimore	61.7	16	9	28	7	5	12	3.1	Yes	3.0%
29	Riley Hospital for Children at IU Health, Indianapolis	60.2	16	9	29	4	7	17	3.1	Yes	3.1%
30	Johns Hopkins All Children's Hospital, St. Petersburg, Fla.	60.1	18	11	31	4	6	14	3.3	No	3.7%
30	University of Iowa Children's Hospital, Iowa City	60.1	18	11	28	6	4	14	2.9	Yes	0.3%
32	Rady Children's Hospital, San Diego	57.1	20	11	33	6	7	24	3.1	No	3.7%
33	Children's Hospital and Medical Center, Omaha	56.5	20	12	28	4	6	17	3.2	Yes	0.9%
34	SSM Health Cardinal Glennon Children's Hospital, St. Louis	56.2	20	10	28	4	6	13	2.9	No	0.7%
35	Levine Children's Hospital, Charlotte, N.C.	55.9	21	11	24	6	6	17	2.3	Yes	1.5%
36	Advocate Children's Heart Institute, Oak Lawn, Ill.	55.3	22	9	27	7	7	20	3.2	Yes	0.3%
37	University of Virginia Children's Hospital, Charlottesville	55.1	18	9	27	6	4	15	2.6	Yes	0.9%
38	UCSF Benioff Children's Hospitals, San Francisco and Oakland	54.6	16	9	31	5	6	22	3.0	Yes	7.2%
39	Le Bonheur Children's Hospital, Memphis	53.7	22	8	29	5	6	20	2.9	Yes	2.5%
40	Nicklaus Children's Hospital, Miami	53.6	19	10	29	5	6	26	3.0	Yes	5.7%
41	Children's Hospital of Alabama at UAB, Birmingham	53.1	17	8	26	8	6	21	3.0	No	1.5%
42	Children's Mercy Kansas City, Mo.	52.8	17	8	32	3	8	20	4.2	Magnet	2.8%
43	Children's Hospital at Montefiore, New York	52.1	17	3	33	7	4	13	3.6	No	1.4%
44	Holtz Children's Hospital at UM-Jackson Memorial Med. Cen., Miami	51.8	19	12	22	10	4	8	3.0	No	1.1%
45	Mount Sinai Kravis Children's Hospital, New York	51.6	19	7	32	5	4	15	3.5	Yes	0.7%
46	Children's Hospital of Michigan, Detroit	51.4	20	5	33	4	6	18	3.0	No	2.7%
47	Nemours Alfred I. duPont Hospital for Children, Wilmington, Del.	51.2	20	10	29	2	5	11	3.8	Yes	1.0%
48	Arnold Palmer Children's Hospital, Orlando, Fla.	51.1	20	12	26	8	4	17	3.2	Yes	0.5%
49	Joe DiMaggio Children's Hospital at Memorial, Hollywood, Fla.	49.5	15	7	28	5	4	15	3.4	No	0.6%
50	Rainbow Babies and Children's Hospital, Cleveland	48.4	16	8	30	10	4	9	3.1	Yes	1.6%

Terms are explained on Page 142.

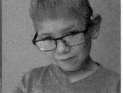

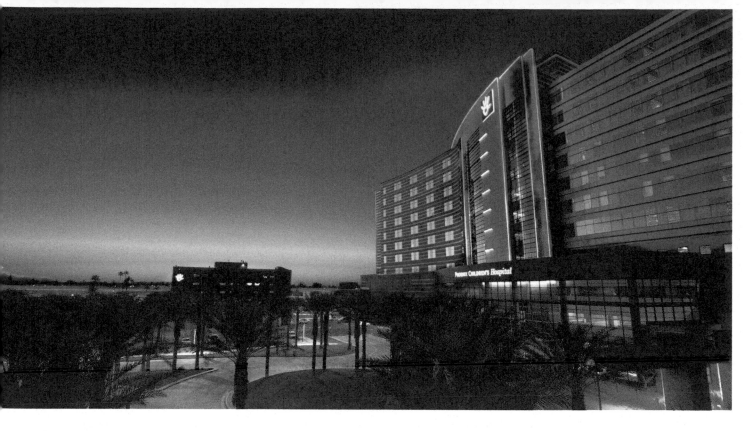

Arizona's only nationally ranked children's hospital lives in the heart of Phoenix.

Phoenix Children's Hospital provides the most comprehensive pediatric care in the Southwest region, capturing the attention of national experts like The Leapfrog Group and *U.S. News & World Report* in their 2016-17 Best Children's Hospitals ranking—one of only 25 hospitals in the country to be recognized in 10 out of 10 specialties.

With our deep expertise across more than 75 pediatric subspecialties, including Barrow Neurological Institute at Phoenix Children's and other elite programs in cancer, orthopedics, fetal and newborn

care, trauma, and cardiac services, we provide exceptional care for children with conditions from routine to rare.

Phoenix Children's is also a leader in the Cancer MoonShot 2020 Pediatrics Consortium, conducting breakthrough genomic research to accelerate lifesaving, personalized treatments for the very sickest children.

PhoenixChildrens.org

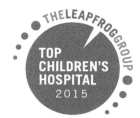
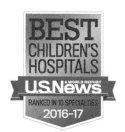
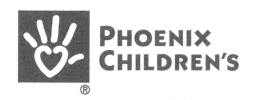

DIABETES & ENDOCRINOLOGY

Rank	Hospital	U.S. News score	Diabetes management score (36=best)	Hypothyroid management score (3=best)	Overall infection prevention score (28=best)	Patient volume score (48=best)	Procedure volume score (42=best)	Nurse-patient ratio (higher is better)	Nurse Magnet status	Best practices (108=best)	Specialists recommending
1	Children's Hospital of Philadelphia	100.0	31	3	28	45	40	3.2	Yes	104	69.6%
2	Boston Children's Hospital	96.2	29	3	23	47	40	3.9	Yes	100	69.3%
3	Cincinnati Children's Hospital Medical Center	92.4	30	3	25	45	32	3.1	Yes	103	38.2%
4	Children's Hospital Colorado, Aurora	89.7	28	3	24	43	38	3.6	Yes	97	39.8%
5	Children's Hospital of Pittsburgh of UPMC	89.3	27	3	27	44	37	3.3	Yes	104	32.6%
6	Seattle Children's Hospital	86.7	31	3	27	45	40	2.9	Yes	103	14.2%
7	Yale-New Haven Children's Hospital, New Haven, Conn.	86.1	32	3	22	40	35	2.4	Yes	105	25.1%
8	Children's Hospital Los Angeles	86.0	33	2	26	48	31	3.7	Yes	96	28.7%
9	NY-Presby. Morgan Stanley-Komansky Children's Hosp., N.Y.	85.9	33	3	28	43	32	2.9	No	106	16.5%
10	UCSF Benioff Children's Hospitals, San Francisco and Oakland	85.0	29	3	24	45	33	3.0	Yes	101	18.6%
11	Texas Children's Hospital, Houston	84.1	27	3	26	43	35	3.3	Yes	95	21.9%
12	Lucile Packard Children's Hospital at Stanford, Palo Alto, Calif.	82.1	32	3	26	34	22	3.5	No	93	16.7%
13	Children's National Medical Center, Washington, D.C.	80.0	29	3	27	43	31	3.1	Yes	103	3.9%
14	Nationwide Children's Hospital, Columbus, Ohio	79.8	26	3	26	46	32	3.0	Yes	98	12.0%
15	Johns Hopkins Children's Center, Baltimore	76.6	26	3	23	33	23	3.1	Yes	99	20.3%
16	Rady Children's Hospital, San Diego	76.3	33	3	26	43	28	3.1	No	98	3.0%
17	Children's Healthcare of Atlanta	75.6	30	3	27	44	38	4.2	No	89	2.7%
18	Mayo Clinic Children's Center, Rochester, Minn.	75.0	31	3	22	32	32	3.6	Yes	94	3.5%
18	UF Health Shands Children's Hospital, Gainesville, Fla.	75.0	26	3	25	29	20	2.6	Yes	100	9.1%
20	Riley Hospital for Children at IU Health, Indianapolis	74.9	23	3	22	43	31	3.1	Yes	95	14.5%
21	Mattel Children's Hospital UCLA, Los Angeles	74.8	30	3	24	26	31	3.8	Yes	105	5.4%
22	Rainbow Babies and Children's Hospital, Cleveland	74.7	25	3	25	39	26	3.1	Yes	107	5.2%
23	University of Iowa Children's Hospital, Iowa City	73.5	31	3	24	33	23	2.9	Yes	89	1.6%
24	North Carolina Children's Hospital at UNC, Chapel Hill	73.4	26	3	28	38	27	3.8	Yes	100	3.4%
25	Children's Medical Center Dallas	73.3	24	3	26	44	32	3.0	Yes	83	8.5%
26	Duke Children's Hospital and Health Center, Durham, N.C.	73.1	26	3	23	39	29	3.0	Yes	100	4.7%
27	Ann and Robert H. Lurie Children's Hospital of Chicago	72.6	25	3	24	44	27	3.5	Yes	91	4.8%
28	Children's Mercy Kansas City, Mo.	72.5	22	3	25	48	32	4.2	Yes	97	3.2%
29	University of California Davis Children's Hospital, Sacramento	72.0	30	3	26	28	18	6.0	Yes	104	0.9%
29	Winthrop-Univ. Hosp. Children's Medical Center, Mineola, N.Y.	72.0	33	3	26	30	11	4.2	No	106	1.2%
31	Monroe Carell Jr. Children's Hospital at Vanderbilt, Nashville	71.5	24	3	23	42	26	3.4	Yes	89	5.2%
32	Akron Children's Hospital, Ohio	71.2	29	3	26	37	27	3.2	Yes	100	2.0%
33	Children's Hospital of Alabama at UAB, Birmingham	70.9	31	3	21	42	34	3.0	No	96	1.3%
33	MassGeneral Hospital for Children, Boston	70.9	30	3	18	29	21	3.0	Yes	91	8.0%
33	Phoenix Children's Hospital	70.9	29	3	23	45	35	3.3	No	105	1.8%
36	Holtz Children's Hospital at UM-Jackson Memorial Med. Cen., Miami	70.7	36	3	19	34	34	3.0	No	106	1.6%
37	Nicklaus Children's Hospital, Miami	70.6	29	3	24	39	18	3.0	Yes	102	3.3%
38	Mount Sinai Kravis Children's Hospital, New York	70.4	23	3	27	40	33	3.5	Yes	106	2.8%
39	Children's Hospital of Wisconsin, Milwaukee	69.6	26	3	22	34	26	4.2	Yes	91	2.9%
40	CHOC Children's Hospital, Orange, Calif.	68.9	26	3	26	44	31	2.9	Yes	90	2.4%
41	Doernbecher Children's Hospital, Portland, Ore.	68.7	25	3	24	34	27	3.4	Nurse	87	6.0%
42	St. Louis Children's Hospital-Washington University	68.3	22	3	22	40	24	3.4	Yes	83	5.2%
43	Children's Hospital at Montefiore, New York	67.4	20	3	28	36	25	3.6	No	105	2.4%
44	Primary Children's Hospital, Salt Lake City	66.8	29	3	26	37	20	3.9	No	80	0.0%
45	Arnold Palmer Children's Hospital, Orlando, Fla.	66.2	28	3	20	37	33	3.2	Yes	104	0.5%
46	Cleveland Clinic Children's Hospital	65.9	25	3	20	39	29	3.2	Yes	91	1.1%
47	Medical Univ. of South Carolina Children's Hosp., Charleston	65.0	28	3	23	31	18	2.7	Yes	100	1.5%
48	Kosair Children's Hospital, Louisville, Ky.	64.3	23	3	25	40	26	2.1	Yes	91	0.9%
49	Children's Hospitals and Clinics of Minnesota, Minneapolis	64.2	32	3	19	40	21	3.4	No	83	0.7%
50	Cook Children's Medical Center, Fort Worth	64.1	25	3	20	45	28	3.4	Yes	93	2.1%

Terms are explained on Page 142.

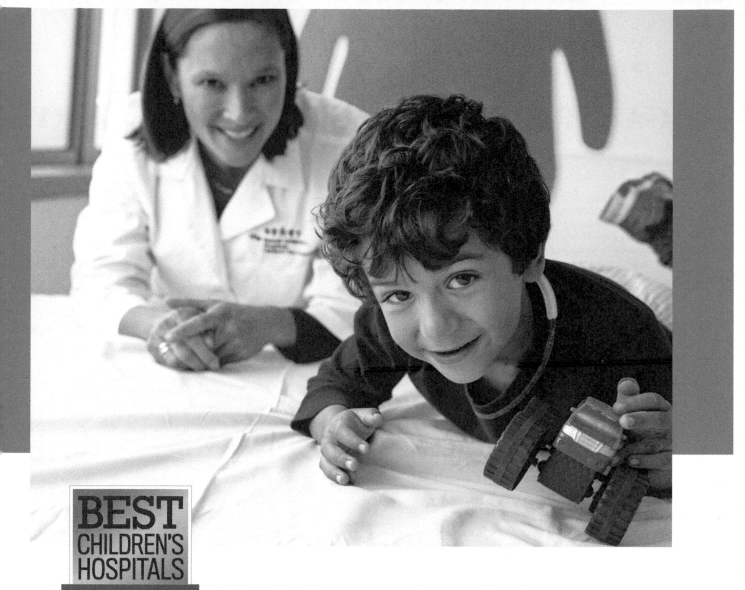

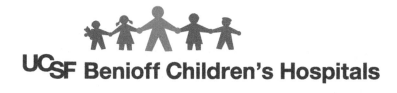

GASTROENTEROLOGY & GI SURGERY

Rank	Hospital	U.S. News score	Selected treatments success score (9=best)	Liver transplant survival score (6=best)	Overall infection prevention score (34=best)	ICU infection prevention score (10=best)	Patient volume score (63=best)	Surgery volume score (16=best)	Nonsurgical procedure volume score (24=best)	Nurse-patient ratio (higher is better)	Nurse Magnet status	Specialists recom-mending
1	Boston Children's Hospital	100.0	7	6	31	6	62	13	22	3.9	Yes	70.9%
2	Cincinnati Children's Hospital Medical Center	94.5	8	4	32	6	60	15	21	3.1	Yes	71.7%
3	Children's Hospital of Philadelphia	92.5	7	5	34	3	63	15	24	3.2	Yes	68.4%
4	Ann and Robert H. Lurie Children's Hospital of Chicago	90.8	8	6	32	7	59	13	16	3.5	Yes	21.2%
5	Children's Hospital of Pittsburgh of UPMC	90.0	9	5	32	5	63	16	10	3.3	Yes	29.6%
6	Texas Children's Hospital, Houston	89.5	6	5	33	7	55	14	22	3.3	Yes	42.1%
7	Children's Medical Center Dallas	85.0	8	6	34	7	56	14	18	3.0	Yes	7.4%
8	Nationwide Children's Hospital, Columbus, Ohio	84.2	9	NA	32	7	60	16	14	3.0	Yes	49.4%
9	Children's Hospital Los Angeles	83.3	8	6	34	6	52	13	22	3.7	Yes	13.0%
10	Children's Hospital Colorado, Aurora	82.3	7	4	30	3	52	14	20	3.6	Yes	37.8%
11	Children's Healthcare of Atlanta	82.0	8	5	34	6	63	15	21	4.2	No	8.4%
12	Children's National Medical Center, Washington, D.C.	77.7	7	6	34	6	43	16	13	3.1	Yes	4.2%
13	Seattle Children's Hospital	77.0	5	6	32	6	52	10	13	2.9	Yes	19.9%
13	St. Louis Children's Hospital-Washington University	77.0	8	5	31	7	36	11	13	3.4	Yes	9.1%
15	Riley Hospital for Children at IU Health, Indianapolis	76.6	9	6	30	4	52	12	17	3.1	Yes	5.0%
16	Johns Hopkins Children's Center, Baltimore	76.4	8	2	29	7	57	14	21	3.1	Yes	11.7%
17	Lucile Packard Children's Hospital at Stanford, Palo Alto, Calif.	75.5	6	6	32	6	55	15	12	3.5	No	13.3%
18	UCSF Benioff Children's Hospitals, San Francisco and Oakland	73.2	5	6	29	5	51	13	11	3.0	Yes	9.6%
19	Cleveland Clinic Children's Hospital	72.5	6	4	26	9	49	13	15	3.2	Yes	8.9%
20	Children's Hospital of Wisconsin, Milwaukee	70.8	7	2	29	8	50	10	20	4.2	Yes	6.8%
21	NY-Presby. Morgan Stanley-Komansky Children's Hosp., N.Y.	70.7	7	5	34	4	54	13	15	2.9	No	6.8%
22	MassGeneral Hospital for Children, Boston	70.6	5	6	27	9	49	7	10	3.0	Yes	5.4%
22	Monroe Carell Jr. Children's Hospital at Vanderbilt, Nashville	70.6	9	1	30	7	49	10	17	3.4	Yes	2.3%
22	Nemours Alfred I. duPont Hosp. for Children, Wilmington, Del.	70.6	8	4	31	2	45	12	8	3.8	Yes	2.3%
25	Mattel Children's Hospital UCLA, Los Angeles	68.7	6	4	30	5	34	9	12	3.8	Yes	9.9%
26	University of Michigan C.S. Mott Children's Hospital, Ann Arbor	67.9	7	6	27	6	52	9	13	3.6	No	2.9%
27	Mount Sinai Kravis Children's Hospital, New York	67.7	8	3	33	5	34	9	9	3.5	Yes	3.5%
28	Rady Children's Hospital, San Diego	66.4	8	3	33	6	42	14	14	3.1	No	3.1%
29	Children's Mercy Kansas City, Mo.	65.9	5	6	31	3	53	11	11	4.2	Yes	3.1%
30	Children's Hospital at Montefiore, New York	65.1	6	6	34	7	29	11	8	3.6	No	2.5%
31	Rainbow Babies and Children's Hospital, Cleveland	64.4	8	0	31	10	44	10	13	3.1	Yes	2.8%
32	North Carolina Children's Hospital at UNC, Chapel Hill	63.9	7	3	34	7	33	9	11	3.8	Yes	1.7%
33	Primary Children's Hospital, Salt Lake City	63.5	7	5	32	3	53	13	13	3.9	No	1.4%
34	American Family Children's Hospital, Madison, Wis.	62.4	6	6	25	8	19	8	6	4.6	Yes	0.3%
35	SSM Health Cardinal Glennon Children's Hospital, St. Louis	61.6	7	6	28	4	25	11	8	2.9	No	0.7%
36	Duke Children's Hospital and Health Center, Durham, N.C.	61.2	6	6	31	7	27	9	8	3.0	Yes	2.6%
37	Steven & Alexandra Cohen Children's Hosp., New Hyde Park, N.Y.	59.6	8	NA	33	8	40	10	13	3.3	No	1.3%
38	Yale-New Haven Children's Hospital, New Haven, Conn.	59.4	6	6	28	2	21	10	6	2.4	Yes	1.8%
39	Medical Univ. of South Carolina Children's Hosp., Charleston	58.5	6	4	29	8	29	7	7	2.7	Yes	1.2%
40	UF Health Shands Children's Hospital, Gainesville, Fla.	58.3	6	3	31	7	22	8	9	2.6	Yes	0.8%
41	University of Minnesota Masonic Children's Hospital, Minneapolis	56.9	6	5	19	7	33	14	10	2.8	No	1.2%
42	Phoenix Children's Hospital	56.1	6	2	30	6	41	13	17	3.3	No	2.2%
43	Children's Hospital and Medical Center, Omaha	54.7	9	NA	24	4	31	14	9	3.2	Yes	2.3%
44	Le Bonheur Children's Hospital, Memphis	54.4	5	3	30	5	31	8	8	2.9	Yes	0.8%
45	Arnold Palmer Children's Hospital, Orlando, Fla.	53.0	6	NA	27	8	42	11	15	3.2	Yes	0.5%
46	Wolfson Children's Hospital, Jacksonville, Fla.	52.6	9	NA	21	3	32	12	13	2.0	Yes	0.7%
47	Mayo Clinic Children's Center, Rochester, Minn.	52.1	5	2	27	1	36	9	13	3.6	Yes	3.3%
47	Nicklaus Children's Hospital, Miami	52.1	8	NA	30	5	36	14	8	3.0	Yes	2.5%
49	CHOC Children's Hospital, Orange, Calif.	51.9	6	NA	32	8	49	11	14	2.9	Yes	0.7%
50	Children's Hospital of Alabama at UAB, Birmingham	50.8	7	1	25	8	44	14	11	3.0	No	0.7%

NA=not applicable. Terms are explained on Page 142.

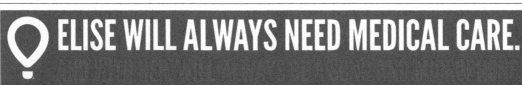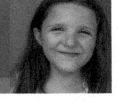

Give them tomorrow

Premature birth is the #1 killer of babies. Every baby deserves a fighting chance.

DO SOMETHING TODAY

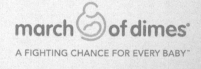
march of dimes
A FIGHTING CHANCE FOR EVERY BABY™

marchofdimes.org/tomorrow

© 2016 March of Dimes Foundation

Thank you to our partners who help save babies' lives.

  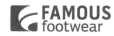 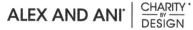

NEONATOLOGY

Rank	Hospital	U.S. News score	Breast milk score (3=best)	Readmissions prevention score (3=best)	Overall infection prevention score (25=best)	NICU infection prevention score (5=best)	Patient volume score (30=best)	Nurse-patient ratio (higher is better)	Nurse Magnet status	Best practices (81=best)	Specialists recommending
1	Boston Children's Hospital	100.0	3	3	22	3	23	3.8	Yes	80	52.7%
2	Children's Hospital of Philadelphia	99.4	3	3	25	2	30	3.6	Yes	78	57.4%
3	Children's National Medical Center, Washington, D.C.	97.5	3	3	25	5	27	2.9	Yes	78	19.6%
4	Rainbow Babies and Children's Hospital, Cleveland	92.9	3	3	22	4	17	3.8	Yes	78	29.0%
5	Seattle Children's Hospital	88.0	3	3	25	3	26	3.6	Yes	71	16.4%
6	Ann & Robert H. Lurie Children's Hosp.-Prentice Women's Hosp.,Chicago	84.9	3	2	23	4	19	3.1	Yes	71	12.7%
7	Children's Hospital Los Angeles	84.5	2	2	24	4	25	4.0	Yes	75	16.2%
8	Children's Hospital of Pittsburgh of UPMC	84.2	3	3	24	4	20	3.0	Yes	77	12.1%
9	NY-Presby. Morgan Stanley-Komansky Children's Hosp., N.Y.	83.7	3	3	25	3	23	2.5	No	75	18.6%
10	Nationwide Children's Hospital, Columbus, Ohio	81.9	2	3	23	5	26	2.7	Yes	73	15.5%
11	Children's Hospital of Wisconsin, Milwaukee	80.9	3	3	22	5	19	2.5	Yes	76	1.4%
12	Cincinnati Children's Hospital Medical Center	80.8	3	2	22	1	29	3.6	Yes	79	42.7%
13	St. Louis Children's Hospital-Washington University	80.6	3	3	23	3	22	3.1	Yes	74	12.9%
14	Texas Children's Hospital, Houston	80.5	3	3	25	1	28	3.0	Yes	78	27.7%
15	Duke Children's Hospital and Health Center, Durham, N.C.	78.8	2	2	23	5	22	2.5	Yes	72	9.3%
16	Children's Healthcare of Atlanta	77.7	2	3	25	4	27	3.1	No	74	7.1%
17	UCSF Benioff Children's Hospitals, San Francisco and Oakland	77.5	3	3	23	1	27	3.4	Yes	76	13.9%
18	Rady Children's Hospital, San Diego	76.8	3	3	25	3	24	3.0	No	72	6.7%
19	Johns Hopkins Children's Center, Baltimore	76.5	2	2	19	3	26	2.9	Yes	66	28.2%
19	University of California Davis Children's Hospital, Sacramento	76.5	3	3	24	4	23	3.0	Yes	76	0.5%
21	Lucile Packard Children's Hospital at Stanford, Palo Alto, Calif.	76.2	3	2	23	1	22	4.0	No	74	27.8%
22	Children's Mercy Kansas City, Mo.	75.8	2	3	24	3	26	3.9	Yes	77	6.7%
23	UF Health Shands Children's Hospital, Gainesville, Fla.	75.0	2	3	22	4	17	2.8	Yes	75	1.5%
24	Akron Children's Hospital, Ohio	73.9	2	3	24	5	16	3.2	Yes	75	1.6%
25	Nicklaus Children's Hospital, Miami	73.3	2	3	21	4	17	3.2	Yes	69	5.4%
26	Children's Hospital Colorado, Aurora	73.0	3	2	22	1	25	3.3	Yes	77	19.8%
26	Monroe Carell Jr. Children's Hospital at Vanderbilt, Nashville	73.0	2	3	21	4	22	2.7	Yes	72	5.0%
28	University of Iowa Children's Hospital, Iowa City	71.5	3	3	22	3	17	2.5	Yes	66	4.9%
29	Steven & Alexandra Cohen Children's Hosp., New Hyde Park, N.Y.	71.1	3	3	24	5	17	2.5	No	74	0.4%
30	Doernbecher Children's Hospital, Portland, Ore.	70.8	3	3	22	3	16	2.5	Yes	76	1.4%
30	University of Minnesota Masonic Children's Hospital, Minneapolis	70.8	3	3	12	5	17	3.2	No	69	3.0%
32	CHOC Children's Hospital, Orange, Calif.	70.7	3	3	22	3	18	2.6	Yes	79	1.8%
33	University of Michigan C.S. Mott Children's Hospital, Ann Arbor	68.9	3	2	18	5	22	2.7	No	67	5.3%
34	Children's Medical Center Dallas-Parkland Memorial Hospital	68.1	2	3	25	3	22	2.3	Yes	74	3.8%
35	Riley Hospital for Children at IU Health, Indianapolis	67.4	3	3	21	1	26	2.8	Yes	68	4.9%
36	Primary Children's Hospital, Salt Lake City	67.0	2	2	25	3	30	2.9	No	77	3.2%
37	Mattel Children's Hospital UCLA, Los Angeles	66.9	3	3	21	1	13	4.0	Yes	76	3.9%
38	University of Virginia Children's Hospital, Charlottesville	66.3	2	3	19	4	15	2.6	Yes	70	0.9%
39	Johns Hopkins All Children's Hospital, St. Petersburg, Fla.	66.0	3	3	23	3	15	2.6	No	73	3.1%
40	North Carolina Children's Hospital at UNC, Chapel Hill	65.2	2	3	25	3	20	2.7	Yes	70	1.6%
41	Phoenix Children's Hospital	64.0	3	3	21	3	24	2.9	No	73	0.3%
42	Cook Children's Medical Center, Fort Worth	63.6	2	2	19	5	18	3.0	Yes	62	2.1%
43	Penn State Children's Hospital, Hershey, Pa.	63.2	2	2	19	4	17	2.6	Yes	70	1.1%
44	Kosair Children's Hospital, Louisville, Ky.	62.9	2	2	24	4	20	2.0	Yes	70	1.4%
45	Inova Children's Hospital, Falls Church, Va.	62.8	3	3	19	4	13	2.8	No	69	3.4%
46	Arkansas Children's Hospital, Little Rock	61.0	2	2	20	4	25	2.4	No	67	1.5%
47	Yale-New Haven Children's Hospital, New Haven, Conn.	60.9	2	2	19	4	14	2.5	Yes	72	1.5%
48	Children's Hospital at Montefiore, New York	60.0	2	2	25	4	10	2.5	No	75	0.9%
49	Valley Children's Healthcare and Hospital, Madera, Calif.	59.9	2	2	23	4	21	2.6	Yes	65	1.1%
50	Children's Hospital of Alabama at UAB, Birmingham	59.7	3	3	18	1	24	3.2	No	74	4.3%

Terms are explained on Page 142.

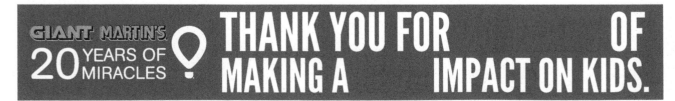

Here, this is
HUGE

Abnormalities in a gene called MLL cause 70 percent of infant leukemia and often result in a devastating prognosis for children of all ages. Hematologist-oncologist Kathrin Bernt, MD, helped discover a way to block MLL, and trials based on her research completely eradicated leukemia in some patients. Now, her team is looking for a way to completely eradicate it in every patient.

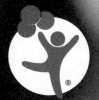

Children's Hospital Colorado
Here, it's different.™

BEST CHILDREN'S HOSPITALS
U.S.News & WORLD REPORT
HONOR ROLL 2016–17

100+
Years Dedicated to Kids

TOP 10
Hospital in the Nation

2000+
Pediatric Specialists

3x
Magnet Recognized

NEPHROLOGY

Rank	Hospital	U.S. News score	Kidney transplant survival score (24=best)	Biopsy complications prevention score (6=best)	Dialysis management score (20=best)	Overall infection prevention score (49=best)	ICU infection prevention score (10=best)	Dialysis infection prevention score (9=best)	Patient volume score (36=best)	Nurse-patient ratio (higher is better)	Nurse Magnet status	Specialists recommending
1	Boston Children's Hospital	100.0	24	5	19	46	6	9	31	3.9	Yes	63.8%
2	Cincinnati Children's Hospital Medical Center	96.8	24	6	18	47	6	9	35	3.1	Yes	64.6%
3	Texas Children's Hospital, Houston	94.9	24	6	18	48	7	8	29	3.3	Yes	40.5%
4	Seattle Children's Hospital	93.4	23	6	20	49	6	7	36	2.9	Yes	52.6%
5	Lucile Packard Children's Hospital at Stanford, Palo Alto, Calif.	91.6	24	6	20	48	6	9	30	3.5	No	36.8%
6	Children's Mercy Kansas City, Mo.	90.8	24	6	20	48	3	9	32	4.2	Yes	26.9%
7	Children's Hospital of Philadelphia	90.0	23	6	15	49	3	7	36	3.2	Yes	52.4%
8	Mattel Children's Hospital UCLA, Los Angeles	88.1	23	6	18	45	5	9	28	3.8	Yes	26.4%
9	Children's Healthcare of Atlanta	86.7	24	6	15	49	6	9	33	4.2	No	23.9%
10	Ann and Robert H. Lurie Children's Hospital of Chicago	85.4	21	6	20	47	7	6	29	3.5	Yes	15.8%
11	Children's Medical Center Dallas	84.7	23	6	19	49	7	8	27	3.0	Yes	12.1%
12	Nationwide Children's Hospital, Columbus, Ohio	82.8	23	4	20	47	7	7	30	3.0	Yes	20.4%
13	Children's National Medical Center, Washington, D.C.	81.9	22	6	18	49	6	9	29	3.1	Yes	6.3%
14	Johns Hopkins Children's Center, Baltimore	80.0	23	6	18	43	7	4	21	3.1	Yes	15.3%
15	Children's Hospital of Pittsburgh of UPMC	78.4	24	6	14	46	5	8	28	3.3	Yes	14.5%
16	UCSF Benioff Children's Hospitals, San Francisco and Oakland	77.0	24	5	17	47	5	7	27	3.0	Yes	7.4%
17	Children's Hospital at Montefiore, New York	76.4	23	6	18	49	7	7	24	3.6	No	7.9%
18	Children's Hospital of Wisconsin, Milwaukee	76.3	24	6	17	44	8	7	27	4.2	Yes	3.4%
19	Phoenix Children's Hospital	75.1	24	6	18	44	6	9	31	3.3	No	2.8%
20	Rady Children's Hospital, San Diego	73.1	24	6	15	48	6	9	30	3.1	No	4.1%
21	Rainbow Babies and Children's Hospital, Cleveland	72.7	20	6	17	46	10	5	35	3.1	Yes	2.8%
22	Medical Univ. of South Carolina Children's Hosp., Charleston	72.2	23	6	18	47	8	9	27	2.7	Yes	0.7%
23	University of Michigan C.S. Mott Children's Hospital, Ann Arbor	71.8	22	5	16	42	6	7	27	3.6	No	9.6%
24	Children's Hospital Los Angeles	71.7	24	6	10	45	6	7	28	3.7	Yes	7.8%
25	American Family Children's Hospital, Madison, Wis.	71.5	24	6	19	38	8	9	22	4.6	Yes	1.1%
26	University of Iowa Children's Hospital, Iowa City	71.4	20	6	14	45	6	6	30	2.9	Yes	9.4%
27	Doernbecher Children's Hospital, Portland, Ore.	71.0	23	6	18	46	8	7	34	3.4	Yes	1.2%
28	Children's Hospital of Alabama at UAB, Birmingham	70.8	23	6	19	42	8	7	34	3.0	No	2.9%
29	Mount Sinai Kravis Children's Hospital, New York	70.4	23	6	20	48	5	5	24	3.5	Yes	2.2%
30	Monroe Carell Jr. Children's Hospital at Vanderbilt, Nashville	70.3	20	4	17	44	7	9	29	3.4	Yes	1.4%
31	Le Bonheur Children's Hospital, Memphis	69.8	20	6	13	45	5	7	27	2.9	Yes	5.4%
32	Nemours Alfred I. duPont Hosp. for Children, Wilmington, Del.	68.6	24	6	15	44	2	6	23	3.8	Yes	2.4%
32	UF Health Shands Children's Hospital, Gainesville, Fla.	68.6	23	6	15	44	7	5	23	2.6	Yes	0.9%
34	Riley Hospital for Children at IU Health, Indianapolis	68.5	23	6	15	44	4	7	27	3.1	Yes	3.3%
34	St. Louis Children's Hospital-Washington University	68.5	21	6	14	46	7	5	23	3.4	Yes	3.3%
36	Children's Hospital Colorado, Aurora	67.5	24	6	12	45	3	7	27	3.6	Yes	2.0%
37	Children's Memorial Hermann Hospital, Houston	67.4	22	6	20	41	6	8	20	2.6	Yes	1.0%
37	Cleveland Clinic Children's Hospital	67.4	10	6	18	41	9	9	23	3.2	Yes	1.3%
37	Duke Children's Hospital and Health Center, Durham, N.C.	67.4	24	6	14	47	7	9	24	3.0	Yes	2.1%
40	Levine Children's Hospital, Charlotte, N.C.	66.8	21	6	19	41	6	8	27	2.3	Yes	1.9%
41	University of Minnesota Masonic Children's Hospital, Minneapolis	66.7	23	6	17	36	7	6	29	2.8	No	5.7%
42	Primary Children's Hospital, Salt Lake City	66.3	23	6	17	48	3	5	30	3.9	No	1.3%
43	Univ. of California Davis Children's Hospital, Sacramento	66.1	22	5	10	47	7	9	24	6.0	Yes	1.0%
44	North Carolina Children's Hospital at UNC, Chapel Hill	65.9	24	6	17	43	7	5	29	3.8	Yes	0.8%
45	Children's Hospital of Michigan, Detroit	65.4	16	6	18	49	4	8	24	3.0	No	2.5%
45	Holtz Children's Hospital at UM-Jackson Memorial Med. Cen., Miami	65.4	23	6	20	38	10	8	22	3.0	No	1.4%
47	NY-Presby. Morgan Stanley-Komansky Children's Hosp., N.Y.	65.1	24	6	14	48	4	8	18	2.9	No	0.6%
48	Spectrum Hlth. Helen DeVos Children's Hosp., Grand Rapids, Mich.	63.6	24	6	10	46	4	9	27	2.6	Yes	0.1%
49	University of Virginia Children's Hospital, Charlottesville	63.2	24	6	13	40	6	9	18	2.6	Yes	1.0%
50	MassGeneral Hospital for Children, Boston	62.7	18	6	15	42	9	8	29	3.0	Yes	1.2%

Terms are explained on Page 142.

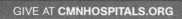
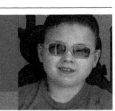

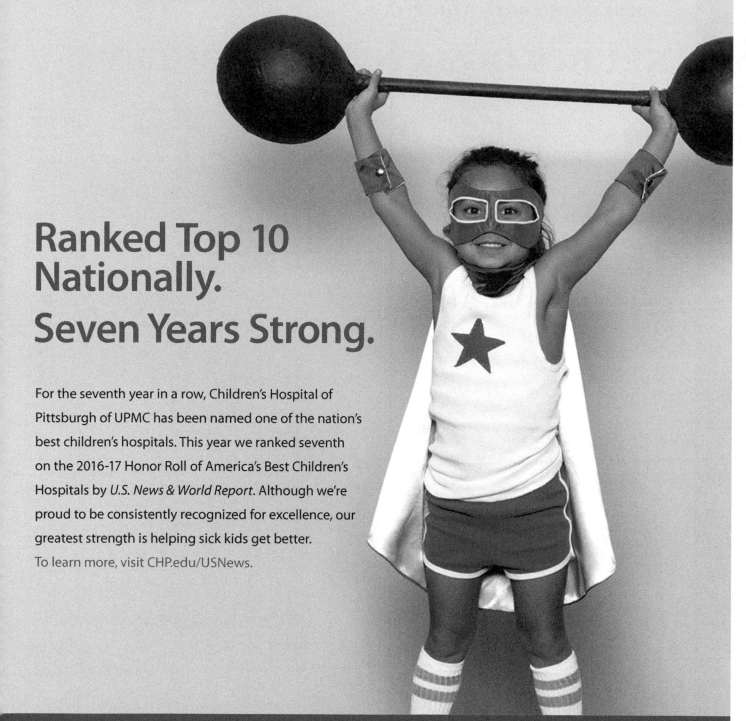

Ranked Top 10 Nationally.
Seven Years Strong.

For the seventh year in a row, Children's Hospital of Pittsburgh of UPMC has been named one of the nation's best children's hospitals. This year we ranked seventh on the 2016-17 Honor Roll of America's Best Children's Hospitals by *U.S. News & World Report*. Although we're proud to be consistently recognized for excellence, our greatest strength is helping sick kids get better.

To learn more, visit CHP.edu/USNews.

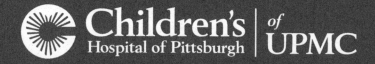
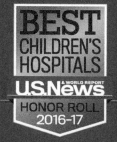

NEUROLOGY & NEUROSURGERY

Rank	Hospital	U.S. News score	Surgical survival score (14=best)	Surgical complications prevention score (22=best)	Epilepsy manage-ment score (10=best)	Overall infection prevention score (32=best)	Clinic patient volume score (60=best)	Surgery volume score (45=best)	Nurse-patient ratio (higher is better)	Nurse Magnet status	Specialists recom-mending
1	Boston Children's Hospital	100.0	12	21	9	29	60	40	3.9	Yes	68.6%
2	Texas Children's Hospital, Houston	97.8	14	22	10	30	57	35	3.3	Yes	33.5%
3	Children's Hospital of Philadelphia	95.2	14	20	7	32	56	38	3.2	Yes	56.1%
4	Cincinnati Children's Hospital Medical Center	93.0	14	20	8	30	58	34	3.1	Yes	32.1%
5	St. Louis Children's Hospital-Washington University	87.4	12	17	10	30	49	26	3.4	Yes	29.6%
6	Ann and Robert H. Lurie Children's Hospital of Chicago	87.1	12	22	7	30	50	35	3.5	Yes	19.9%
7	Johns Hopkins Children's Center, Baltimore	86.6	12	19	8	27	48	30	3.1	Yes	35.6%
8	Children's National Medical Center, Washington, D.C.	85.9	12	18	8	32	60	32	3.1	Yes	21.6%
9	Seattle Children's Hospital	84.8	11	17	9	32	55	28	2.9	Yes	26.7%
10	Primary Children's Hospital, Salt Lake City	84.6	14	19	10	31	52	28	3.9	No	10.8%
11	Children's Hospital of Pittsburgh of UPMC	83.5	13	20	7	29	47	37	3.3	Yes	12.4%
12	Monroe Carell Jr. Children's Hospital at Vanderbilt, Nashville	83.4	14	20	10	28	49	27	3.4	Yes	4.9%
13	Nicklaus Children's Hospital, Miami	83.1	12	22	8	28	56	31	3.0	Yes	13.6%
14	Nationwide Children's Hospital, Columbus, Ohio	82.8	12	21	6	30	54	27	3.0	Yes	21.5%
15	Children's Hospital Colorado, Aurora	82.6	11	20	7	28	52	30	3.6	Yes	19.1%
16	Children's Hospital Los Angeles	82.0	12	19	8	31	54	32	3.7	Yes	10.9%
17	Le Bonheur Children's Hospital, Memphis	81.1	12	21	9	28	40	24	2.9	Yes	7.7%
18	Children's Medical Center Dallas	80.5	12	21	9	32	50	33	3.0	Yes	3.4%
19	Cleveland Clinic Children's Hospital	79.6	12	19	8	24	55	29	3.2	Yes	19.6%
20	Phoenix Children's Hospital	78.5	12	21	10	28	48	34	3.3	No	4.1%
21	UCSF Benioff Children's Hospitals, San Francisco and Oakland	78.4	12	14	7	30	49	27	3.0	Yes	19.6%
22	Rady Children's Hospital, San Diego	77.4	11	22	10	32	53	41	3.1	No	2.7%
23	NY-Presby. Morgan Stanley-Komansky Children's Hospital, N.Y.	75.5	12	21	7	31	31	28	2.9	No	8.4%
24	Children's Hospital of Wisconsin, Milwaukee	75.2	14	15	9	28	52	27	4.2	Yes	1.1%
25	Duke Children's Hospital and Health Center, Durham, N.C.	74.1	11	18	10	30	37	33	3.0	Yes	1.8%
26	Children's Healthcare of Atlanta	73.9	12	17	8	32	48	34	4.2	No	2.6%
27	Rainbow Babies and Children's Hospital, Cleveland	73.7	12	16	8	29	46	19	3.1	Yes	7.6%
28	Mayo Clinic Children's Center, Rochester, Minn.	73.6	12	19	7	27	34	21	3.6	Yes	7.3%
29	Children's Hospital of Alabama at UAB, Birmingham	73.1	12	18	9	23	43	31	3.0	No	10.1%
30	Mount Sinai Kravis Children's Hospital, New York	73.0	12	22	8	30	28	22	3.5	Yes	0.2%
31	Mattel Children's Hospital UCLA, Los Angeles	71.7	12	19	5	27	32	12	3.8	Yes	10.1%
32	Doernbecher Children's Hospital, Portland, Ore.	70.9	12	17	8	29	39	24	3.4	Yes	0.8%
33	Children's Hospital of Michigan, Detroit	70.7	12	16	9	31	48	27	3.0	No	1.9%
34	Children's Hospital at Montefiore, New York	69.8	12	20	4	32	46	18	3.6	No	3.5%
35	Riley Hospital for Children at IU Health, Indianapolis	69.7	11	18	6	28	41	36	3.1	Yes	2.0%
36	University of Michigan C.S. Mott Children's Hospital, Ann Arbor	69.0	14	21	7	25	29	20	3.6	No	3.4%
37	Cook Children's Medical Center, Fort Worth	68.9	12	20	6	26	38	31	3.4	Yes	3.3%
37	Lucile Packard Children's Hospital at Stanford, Palo Alto, Calif.	68.9	10	17	5	31	47	19	3.5	No	11.0%
39	Steven & Alexandra Cohen Children's Hosp., New Hyde Park, N.Y.	68.8	12	22	7	31	33	28	3.3	No	1.6%
40	CHOC Children's Hospital, Orange, Calif.	68.6	9	14	10	30	36	28	2.9	Yes	2.3%
41	Children's Mercy Kansas City, Mo.	68.4	11	15	5	31	47	32	4.2	Nurse	1.1%
42	Akron Children's Hospital, Ohio	67.2	12	17	6	31	49	27	3.2	Yes	1.2%
43	Kosair Children's Hospital, Louisville, Ky.	65.3	12	21	4	31	31	22	2.1	Yes	1.0%
44	Children's Memorial Hermann Hospital, Houston	64.6	14	21	7	24	3	25	2.6	Yes	0.5%
45	MassGeneral Hospital for Children, Boston	64.0	12	17	4	24	32	18	3.0	Yes	4.3%
46	UF Health Shands Children's Hospital, Gainesville, Fla.	63.8	12	18	6	29	25	16	2.6	Yes	0.2%
47	Yale-New Haven Children's Hospital, New Haven, Conn.	63.5	10	21	6	26	27	14	2.4	Yes	1.5%
48	Wolfson Children's Hospital, Jacksonville, Fla.	63.4	12	19	6	22	35	16	2.0	Yes	1.2%
49	Levine Children's Hospital, Charlotte, N.C.	62.7	12	19	7	24	22	21	2.3	Yes	0.4%
50	Penn State Children's Hospital, Hershey, Pa.	62.6	12	20	4	26	35	18	2.6	Yes	0.3%

Terms are explained on Page 142.

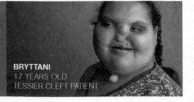

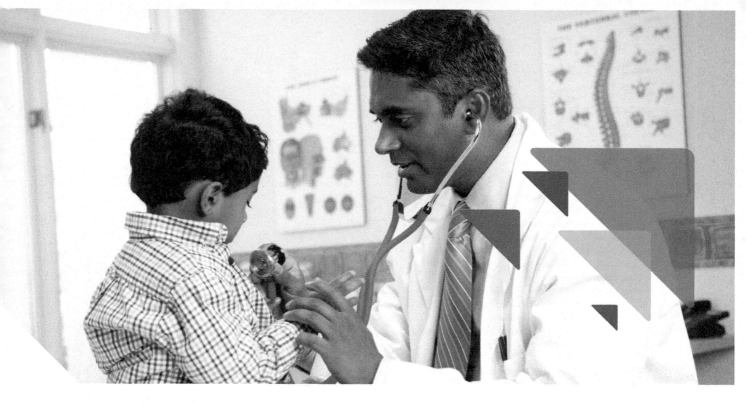

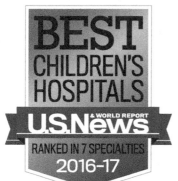
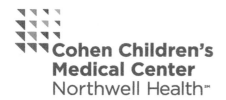

ORTHOPEDICS

Rank	Hospital	U.S. News score	Fracture repair score (6=best)	Surgical complications prevention score (18=best)	Overall infection prevention score (29=best)	Patient volume score (57=best)	Procedure volume score (24=best)	Nurse-patient ratio (higher is better)	Nurse Magnet status	Best practices (60=best)	Specialists recom-mending
1	Boston Children's Hospital	100.0	6	18	26	57	22	3.9	Yes	60	73.8%
2	Children's Hospital of Philadelphia	97.2	6	17	29	50	21	3.2	Yes	58	66.7%
3	Cincinnati Children's Hospital Medical Center	92.3	6	18	27	35	19	3.1	Yes	59	37.8%
4	Rady Children's Hospital, San Diego	90.7	6	18	29	43	13	3.1	No	57	58.4%
5	Nemours Alfred I. duPont Hospital for Children, Wilmington, Del.	90.2	6	18	26	48	17	3.8	Yes	58	26.5%
6	Children's Med. Center Dallas-Texas Scottish Rite Hosp. for Children	87.1	5	16	29	40	21	3.0	Y/N*	52	60.5%
7	Children's Hospital Colorado, Aurora	85.0	5	18	26	44	15	3.6	Yes	55	25.8%
8	Children's Hospital Los Angeles	82.7	4	16	29	51	19	3.7	Yes	55	35.3%
9	Children's National Medical Center, Washington, D.C.	81.8	6	18	29	44	15	3.1	Yes	59	3.4%
10	Johns Hopkins Children's Center, Baltimore	80.2	6	18	24	44	18	3.1	Yes	57	5.9%
11	St. Louis Children's Hospital-Washington Univ.-Shriners Hospital	79.3	6	15	27	41	16	3.4	Y/N*	49	20.6%
12	Children's Healthcare of Atlanta	79.1	5	17	29	43	17	4.2	No	54	16.4%
13	Children's Hospital of Wisconsin, Milwaukee	78.8	6	18	25	42	19	4.2	Yes	57	2.0%
14	Monroe Carell Jr. Children's Hospital at Vanderbilt, Nashville	78.4	6	18	25	36	17	3.4	Yes	50	4.5%
15	Le Bonheur Children's Hospital, Memphis	77.8	6	17	25	32	13	2.9	Yes	58	6.3%
16	Ann and Robert H. Lurie Children's Hospital of Chicago	77.1	5	17	27	33	12	3.5	Yes	55	9.0%
16	Primary Children's Hospital-Shriners Hospitals Salt Lake City	77.1	6	16	29	31	18	3.9	No	53	8.3%
18	Rainbow Babies and Children's Hospital, Cleveland	77.0	5	18	26	37	17	3.1	Yes	55	8.2%
19	Mattel Children's Hospital UCLA, Los Angeles	76.4	6	18	25	32	14	3.8	Yes	55	2.6%
20	Children's Mercy Kansas City, Mo.	75.4	6	14	28	41	16	4.2	Yes	58	2.2%
21	Texas Children's Hospital, Houston	74.7	5	14	28	40	17	3.3	Yes	54	8.3%
22	Children's Hospital at Montefiore, New York	74.4	6	18	29	25	15	3.6	No	56	0.8%
23	Nationwide Children's Hospital, Columbus, Ohio	74.2	4	18	27	48	16	3.0	Yes	52	7.4%
24	Riley Hospital for Children at IU Health, Indianapolis	73.5	6	18	25	33	13	3.1	Yes	50	1.5%
25	North Carolina Children's Hospital at UNC, Chapel Hill	72.4	6	16	29	23	15	3.8	Yes	49	0.2%
26	Phoenix Children's Hospital	72.2	6	18	25	39	16	3.3	No	55	0.9%
27	Cleveland Clinic Children's Hospital	72.1	6	18	21	33	6	3.2	Yes	53	3.0%
28	Children's Hospital of Michigan, Detroit	71.9	6	17	29	41	15	3.0	No	54	0.9%
29	CHOC Children's Hospital, Orange, Calif.	71.4	6	16	27	26	13	2.9	Yes	57	1.9%
30	Johns Hopkins All Children's Hospital, St. Petersburg, Fla.	71.3	6	18	27	28	13	3.3	No	59	1.3%
31	American Family Children's Hospital, Madison, Wis.	70.6	6	18	21	23	13	4.6	Yes	49	0.2%
32	Nicklaus Children's Hospital, Miami	70.4	5	18	25	36	12	3.0	Yes	48	3.5%
33	Mayo Clinic Children's Center, Rochester, Minn.	69.9	5	16	25	27	14	3.6	Yes	58	2.5%
34	NY-Presby. Morgan Stanley-Komansky Children's Hospital, N.Y.	69.4	5	15	29	24	13	2.9	No	49	9.3%
35	Cook Children's Medical Center, Fort Worth	69.3	6	18	23	28	12	3.4	Yes	50	0.1%
35	University of Iowa Children's Hospital, Iowa City	69.3	6	17	25	26	6	2.9	Yes	45	2.1%
37	Lucile Packard Children's Hospital at Stanford, Palo Alto, Calif.	69.2	4	18	28	41	17	3.5	No	56	3.1%
38	UC Davis Children's Hospital-Shriners Hosp., Sacramento	68.9	4	18	28	36	15	6.0	Y/N*	58	3.4%
39	Arnold Palmer Children's Hospital, Orlando, Fla.	68.4	6	18	22	16	9	3.2	Yes	51	1.9%
40	Duke Children's Hospital and Health Center, Durham, N.C.	68.2	6	17	27	21	7	3.0	Yes	42	0.0%
40	Steven & Alexandra Cohen Children's Hosp., New Hyde Park, N.Y.	68.2	5	18	28	25	13	3.3	No	59	0.3%
42	Penn State Children's Hospital, Hershey, Pa.	67.7	6	18	23	24	4	2.6	Yes	40	0.0%
43	Seattle Children's Hospital	67.1	4	15	29	31	10	2.9	Yes	36	14.7%
43	University of Michigan C.S. Mott Children's Hospital, Ann Arbor	67.1	5	17	22	35	12	3.6	No	43	5.1%
45	Joe DiMaggio Children's Hospital at Memorial, Hollywood, Fla.	66.8	6	18	24	46	18	3.4	No	57	0.5%
46	Children's Hospital and Medical Center, Omaha	66.7	6	17	24	22	8	3.2	Yes	42	1.0%
47	UCSF Benioff Children's Hospitals, San Francisco and Oakland	66.6	4	18	27	27	14	3.0	Yes	47	1.3%
48	Yale-New Haven Children's Hospital, New Haven, Conn.	66.5	6	18	23	15	8	2.4	Yes	46	0.4%
49	Dell Children's Medical Center of Central Texas, Austin	66.4	6	18	23	16	8	2.9	Yes	49	0.2%
50	Levine Children's Hospital, Charlotte, N.C.	65.5	6	17	21	28	12	2.3	Yes	48	0.5%

Terms are explained on Page 142.
*The second hospital in this combination does not have Nurse Magnet status.

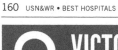
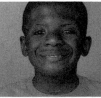

Dylan & Levi

Age 4, Pulmonary Atresia

Comprehensive cardiac expertise and state-of-the-art techniques – that's our *twin-ning* combination and we put it to work for children every day.

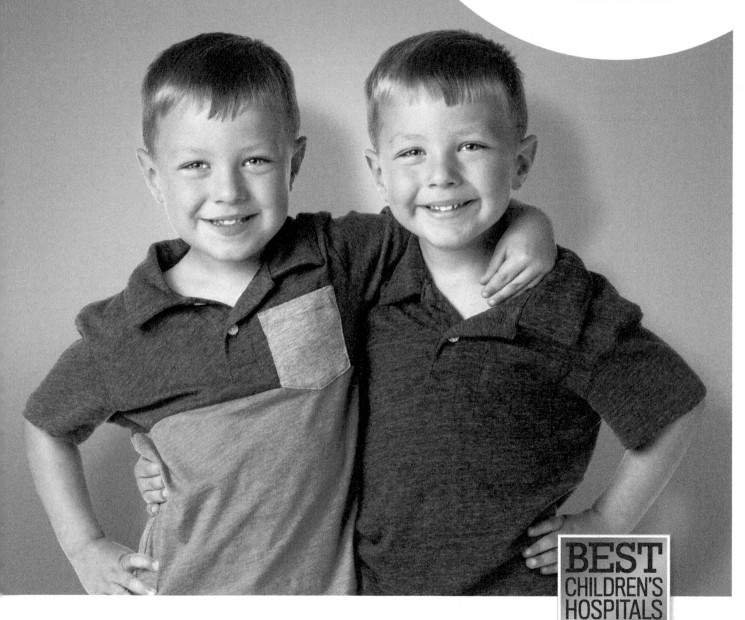

Experienced, unparalleled care for a full spectrum of pediatric and adult congenital cardiac conditions brings families from across the Midwest and the United States to Children's Hospital & Medical Center in Omaha. Our Dr. C.C. and Mabel L. Criss Heart Center specializes in pediatric heart transplantation, cardiac surgery, treatment of congenital or acquired heart disease and other cardiac conditions.

For a pediatric cardiology specialist, call **1.800.833.3100.** Find more at **ChildrensOmaha.org/HeartCenter.**

PULMONOLOGY

Rank	Hospital	U.S. News score	Asthma inpatient score (5=best)	Cystic fibrosis management score (16=best)	Overall infection prevention score (42=best)	ICU infection prevention score (10=best)	Patient volume score (21=best)	Nurse-patient ratio (higher is better)	Nurse Magnet status	Lung transplant survival score (6=best)	Specialists recom-mending
1	Texas Children's Hospital, Houston	100.0	4	12	41	7	20	3.3	Yes	5	52.5%
2	Boston Children's Hospital	98.4	4	10	39	6	17	3.9	Yes	3	62.8%
3	Cincinnati Children's Hospital Medical Center	97.3	5	13	39	6	18	3.1	Yes	3	66.1%
4	Children's Hospital of Philadelphia	95.3	4	12	41	3	21	3.2	Yes	3	67.9%
5	Children's Hospital of Pittsburgh of UPMC	91.6	4	13	41	5	16	3.3	Yes	5	34.3%
6	Nationwide Children's Hospital, Columbus, Ohio	90.7	4	13	40	7	19	3.0	Yes	4	18.3%
7	Lucile Packard Children's Hospital at Stanford, Palo Alto, Calif.	84.8	5	12	41	6	14	3.5	No	3	17.0%
8	Rainbow Babies and Children's Hospital, Cleveland	83.3	5	12	39	10	16	3.1	Yes	0	21.1%
9	St. Louis Children's Hospital-Washington University	81.0	5	9	38	7	14	3.4	Yes	2	26.1%
10	Johns Hopkins Children's Center, Baltimore	80.8	4	12	35	7	16	3.1	Yes	NA	28.3%
11	Seattle Children's Hospital	80.0	4	10	41	6	17	2.9	Yes	NA	37.0%
12	Children's Hospital Colorado, Aurora	78.7	4	9	38	3	18	3.6	Yes	NA	54.0%
13	North Carolina Children's Hospital at UNC, Chapel Hill	73.9	4	10	42	7	9	3.8	Yes	1	18.8%
14	NY-Presby. Morgan Stanley-Komansky Children's Hospital, N.Y.	70.8	4	9	42	4	16	2.9	No	6	7.2%
15	Ann and Robert H. Lurie Children's Hospital of Chicago	69.1	4	12	37	7	16	3.5	Yes	NA	14.1%
15	Children's National Medical Center, Washington, D.C.	69.1	5	11	42	6	17	3.1	Yes	NA	4.8%
17	Children's Hospital of Wisconsin, Milwaukee	68.9	5	14	37	8	15	4.2	Yes	NA	2.6%
17	Monroe Carell Jr. Children's Hospital at Vanderbilt, Nashville	68.9	5	11	36	7	14	3.4	Yes	NA	5.7%
19	Children's Hospital Los Angeles	65.8	5	5	42	6	16	3.7	Yes	NA	13.7%
20	Riley Hospital for Children at IU Health, Indianapolis	63.0	4	10	38	4	19	3.1	Yes	NA	12.1%
21	Mount Sinai Kravis Children's Hospital, New York	62.2	5	14	41	5	8	3.5	Yes	NA	0.0%
22	Children's Medical Center Dallas	61.5	5	11	40	7	15	3.0	Yes	NA	3.0%
23	Cleveland Clinic Children's Hospital	60.3	3	12	34	9	12	3.2	Yes	NA	2.6%
24	Children's Healthcare of Atlanta	59.6	5	11	40	6	19	4.2	No	NA	2.6%
25	UCSF Benioff Children's Hospitals, San Francisco and Oakland	59.1	4	12	35	5	12	3.0	Yes	NA	4.8%
26	CHOC Children's Hospital, Orange, Calif.	58.7	5	11	40	8	12	2.9	Yes	NA	1.0%
27	UF Health Shands Children's Hospital, Gainesville, Fla.	58.4	5	11	39	7	8	2.6	Yes	1	0.3%
28	Nicklaus Children's Hospital, Miami	57.6	4	12	38	5	14	3.0	Yes	NA	1.3%
29	American Family Children's Hospital, Madison, Wis.	57.3	4	12	28	8	12	4.6	Yes	NA	1.3%
30	Children's Hospital of Alabama at UAB, Birmingham	56.9	5	12	34	8	15	3.0	No	NA	5.5%
31	University of Michigan C.S. Mott Children's Hospital, Ann Arbor	55.3	4	12	32	6	13	3.6	No	NA	4.8%
32	Rady Children's Hospital, San Diego	55.2	5	12	39	6	16	3.1	No	NA	3.3%
33	Children's Hospitals and Clinics of Minnesota, Minneapolis	55.1	5	11	33	8	17	3.4	No	NA	2.3%
33	University of Minnesota Masonic Children's Hospital, Minneapolis	55.1	5	12	26	7	10	2.8	No	3	1.8%
35	Doernbecher Children's Hospital, Portland, Ore.	54.9	5	10	38	8	11	3.4	Yes	NA	0.6%
35	University of Iowa Children's Hospital, Iowa City	54.9	4	11	37	6	9	2.9	Yes	NA	1.9%
37	MassGeneral Hospital for Children, Boston	54.5	3	8	33	9	9	3.0	Yes	NA	3.2%
38	Le Bonheur Children's Hospital, Memphis	54.3	4	9	37	5	12	2.9	Yes	NA	3.3%
39	Mattel Children's Hospital UCLA, Los Angeles	53.3	4	9	38	5	8	3.8	Yes	NA	2.1%
40	Steven & Alexandra Cohen Children's Hosp., New Hyde Park, N.Y.	53.2	3	10	41	8	12	3.3	No	NA	0.4%
41	Akron Children's Hospital, Ohio	53.0	4	10	37	5	15	3.2	Yes	NA	1.1%
42	Children's Mercy Kansas City, Mo.	52.7	4	10	37	3	18	4.2	Yes	NA	2.0%
43	Mayo Clinic Children's Center, Rochester, Minn.	50.7	3	13	37	1	8	3.6	Yes	NA	1.7%
44	Maria Fareri Children's Hospital, Valhalla, N.Y.	50.6	4	14	33	4	20	2.9	No	NA	1.1%
45	Phoenix Children's Hospital	48.6	5	8	37	6	17	3.3	No	NA	0.2%
46	Nemours Alfred I. duPont Hosp. for Children, Wilmington, Del.	48.5	3	8	39	2	14	3.8	Yes	NA	1.1%
47	Arkansas Children's Hospital, Little Rock	48.1	5	12	33	6	10	3.3	No	NA	2.1%
48	Duke Children's Hospital and Health Center, Durham, N.C.	47.8	3	8	39	7	10	3.0	Yes	1	0.4%
49	Johns Hopkins All Children's Hospital, St. Petersburg, Fla.	47.6	4	13	36	4	10	3.3	No	NA	0.2%
50	Winthrop-Univ. Hosp. Children's Medical Center, Mineola, N.Y.	47.3	3	9	39	6	8	4.2	No	NA	1.3%

NA=not applicable. Terms are explained on Page 142.

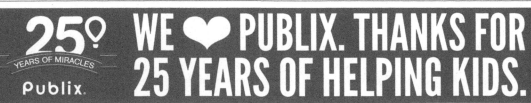

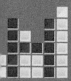
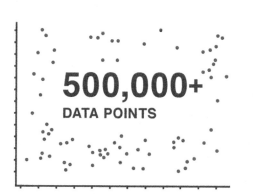
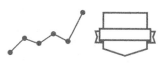

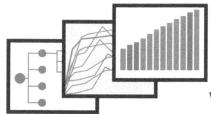
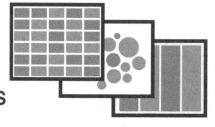
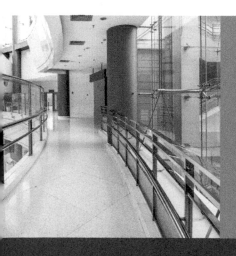

UROLOGY

Rank	Hospital	U.S. News score	Surgical complications prevention score (27=best)	Testicular torsion care score (2=best)	Urinary-tract infection prevention score (5=best)	Overall infection prevention score (23=best)	Patient volume score (24=best)	Surgery volume score (28=best)	Minimally invasive volume score (12=best)	Nurse-patient ratio (higher is better)	Nurse Magnet status	Specialists recommending
1	Boston Children's Hospital	100.0	23	2	4	20	21	23	11	3.9	Yes	79.7%
2	Children's Hospital of Philadelphia	94.8	22	2	2	23	23	24	10	3.2	Yes	80.5%
3	Cincinnati Children's Hospital Medical Center	93.8	23	2	4	21	20	20	11	3.1	Yes	45.4%
4	Monroe Carell Jr. Children's Hospital at Vanderbilt, Nashville	92.1	22	2	4	19	24	22	12	3.4	Yes	45.9%
5	Texas Children's Hospital, Houston	91.8	19	2	4	22	23	24	12	3.3	Yes	38.9%
6	Seattle Children's Hospital	90.0	19	2	5	23	17	17	10	2.9	Yes	37.1%
7	Ann and Robert H. Lurie Children's Hospital of Chicago	89.2	22	2	3	21	22	23	11	3.5	Yes	39.0%
8	Riley Hospital for Children at IU Health, Indianapolis	84.5	24	2	1	19	22	25	8	3.1	Yes	57.1%
9	Nationwide Children's Hospital, Columbus, Ohio	84.3	21	2	5	21	23	23	10	3.0	Yes	18.2%
10	Children's Hospital Los Angeles	83.9	24	2	4	23	17	22	12	3.7	Yes	10.5%
11	Johns Hopkins Children's Center, Baltimore	81.3	22	2	4	18	16	18	8	3.1	Yes	26.3%
12	Children's Medical Center Dallas	77.9	19	2	4	23	23	18	12	3.0	Yes	13.3%
13	Steven & Alexandra Cohen Children's Hosp., New Hyde Park, N.Y.	75.0	27	2	3	22	22	24	12	3.3	No	6.9%
14	Children's Hospital of Pittsburgh of UPMC	74.7	21	2	2	22	18	19	11	3.3	Yes	11.0%
15	UCSF Benioff Children's Hospitals, San Francisco and Oakland	73.0	19	2	4	21	15	13	7	3.0	Yes	9.7%
16	Children's Mercy Kansas City, Mo.	72.6	24	2	3	22	17	17	6	4.2	Yes	2.0%
17	St. Louis Children's Hospital-Washington University	72.4	20	2	4	21	13	19	8	3.4	Yes	6.1%
18	Lucile Packard Children's Hospital at Stanford, Palo Alto, Calif.	71.1	19	2	5	22	16	13	3	3.5	No	5.0%
19	Children's National Medical Center, Washington, D.C.	70.6	19	1	3	23	16	16	12	3.1	Yes	19.8%
19	Rainbow Babies and Children's Hospital, Cleveland	70.6	25	2	5	20	9	12	5	3.1	Yes	2.3%
21	Mount Sinai Kravis Children's Hospital, New York	70.2	26	2	4	22	9	12	5	3.5	Yes	0.5%
22	CHOC Children's Hospital, Orange, Calif.	69.1	23	2	4	21	17	16	8	2.9	Yes	3.0%
23	American Family Children's Hospital, Madison, Wis.	68.0	26	2	3	15	16	17	7	4.6	Yes	2.7%
24	University of Iowa Children's Hospital, Iowa City	67.9	20	2	5	19	16	16	5	2.9	Yes	4.6%
25	Children's Hospital Colorado, Aurora	67.7	20	2	2	20	17	17	6	3.6	Yes	7.0%
26	Cleveland Clinic Children's Hospital	67.3	27	2	4	15	11	13	7	3.2	Yes	0.9%
27	Bristol-Myers Squibb Children's Hosp., New Brunswick, N.J.	67.0	25	2	5	16	16	16	7	2.4	Yes	0.6%
28	NY-Presby. Morgan Stanley-Komansky Children's Hosp., N.Y.	65.6	24	2	2	23	16	21	8	2.9	No	3.8%
29	Medical Univ. of South Carolina Children's Hosp., Charleston	65.3	21	2	5	21	11	15	7	2.7	Yes	1.1%
30	Children's Hospital of Wisconsin, Milwaukee	64.0	16	2	3	19	19	20	10	4.2	Yes	2.7%
31	Arnold Palmer Children's Hospital, Orlando, Fla.	62.3	27	2	5	16	5	14	8	3.2	Yes	0.5%
32	Mattel Children's Hospital UCLA, Los Angeles	62.0	24	2	1	19	10	13	4	3.8	Yes	5.5%
32	UC Davis Children's Hosp.-Shriners Hosp., Sacramento	62.0	25	2	3	22	12	11	6	6.0	Y/N*	0.8%
34	Children's Healthcare of Atlanta	61.9	19	1	3	23	20	19	11	4.2	No	10.7%
35	University of Virginia Children's Hospital, Charlottesville	61.7	22	2	5	17	6	13	9	2.6	Yes	1.8%
36	Children's Hospital of Illinois, Peoria	60.8	25	2	4	19	11	15	9	2.4	Yes	0.7%
36	Le Bonheur Children's Hospital, Memphis	60.8	19	2	2	19	17	15	6	2.9	Yes	2.0%
38	Primary Children's Hospital, Salt Lake City	60.4	16	2	1	23	21	21	8	3.9	No	9.8%
39	Nicklaus Children's Hospital, Miami	59.1	21	2	2	19	10	19	8	3.0	Yes	3.9%
40	UF Health Shands Children's Hospital, Gainesville, Fla.	59.0	24	2	4	20	10	10	3	2.6	Yes	0.8%
41	Akron Children's Hospital, Ohio	58.8	23	2	1	22	18	12	6	3.2	Yes	1.3%
42	Doernbecher Children's Hospital, Portland, Ore.	58.7	23	1	4	20	8	16	6	3.4	Yes	2.5%
43	Mayo Clinic Children's Center, Rochester, Minn.	57.9	23	2	1	19	17	11	5	3.6	Yes	2.2%
44	Phoenix Children's Hospital	57.5	20	2	2	19	24	15	6	3.3	No	3.3%
45	Penn State Children's Hospital, Hershey, Pa.	57.2	20	2	4	17	11	13	6	2.6	Yes	1.7%
46	Johns Hopkins All Children's Hospital, St. Petersburg, Fla.	56.5	24	2	4	21	8	18	4	3.3	No	1.3%
47	Spectrum Hlth. Helen DeVos Children's Hosp., Grand Rapids, Mich.	55.9	24	2	1	20	14	15	7	2.6	Yes	0.2%
48	Winthrop-Univ. Hosp. Children's Medical Center, Mineola, N.Y.	54.9	21	2	5	21	3	7	4	4.2	No	0.2%
49	Children's Hospital of Alabama at UAB, Birmingham	54.6	22	1	5	16	14	13	7	3.0	No	3.0%
50	Duke Children's Hospital and Health Center, Durham, N.C.	54.4	18	1	4	21	13	13	7	3.0	Yes	3.7%

Terms are explained on Page 142.
*The second hospital in this combination does not have Nurse Magnet status.

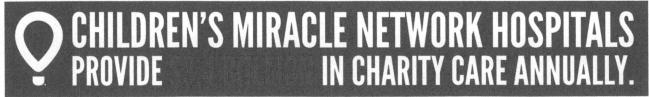

CHILDREN'S MIRACLE NETWORK HOSPITALS PROVIDE   IN CHARITY CARE ANNUALLY.

Our Partners
PUT THE MONEY
WHERE THE MIRACLES ARE.

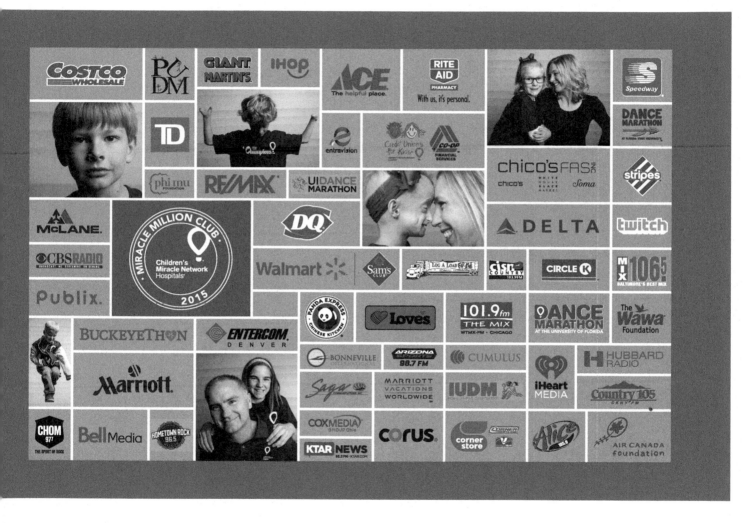

Thanks to all of our partners, we raised more than
$360 million last year for children's hospitals.

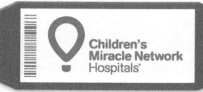

Children's
Miracle Network
Hospitals

cmnhospitals.org

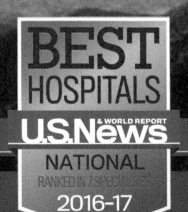

7

BEST REGIONAL HOSPITALS

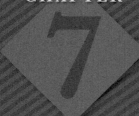

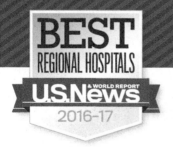

Atlanta • Austin, Texas • Baltimore • Birmingham, Ala. • Boston • Buffalo, N.Y. • Charlotte, N.C. • Chicago • Cincinnati • Cleveland • Columbus, Ohio • Dallas-Fort Worth • Denver • Detroit • Hartford, Conn. • Houston • Indianapolis • Jacksonville, Fla. • Kansas City • Las Vegas • Los Angeles • Louisville, Ky. • Memphis, Tenn. • Miami-Fort Lauderdale • Milwaukee • Minneapolis-St. Paul • Nashville, Tenn. • New Orleans • New York • Oklahoma City • Orlando, Fla. • Philadelphia • Phoenix • Pittsburgh • Portland, Ore. • Providence, R.I. • Raleigh-Durham, N.C. • Richmond, Va. • Riverside-San Bernardino, Calif. • Rochester, N.Y. • Sacramento, Calif. • Salt Lake City • San Antonio • San Diego • San Francisco • San Jose, Calif. • Seattle • St. Louis • Tampa-St. Petersburg, Fla. • Virginia Beach-Norfolk-Newport News, Va. • Washington, D.C.

INSIDE THE RANKINGS

How we identified great care in 51 metro areas

BY AVERY COMAROW

If you're like most people facing hospitalization, you have a strong preference for staying close to home. It's easier on everybody – you'll feel more comfortable, and lower stress can lead to faster recovery. Your family can visit without racking up massive hotel bills. And a battle with your health insurer over coverage at an out-of-network facility might be avoided as well.

Since 2011, our Best Regional Hospitals listings have showcased hundreds of facilities around the U.S. that, while they may not be among the nationally ranked Best Hospitals (Page 89), offer the kind of care that nearly matches those tough standards. These regional rankings, which can be found at usnews.com/best-hospitals/area in their entirety, have multiplied the number of high-quality choices that are apt to be convenient and in-network. This year their usefulness has taken another jump.

Our latest regional evaluations include ratings of how well hospitals handle nine relatively common procedures and conditions in addition to their assessments in 12 specialties. This continues our shift toward emphasizing performance in the sorts of care that most hospitals provide day in and day out, and thus matter most to large numbers of consumers. The nine areas of care are heart bypass surgery, aortic valve surgery, abdominal aortic aneurysm repair, heart failure, hip replacement, knee replacement, colon cancer surgery, lung cancer surgery and chronic obstructive pulmonary disease. Hospitals are assigned a rating of "high performing," "average" or "below average" in each of the nine areas in which they see enough patients to be evaluated.

Recognition as a 2016-17 Best Regional Hospital means a hospital was nationally ranked in at least one of the 12 Best Hospitals specialties that use objective data* or that it earned at least four "high performing" ratings across the nine procedures and conditions and the 12 specialties. In the specialties, high performing signifies a score below those of the 50 top hospitals but within the highest 10 percent. (An FAQ at usnews.com/best-hospitals offers more details.)

THIS YEAR 505 HOSPITALS merited Best Regional Hospitals status. Those in the 51 metropolitan areas of 1 million or more are displayed on the following pages. Three of the 51 metro areas have a single Best Regional Hospital; hospitals are ranked in the other 48 areas.

Within each of the 48, hospitals are numerically ordered according to the following rules:

1. The higher rank went to the hospital with the better status in the Best Hospitals Honor Roll ranking, if any.

2. Next, a higher rank went to the hospital that

NEED ROUTINE CARE?

U.S. News evaluated more than 4,500 hospitals for excellence at handling nine surgical procedures and chronic conditions: colon cancer surgery, lung cancer surgery, heart bypass surgery, aortic valve surgery, abdominal aortic aneurysm surgery, hip replacement, knee replacement, heart failure and COPD. Of that total, 1,628 earned at least one top rating of "high performing." But only the following 63 standouts got the top rating in all nine:

- Abbott Northwestern Hospital, Minneapolis
- Advocate Christ Medical Center, Oak Lawn, Ill.
- Aspirus Wausau Hospital, Wausau, Wis.
- Aurora St. Luke's Medical Center, Milwaukee
- Baptist Health Louisville, Ky.
- Barnes-Jewish Hospital/Washington University, St. Louis
- Baystate Medical Center, Springfield, Mass.

- Beaumont Hospital-Royal Oak, Mich.
- Boone Hospital Center, Columbia, Mo.
- Brigham and Women's Hospital, Boston
- Carilion Roanoke Memorial Hospital, Roanoke, Va.
- Cedars-Sinai Medical Center, Los Angeles
- Christ Hospital, Cincinnati
- Christiana Care Christiana Hospital, Newark, Del.
- Cleveland Clinic

- Duke University Hospital, Durham, N.C.
- Eisenhower Medical Center, Rancho Mirage, Calif.
- Emory St. Joseph's Hospital, Atlanta
- Emory University Hospital, Atlanta
- Florida Hospital Orlando
- Hackensack University Medical Center, Hackensack, N.J.
- Hoag Memorial Hospital Presbyterian, Newport Beach, Calif.
- Holy Cross Hospital, Fort Lauderdale, Fla.
- Hospitals of the University of Pennsylvania-Penn Presbyterian, Philadelphia
- Houston Methodist Hospital
- IU Health Academic Health Center, Indianapolis
- Lancaster General Hospital, Lancaster, Pa.

earned more spots, if any, in the 12 data-driven Best Hospitals specialties.

3. A higher rank next went to the hospital with more ratings of "high performing" across both specialties and procedures and conditions.

4. Finally, a higher rank went to the hospital with fewer ratings of "below average" across the nine procedures and conditions.

Of the 505 Best Regional Hospitals, 311 are inside the cities at the hearts of the metro areas featured here or within an hour or so drive at most. That's to be expected, given that more than 54 percent of all Americans live in these 51 population magnets. The nearly 200 others are scattered around the country in smaller cities and towns.

One of these, Mission Hospital in Asheville, North Carolina, illustrates the sort of powerhouse that can often be found close to home. Asheville, a city of about 85,000 tucked into the Blue Ridge mountains at the far western edge of the state, is more than two hours from a number of large hospitals in Charlotte and more than four hours from the big academic centers in Raleigh and Durham. But Mission, which has more than 750 beds, is one of just 63 hospitals in the country to be rated high performing in all nine procedures and conditions (box, below). It also earned that recognition in three specialties.

And consider St. Luke's Regional Medical Center in Idaho's capital city of Boise. The nearest cluster of big-city medical centers is in Portland, Oregon, more than 425 miles away. Most of the time there's no need to go there. St. Luke's has more than 550 beds and, like Mission, excels in nine out of nine procedures and conditions. It was also nationally ranked in pulmonology and rated "high performing" in two other specialties.

> " THIS YEAR 505 *HOSPITALS* MERITED *BEST REGIONAL HOSPITAL* STATUS. "

Beyond the options in the largest metro areas on the following pages, our website displays Best Regional Hospitals in the 37 metro areas of 500,000 to 1 million people. Regionally recognized hospitals can also be viewed by state within the 42 states in which at least two hospitals met our standards. In addition, the country has been divided into some 200 U.S. News-defined regions, such as Southern Indiana and Texas Hill Country, to help consumers searching for high-quality care close to home.

Aside from meeting performance standards, hospitals had to fit certain definitions and meet certain standards to be eligible for consideration as a Best Regional Hospital. Those standards have been tightened somewhat in the last two years. Until last year, a rating of high performing in one of the 12 specialties required a score in the top 25 percent of the hospitals evaluated. It was changed to the top 10 percent.

A hospital's performance in four specialties – ophthalmology, psychiatry, rehabilitation and rheumatology – also is no longer considered. Ranking in these specialties is solely determined by a hospital's reputation with specialists rather than by hard data, based on three years of national physician surveys.

That these specialties are important is undeniable. Hospitals that are nationally ranked or high performing in one or more are recognized as such on their online profile pages. But the absence of objective performance measures critically limits the information available about such hospitals, so we could not justify including the specialties in our formula.

In addition, only hospitals that deliver a wide range of clinical services can get Best Regional status. Specialty hospitals have indisputable but narrow value; such a hospital might only do surgery, say, or only treat heart patients. Our goal with Best Regional Hospitals is to identify general medical-surgical hospitals that offer both high-quality care and breadth of care.

Children's hospitals are excluded from consideration in the regional rankings because so few metro areas have more than one or two. There are fewer than 200 in the entire country. ●

*Cancer; cardiology & heart surgery; diabetes & endocrinology; ear, nose & throat; gastroenterology & GI surgery; geriatrics; gynecology; nephrology; neurology & neurosurgery; orthopedics; pulmonology and urology.

- **Lankenau Medical Center,** Wynnewood, Pa.
- **Lehigh Valley Hospital,** Allentown, Pa.
- **Maine Medical Center,** Portland
- **Massachusetts General Hospital,** Boston
- **Mayo Clinic,** Rochester, Minn.
- **Mission Hospital,** Asheville, N.C.
- **Morristown Medical Center,** Morristown, N.J.
- **Moses H. Cone Memorial Hospital,** Greensboro, N.C.
- **Munson Medical Center,** Traverse City, Mich.
- **Northwestern Memorial Hospital,** Chicago
- **NYU Langone Medical Center,** New York
- **Ohio State University Wexner Medical Center,** Columbus
- **Oregon Health and Science University Hospital,** Portland

- **Penn State Milton S. Hershey Medical Center,** Hershey
- **PinnacleHealth Hospitals,** Harrisburg, Pa.
- **Providence St. Vincent Medical Center,** Portland, Ore.
- **Robert Wood Johnson University Hospital,** New Brunswick, N.J.
- **Sarasota Memorial Hospital,** Fla.
- **Scripps La Jolla Hospitals and Clinics,** La Jolla, Calif.
- **Spectrum Health Hospitals Butterworth-Blodgett Campuses,** Grand Rapids, Mich.
- **St. Cloud Hospital,** St. Cloud, Minn.
- **St. Joseph Hospital,** Orange, Calif.
- **St. Joseph's Hospital Health Center,** Syracuse, N.Y.
- **St. Luke's Regional Medical Center,** Boise, Idaho
- **Stanford Health Care-Stanford Hospital,** Stanford, Calif.

- **UCLA Medical Center,** Los Angeles
- **University of Colorado Hospital,** Aurora
- **University of Michigan Hospitals and Health Centers,** Ann Arbor
- **University of Virginia Medical Center,** Charlottesville
- **University of Wisconsin Hospital and Clinics,** Madison
- **UPMC Presbyterian Shadyside,** Pittsburgh
- **Valley Hospital,** Ridgewood, N.J.
- **Vanderbilt University Medical Center,** Nashville
- **Vidant Medical Center,** Greenville, N.C.
- **Wake Forest Baptist Medical Center,** Winston-Salem, N.C.
- **Yale-New Haven Hospital,** New Haven, Conn.

COMPLEX CARE BY SPECIALTY
- ● Nationally ranked
- ● High performing

COMMON PROCEDURES & CONDITIONS
- ● High performing
- ● Average
- ● Below average

COMPLEX CARE BY SPECIALTY — **COMMON PROCEDURES & CONDITIONS**

Column headings (left to right):
Cancer · Cardiology & Heart Surgery · Diabetes & Endocrinology · Ear, Nose & Throat · Gastroenterology & GI Surgery · Geriatrics · Gynecology · Nephrology · Neurology & Neurosurgery · Orthopedics · Pulmonology · Urology · Colon Cancer Surgery · Lung Cancer Surgery · Heart Bypass Surgery · Heart Failure · Heart Valve Surgery · Abdominal Aortic Aneurysm · Hip Replacement · Knee Replacement · COPD

Metro Rank / Hospital	Can	Card	Diab	ENT	Gast	Ger	Gyn	Neph	Neur	Orth	Pulm	Uro	Colon	Lung	Byp	HF	Valve	AAA	Hip	Knee	COPD
ATLANTA																					
1 Emory University Hospital[1]	●	●	●	–	●	●	–	●	●	●	–	●	●	●	●	●	●	●	●	●	●
2 Emory St. Joseph's Hospital	–	–	–	–	–	–	–	●	–	–	●	–	●	●	●	●	●	●	●	●	●
3 Kennestone Hospital, Marietta	–	–	–	–	–	–	–	–	–	–	–	–	●	●	●	●	●	●	●	●	●
3 Piedmont Atlanta Hospital	–	●	–	–	●	–	–	–	–	–	–	–	●	●	●	●	●	●	●	●	●
5 Emory University Hospital Midtown	–	–	–	–	–	–	–	–	–	–	–	–	●	●	●	●	●	●	●	●	●
AUSTIN, TEXAS																					
1 Seton Medical Center	–	–	–	●	–	–	–	–	–	–	–	–	●	●	●	●	●	●	●	●	●
2 St. David's Medical Center	–	–	–	–	–	–	–	–	–	–	–	–	●	●	●	●	●	●	●	●	●
BALTIMORE																					
1 Johns Hopkins Hospital	●	●	●	●	●	●	●	●	●	●	●	●	●	●	●	●	●	●	–	●	●
2 University of Maryland Medical Center	●	–	●	●	●	●	–	●	–	–	●	●	●	●	●	●	●	●	●	●	●
3 Mercy Medical Center	–	–	–	–	–	–	–	●	–	●	–	–	●	●	–	●	–	●	●	●	●
3 Sinai Hospital of Baltimore	●	–	–	–	●	●	–	●	●	–	–	–	●	●	●	●	●	●	●	●	●
5 MedStar Union Memorial Hospital	–	–	–	–	●	●	–	●	●	–	–	–	●	●	●	●	●	●	●	●	●
5 University of Maryland St. Joseph Medical Center, Towson	–	–	–	–	●	●	–	●	–	●	–	–	●	●	●	●	●	●	●	●	●
7 Anne Arundel Medical Center, Annapolis	–	–	–	–	–	–	–	–	–	–	–	–	●	●	●	●	●	–	●	●	●
7 MedStar Franklin Square Medical Center	–	–	●	–	–	–	–	●	–	–	●	–	●	●	●	●	●	–	●	●	●
9 MedStar Harbor Hospital	–	–	–	●	–	●	–	–	●	●	–	–	●	●	●	●	●	–	●	●	●
10 MedStar Good Samaritan Hospital	–	–	–	●	–	●	–	●	–	●	–	–	●	–	●	●	●	–	●	●	●
11 Greater Baltimore Medical Center	–	–	–	●	–	●	–	●	–	●	–	–	●	●	–	●	●	–	●	●	●
11 Johns Hopkins Bayview Medical Center	–	–	●	–	●	–	●	–	●	–	–	–	●	●	●	●	●	–	●	●	●
BIRMINGHAM, ALA.																					
1 University of Alabama Hospital at Birmingham	●	●	●	●	–	●	●	●	●	●	●	●	●	●	●	●	●	●	●	●	●
2 Trinity Medical Center	–	–	–	–	–	–	–	–	–	–	–	–	●	●	●	●	●	●	●	●	●
BOSTON																					
1 Massachusetts General Hospital[2]	●	●	●	●	●	●	●	●	●	●	●	●	●	●	●	●	●	●	●	●	●
2 Brigham and Women's Hospital[3]	●	●	●	–	●	●	●	●	●	●	●	●	●	●	●	●	●	●	●	●	●
3 Beth Israel Deaconess Medical Center	●	–	●	–	●	●	–	●	–	●	●	–	●	●	●	●	●	●	●	●	●
4 Tufts Medical Center	–	–	●	–	–	–	–	●	●	–	–	●	●	●	●	●	●	●	●	●	●
5 Lahey Hospital and Medical Center, Burlington	–	–	–	–	●	●	–	●	●	–	–	●	●	●	●	●	●	●	●	●	●
6 South Shore Hospital, South Weymouth	–	–	–	–	–	–	–	–	–	–	–	–	●	●	–	●	–	●	●	●	●
7 Cape Cod Hospital, Hyannis	–	–	–	–	–	–	–	–	–	–	–	–	●	●	–	●	–	●	●	●	●
7 Winchester Hospital, Winchester	–	–	–	–	–	–	●	–	–	–	–	–	●	●	–	●	–	●	●	●	●
9 Boston Medical Center	–	–	–	–	●	–	●	–	–	–	–	–	●	●	●	●	●	●	●	●	●
10 Lowell General Hospital, Lowell	–	–	–	–	–	–	–	–	–	–	–	–	●	●	–	●	●	–	●	●	●
10 North Shore Medical Center, Salem	–	–	–	–	–	●	–	–	–	–	–	–	●	●	●	●	●	–	●	●	●
BUFFALO, N.Y.																					
- Buffalo General Medical Center	–	–	–	–	–	–	–	●	–	–	–	–	●	●	●	●	●	●	●	●	●
CHARLOTTE, N.C.																					
1 Carolinas Medical Center	●	–	–	●	–	●	●	●	●	●	–	–	●	●	●	●	●	●	●	●	●
2 Novant Health Presbyterian Medical Center	–	–	–	–	–	–	–	–	–	–	–	–	●	●	●	●	●	●	●	–	●
3 Caromont Regional Medical Center, Gastonia	–	–	–	–	–	–	–	–	–	–	–	–	●	●	●	●	●	●	●	●	●
4 Carolinas Medical Center-Northeast, Concord	–	–	–	–	–	–	–	–	–	–	–	–	●	●	●	●	●	●	●	●	●
4 Carolinas Medical Center-Pineville	–	–	–	–	–	–	–	–	–	–	–	–	●	–	●	●	●	–	●	●	●
4 Novant Health Huntersville Medical Center	–	–	–	–	–	–	–	–	–	–	–	–	●	–	–	●	–	–	●	●	●

A (-) in a complex care specialty indicates hospital is neither nationally ranked nor high performing.
A (-) in a procedure or condition indicates hospital does not offer the indicated care or has too few patients to be rated.

A footnote indicates that another hospital's results were included or that the hospital has a different name in one or more specialties. [1]Emory Wesley Woods Geriatric Hospital (Geriatrics). [2]Massachusetts Eye and Ear Infirmary, Massachusetts General Hospital (Ear, Nose & Throat). [3]Dana-Farber/Brigham and Women's Cancer Center (Cancer).

▶ More @ usnews.com/bestmetrohospitals

COMPLEX CARE BY SPECIALTY
- ● Nationally ranked
- ● High performing

COMMON PROCEDURES & CONDITIONS
- ● High performing
- ● Average
- ● Below average

Legend abbreviations for columns (Complex Care by Specialty): CANCER; CARDIOLOGY & HEART SURGERY; DIABETES & ENDOCRINOLOGY; EAR, NOSE & THROAT; GASTROENTEROLOGY & GI SURGERY; GERIATRICS; GYNECOLOGY; NEPHROLOGY; NEUROLOGY & NEUROSURGERY; ORTHOPEDICS; PULMONOLOGY; UROLOGY. (Common Procedures & Conditions): COLON CANCER SURGERY; LUNG CANCER SURGERY; HEART BYPASS SURGERY; HEART FAILURE; HEART VALVE SURGERY; ABDOMINAL AORTIC ANEURYSM; HIP REPLACEMENT; KNEE REPLACEMENT; COPD.

Metro Rank / Hospital	Cancer	Card. & Heart Surg.	Diabetes & Endo.	Ear, Nose & Throat	Gastro. & GI Surg.	Geriatrics	Gynecology	Nephrology	Neuro. & Neurosurg.	Orthopedics	Pulmonology	Urology	Colon Cancer Surg.	Lung Cancer Surg.	Heart Bypass Surg.	Heart Failure	Heart Valve Surg.	Abd. Aortic Aneurysm	Hip Replacement	Knee Replacement	COPD
CHICAGO																					
1 Northwestern Memorial Hospital	●	●	●	●	●	●	●	●	●	●	●	●	●	●	●	●	●	●	●	●	●
2 Rush University Medical Center	●	●	●	●	●	●	●	●	●	●	●	●	●	●	●	●	●	●	●	●	●
3 University of Chicago Medical Center	●	–	–	●	●	–	●	●	●	●	●	●	●	●	●	●	●	●	●	●	●
4 Advocate Christ Medical Center, Oak Lawn	–	●	●	–	●	●	–	●	●	●	●	●	●	●	●	●	●	●	●	●	●
5 Loyola University Medical Center, Maywood	●	●	●	–	●	●	●	●	●	●	●	●	●	●	●	●	●	●	●	●	●
6 Advocate Lutheran General Hospital, Park Ridge	●	–	–	–	●	●	●	–	–	●	●	●	●	●	●	●	●	●	●	●	●
7 Northwestern Medicine Central DuPage Hospital, Winfield	–	–	–	–	●	–	●	●	–	●	–	●	●	●	●	●	●	●	●	●	●
8 University of Illinois Hospital	–	–	–	●	–	–	●	●	–	●	–	●	●	–	●	●	–	–	●	●	●
9 NorthShore Evanston Hospital, Evanston	–	–	–	–	●	●	–	●	●	●	●	●	●	●	●	●	●	●	●	●	●
10 Elmhurst Memorial Hospital, Elmhurst	–	–	–	–	●	–	–	●	●	●	●	●	●	●	●	●	●	●	●	●	●
11 Advocate Sherman Hospital, Elgin	–	–	●	–	–	–	–	●	●	●	●	●	●	●	●	●	●	●	●	●	●
11 Alexian Brothers Medical Center, Elk Grove Village	–	–	–	–	●	●	–	●	●	●	●	●	●	●	●	●	●	●	●	●	●
13 Edward Hospital, Naperville[4]	–	–	–	●	●	–	–	–	–	–	–	●	●	●	●	●	●	●	●	●	●
14 Advocate Illinois Masonic Medical Center	–	–	–	–	–	–	●	–	●	●	●	●	●	●	●	●	●	●	●	●	●
14 Amita Health Adventist Hinsdale Hospital, Hinsdale	–	–	–	–	●	●	–	●	–	●	●	●	●	●	●	●	●	●	●	●	●
14 Centegra Hospitals McHenry-Woodstock	–	–	–	–	–	–	–	●	●	●	●	●	●	●	●	●	●	●	●	●	●
14 St. Alexius Medical Center, Hoffman Estates	–	–	●	–	●	●	–	●	–	●	●	●	●	–	–	●	●	–	●	●	●
18 Northwest Community Healthcare, Arlington Heights	–	–	–	–	●	–	–	–	–	–	–	●	●	●	●	●	●	●	●	●	●
19 Advocate Good Samaritan Hospital, Downers Grove	–	–	–	–	–	–	–	–	–	–	–	●	●	●	●	●	●	●	●	●	●
19 Advocate Good Shepherd Hospital, Barrington	–	–	–	–	–	–	–	–	–	–	–	●	●	●	●	●	●	●	●	●	●
19 Northwestern Lake Forest Hospital, Lake Forest	–	–	–	–	–	–	–	–	●	–	–	●	●	–	●	●	●	●	●	●	●
19 Northwestern Medicine Delnor Hospital, Geneva	–	–	–	–	–	–	–	–	–	–	–	●	●	●	●	●	●	●	●	●	●
19 Swedish Covenant Hospital	–	–	–	–	–	–	–	–	–	–	–	●	●	●	●	●	●	●	●	●	●
CINCINNATI																					
1 Christ Hospital	–	–	●	–	●	●	●	●	–	●	●	●	●	●	●	●	●	●	●	●	●
2 Good Samaritan Hospital	–	–	●	–	●	●	●	●	●	●	–	●	●	●	●	●	●	●	●	●	●
3 University of Cincinnati Medical Center	–	–	–	●	–	–	–	●	●	–	–	●	●	●	●	●	●	●	●	●	●
4 Bethesda North Hospital	–	–	–	–	●	●	●	–	–	●	●	●	●	●	●	●	●	–	●	●	●
5 St. Elizabeth Edgewood-Covington Hosps., Edgewood, Ky.	–	–	●	–	–	–	–	–	–	–	–	●	●	●	●	●	●	●	●	●	●
CLEVELAND																					
1 Cleveland Clinic	●	●	●	●	●	●	●	●	●	●	●	●	●	●	●	●	●	●	●	●	●
2 University Hospitals Case Medical Center[5]	●	●	●	●	●	●	●	●	●	●	●	●	●	●	●	●	●	●	●	●	●
3 Fairview Hospital	–	●	–	–	●	●	–	●	–	●	–	●	●	●	●	●	●	●	●	●	●
4 MetroHealth Medical Center	–	–	●	–	–	–	●	–	●	–	●	–	●	●	●	●	●	●	●	●	●
5 Hillcrest Hospital	–	●	●	●	●	●	–	●	–	●	●	●	●	●	●	●	●	●	●	●	●
6 Lake Hospital, Concord Township	–	–	–	–	–	–	–	–	–	–	–	●	●	●	●	–	●	●	●	●	●
COLUMBUS, OHIO																					
1 Ohio State University Wexner Medical Center[6]	●	●	●	●	●	●	●	●	●	●	●	●	●	●	●	●	●	●	●	●	●
2 OhioHealth Riverside Hospital	–	●	●	●	●	●	–	●	●	●	●	●	●	●	●	●	●	●	●	●	●
3 Grant Medical Center-Ohio Health	–	–	–	–	●	–	●	–	●	●	–	●	–	●	●	●	●	●	●	●	●
4 Mount Carmel East and West Hospitals	–	–	–	–	–	–	–	–	–	●	–	●	●	●	●	●	●	●	●	●	●
DALLAS-FORT WORTH																					
1 Baylor University Medical Center, Dallas[7]	●	–	●	●	●	●	●	●	●	●	●	●	●	●	●	●	●	●	–	●	●
2 UT Southwestern Medical Center, Dallas	●	–	–	–	●	●	–	●	●	●	–	●	●	●	●	●	●	●	●	●	●
3 Medical City Dallas Hospital	–	–	–	–	–	●	●	●	●	–	–	●	●	●	●	●	●	●	●	●	●

A (-) in a complex care specialty indicates hospital is neither nationally ranked nor high performing.
A (-) in a procedure or condition indicates hospital does not offer the indicated care or has too few patients to be rated.

A footnote indicates that another hospital's results were included or that the hospital has a different name in one or more specialties.
[4] Edward Cancer Center (Cancer); Edward Heart Hospital (Cardiology & Heart Surgery). [5] Seidman Cancer Center at University Hospitals Case Medical (Cancer).
[6] Ohio State University James Cancer Hospital (Cancer). [7] Baylor University Heart and Vascular Hospital (Cardiology & Heart Surgery).

	COMPLEX CARE BY SPECIALTY	COMMON PROCEDURES & CONDITIONS
COMPLEX CARE BY SPECIALTY ● Nationally ranked ● High performing	**COMMON PROCEDURES & CONDITIONS** ● High performing ● Average ● Below average	

COMPLEX CARE BY SPECIALTY — **COMMON PROCEDURES & CONDITIONS**

Metro Rank Hospital	Cancer	Cardiology & Heart Surgery	Diabetes & Endocrinology	Ear, Nose & Throat	Gastroenterology & GI Surgery	Geriatrics	Gynecology	Nephrology	Neurology & Neurosurgery	Orthopedics	Pulmonology	Urology	Colon Cancer Surgery	Lung Cancer Surgery	Heart Bypass Surgery	Heart Failure	Heart Valve Surgery	Abdominal Aortic Aneurysm	Hip Replacement	Knee Replacement	COPD
DALLAS-FORT WORTH (CONTINUED)																					
4 Texas Health Presbyterian Hospital Dallas	–	–	–	–	–	–	–	–	●	●	–	–	●	●	●	●	●	●	●	●	●
5 Texas Health Harris Methodist Hospital Fort Worth	–	–	–	–	–	–	–	–	–	–	–	–	●	●	●	●	●	●	●	●	●
6 Texas Health Presbyterian Hospital Plano	–	–	–	–	–	–	–	–	●	●	–	–	●	●	●	●	●	●	●	●	●
7 Baylor Regional Medical Center, Grapevine	–	–	–	–	–	–	–	–	–	–	–	–	●	●	●	●	●	–	–	●	●
8 Denton Regional Medical Center, Denton	–	–	–	–	–	–	–	–	–	–	–	–	●	●	●	●	●	●	●	●	●
8 Plaza Medical Center, Fort Worth	–	–	–	–	–	–	–	–	–	–	–	–	●	●	●	●	●	●	●	●	●
8 Texas Health Arlington Memorial Hospital, Arlington	–	–	–	–	–	–	–	–	–	–	–	–	●	●	–	●	–	–	●	●	●
DENVER																					
1 University of Colorado Hospital, Aurora[8]	●	●	●	–	●	●	●	●	●	●	●	●	●	●	●	●	●	●	●	●	●
2 Porter Adventist Hospital	–	–	●	●	●	●	–	–	●	●	–	●	●	●	●	●	●	●	●	●	●
3 Sky Ridge Medical Center, Lone Tree	–	–	–	–	–	–	–	●	–	–	–	●	●	●	●	●	●	–	●	●	●
DETROIT																					
1 Univ. of Michigan Hospitals and Health Centers, Ann Arbor	●	●	●	●	●	●	●	●	●	●	●	●	●	●	●	●	●	●	●	●	●
2 Beaumont Hospital-Royal Oak	–	●	●	–	●	●	●	●	●	●	●	●	●	●	●	●	●	●	●	●	●
3 Harper University Hospital	–	–	●	–	●	●	●	–	●	●	●	●	●	●	●	●	●	●	–	●	●
4 Beaumont Hospital-Troy	–	–	–	–	●	●	–	●	●	●	●	●	●	●	●	●	●	●	●	●	●
5 Genesys Regional Medical Center, Grand Blanc	–	–	●	–	–	●	●	–	●	●	–	●	●	●	●	●	●	●	●	●	●
6 St. Joseph Mercy Ann Arbor Hospital, Ypsilanti	–	–	–	–	–	–	–	–	●	●	–	–	●	●	●	●	●	●	●	●	●
7 Beaumont Hospital-Dearborn	–	–	–	–	–	–	–	●	–	–	–	●	●	●	●	●	●	●	●	●	●
7 Providence Hospital, Southfield	–	–	–	–	–	–	–	–	●	–	–	●	●	●	●	●	●	●	●	●	●
9 Beaumont Hospital-Grosse Pointe	–	–	–	–	●	–	–	●	●	–	●	●	●	●	●	●	–	●	●	●	●
9 Henry Ford Hospital	●	–	–	–	–	●	●	–	●	●	●	●	●	●	●	●	●	●	●	●	●
9 Henry Ford Macomb Hospital, Clinton Township	–	–	–	●	–	–	–	–	●	●	●	●	●	●	●	●	●	●	●	●	●
9 St. John Hospital and Medical Center	–	–	–	–	–	–	–	●	–	–	●	●	●	●	●	●	●	●	●	●	●
13 Huron Valley-Sinai Hospital, Commerce Township, Mich.	–	–	–	–	–	–	–	–	–	●	●	●	●	●	–	●	●	●	●	●	●
13 St. Joseph Mercy Oakland, Pontiac	–	–	–	–	–	–	–	–	–	●	●	●	●	●	●	●	●	●	●	●	●
15 McLaren Regional Medical Center, Flint	–	–	–	–	–	–	–	–	–	●	●	●	●	●	●	●	●	●	●	●	●
HARTFORD, CONN.																					
1 Hartford Hospital	–	–	●	–	●	–	●	–	●	●	–	●	●	●	●	●	●	●	●	●	●
2 St. Francis Hospital and Medical Center	–	–	–	–	–	–	–	–	–	–	●	●	●	●	●	●	●	●	●	●	●
3 Middlesex Hospital, Middletown	–	–	–	–	–	–	–	–	–	–	●	●	●	–	●	●	●	●	●	●	●
HOUSTON																					
1 Houston Methodist Hospital	●	●	●	–	●	●	–	●	●	●	●	●	●	●	●	●	●	●	●	●	●
2 Memorial Hermann-Texas Medical Center	–	●	–	–	●	●	●	●	●	●	●	●	●	●	●	●	●	●	●	●	●
3 Baylor St. Luke's Medical Center[9]	–	●	●	–	●	●	●	–	●	–	●	●	●	●	●	●	●	●	●	●	●
4 University of Texas Medical Branch Hospitals, Galveston	–	–	–	–	–	–	●	●	–	–	–	●	●	●	●	●	●	●	●	●	●
5 Clear Lake Regional Medical Center, Webster	–	–	●	–	–	–	●	–	–	–	●	●	●	●	●	●	●	●	●	●	●
6 Memorial Hermann Memorial City Medical Center	–	–	–	–	●	–	–	–	●	●	●	●	–	●	●	●	●	●	●	●	●
7 Memorial Hermann Northwest Complex	–	–	–	–	–	–	●	–	●	–	●	●	●	●	●	●	●	●	●	●	●
8 Houston Methodist Willowbrook Hospital	–	–	–	●	–	–	●	–	●	●	●	●	–	●	●	●	●	●	●	●	●
9 Houston Methodist Sugar Land Hospital	–	–	–	–	●	–	●	–	●	●	●	●	●	●	●	●	●	●	●	●	●
10 Memorial Hermann Northeast Hospital, Humble	–	–	–	–	●	–	●	–	●	●	●	●	●	●	–	●	●	●	●	●	●

A (-) in a complex care specialty indicates hospital is neither nationally ranked nor high performing.
A (-) in a procedure or condition indicates hospital does not offer the indicated care or has too few patients to be rated.

A footnote indicates that another hospital's results were included or that the hospital has a different name in one or more specialties.
[8]National Jewish Health, Denver-University of Colorado Hospital, Aurora (Pulmonology). [9]Texas Heart Institute at Baylor St. Luke's Medical Center (Cardiology & Heart Surgery).

▶ **More @ usnews.com/bestmetrohospitals**

MOST-RECOGNIZED CARE YEAR AFTER YEAR*

Most-Recognized Hospitals in Texas.

More High Performing ratings than any other Texas health care system, according to U.S. News & World Report's 2016-2017 ratings.

At Baylor Scott & White Health, we're proud to lead our state in the number of accolades earned for three consecutive years in *U.S. News & World Report's "Best Hospitals."* Together, 15 Baylor Scott & White hospitals received more national rankings and high-performing ratings than any other health system in Texas. For you, these recognitions confirm our commitment to providing quality health care each day.

It's one way we're Changing Health Care. For Life.®

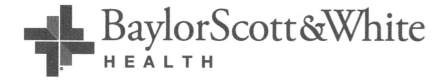

Baylor Scott & White
HEALTH

To find out more about our award winning care, call
1.844.BSWDocs or visit **BaylorScott*and*White.com/Recognition.**

BAYLOR INSTITUTE FOR REHABILITATION

BAYLOR JACK AND JANE HAMILTON HEART & VASCULAR HOSPITAL

CARROLLTON

DALLAS

FORT WORTH

GARLAND

GRAPEVINE

THE HEART HOSPITAL BAYLOR PLANO

IRVING

PLANO

ROUND ROCK

TEMPLE

UPTOWN

WACO

WHITE ROCK

COMPLEX CARE BY SPECIALTY
● Nationally ranked
● High performing

COMMON PROCEDURES & CONDITIONS
● High performing
● Average
● Below average

COMPLEX CARE BY SPECIALTY												COMMON PROCEDURES & CONDITIONS								
Metro Rank / Hospital	Cancer	Cardiology & Heart Surgery	Diabetes & Endocrinology	Ear, Nose & Throat	Gastroenterology & GI Surgery	Geriatrics	Gynecology	Nephrology	Neurology & Neurosurgery	Orthopedics	Pulmonology	Urology	Colon Cancer Surgery	Lung Cancer Surgery	Heart Bypass Surgery	Heart Failure	Heart Valve Surgery	Abdominal Aortic Aneurysm	Hip Replacement	Knee Replacement	COPD
INDIANAPOLIS																					
1 IU Health Academic Health Center	●	●	●	–	●	●	●	●	●	●	●	●	●	●	●	●	●	●	●	●	●
2 St. Vincent Hospital and Health Center	–	–	–	●	●	●	–	●	–	–	–	●	●	●	●	●	●	●	●	●	●
3 IU Health North Hospital, Carmel	–	–	–	–	●	●	●	–	–	–	●	●	●	●	–	–	●	–	–	●	●
4 IU Health West Hospital, Avon	–	–	–	–	●	●	●	–	–	–	●	●	●	–	–	●	–	–	●	●	●
JACKSONVILLE, FLA.																					
1 Mayo Clinic Jacksonville	●	●	–	●	●	●	●	●	●	●	●	●	●	●	●	●	●	●	●	●	●
2 Baptist Medical Center	–	–	●	–	●	–	●	●	●	–	–	–	●	●	●	●	●	●	●	●	●
3 UF Health Jacksonville	–	–	–	–	–	–	●	–	–	–	●	–	●	●	●	●	●	●	●	●	●
KANSAS CITY																					
1 University of Kansas Hospital	●	●	●	●	●	●	●	●	●	●	●	●	●	●	●	●	●	●	●	●	●
2 St. Luke's Hospital, Kansas City, Mo.	●	●	–	–	●	●	●	●	●	●	●	●	●	●	●	●	●	●	●	●	●
LAS VEGAS																					
– St. Rose Dominican Hospitals-Siena Campus, Henderson	–	–	–	–	–	–	–	–	–	–	–	–	●	●	●	●	●	●	●	●	●
LOS ANGELES																					
1 UCLA Medical Center	●	●	●	●	●	●	●	●	●	●	●	●	●	●	●	●	●	●	●	●	●
2 Cedars-Sinai Medical Center	●	●	●	●	●	●	●	●	●	●	●	●	●	●	●	●	●	●	●	●	●
3 Keck Medical Center of USC[10]	●	●	●	–	●	●	–	●	●	●	●	●	●	●	●	●	●	●	●	●	●
4 Huntington Memorial Hospital, Pasadena	–	–	●	–	●	●	●	●	●	●	●	●	●	●	●	●	●	●	●	●	●
5 University of California, Irvine Medical Center, Orange	●	–	–	●	●	●	●	●	●	●	●	●	●	●	●	●	●	●	●	●	●
6 Hoag Memorial Hospital Presbyterian, Newport Beach	–	–	–	–	●	●	●	–	–	●	●	●	●	●	●	●	●	●	●	●	●
7 St. Jude Medical Center, Fullerton	–	–	●	–	●	–	–	–	–	●	–	●	●	●	●	●	●	●	●	●	●
8 Kaiser Permanente Los Angeles Medical Center	–	●	●	–	–	●	–	●	●	–	●	●	●	●	●	●	–	●	●	●	●
8 Providence Holy Cross Medical Center, Mission Hills	–	–	●	–	●	●	–	–	–	●	●	●	●	●	●	●	–	–	●	●	●
8 St. Joseph Hospital, Orange	–	–	–	–	–	–	–	–	●	–	●	●	●	●	●	●	●	●	●	●	●
11 Long Beach Memorial Medical Center, Long Beach	–	–	–	–	–	–	–	●	–	–	●	●	●	●	●	●	●	●	●	●	●
11 Torrance Memorial Medical Center, Torrance	–	–	–	–	●	–	–	–	–	–	●	●	●	●	●	●	●	●	●	●	●
13 Glendale Adventist Medical Center, Glendale	–	–	–	–	–	●	●	–	●	●	●	–	●	–	●	●	●	●	●	●	●
14 Kaiser Permanente Anaheim Medical Center, Anaheim	–	–	–	–	–	–	–	●	–	–	●	●	–	●	–	●	–	●	●	●	●
14 Orange Coast Memorial Medical Center, Fountain Valley	–	–	–	–	–	–	–	–	–	–	●	●	●	●	●	●	–	●	●	●	●
16 Mission Hospitals, Mission Viejo and Laguna Beach	–	–	–	–	●	–	–	–	–	–	●	●	●	●	●	●	●	●	●	●	●
16 PIH Health Hospital-Whittier	–	–	–	–	–	–	–	–	–	–	●	●	●	●	●	●	●	●	●	●	●
18 Henry Mayo Newhall Memorial Hospital, Valencia	–	–	–	–	●	–	–	–	●	–	●	–	●	●	–	–	●	●	●	●	●
18 Providence Tarzana Medical Center, Tarzana	–	–	–	–	●	–	–	–	–	–	●	●	●	●	●	●	●	●	●	●	●
18 Saddleback Memorial Medical Center, Laguna Hills	–	–	–	–	–	–	–	–	–	–	●	●	●	●	●	●	●	●	●	●	●
21 Providence St. Joseph Medical Center, Burbank	–	–	–	–	–	–	–	–	–	–	●	●	●	●	●	●	●	●	●	●	●
LOUISVILLE, KY.																					
1 Baptist Health Louisville	–	–	–	–	–	–	–	–	–	–	●	●	●	●	●	●	●	●	●	●	●
2 Norton Hospital	–	–	–	–	–	–	–	–	–	–	●	●	●	●	●	●	●	●	●	●	●
MEMPHIS, TENN.																					
1 Methodist Hospitals of Memphis	–	–	–	–	–	●	●	–	–	–	●	●	●	●	●	●	●	●	●	●	●
2 Baptist Memorial Hospital-Memphis	–	–	–	–	–	–	–	–	–	–	●	●	●	●	●	●	●	●	●	●	●

A (-) in a complex care specialty indicates hospital is neither nationally ranked nor high performing.
A (-) in a procedure or condition indicates hospital does not offer the indicated care or has too few patients to be rated.

A footnote indicates that another hospital's results were included or that the hospital has a different name in one or more specialties.
[10]USC Norris Cancer Hospital-Keck Medical Center of USC (Cancer).

▶ More @ usnews.com/bestmetrohospitals

U inspire us to be the best

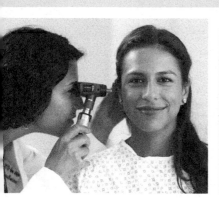
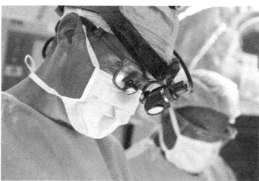
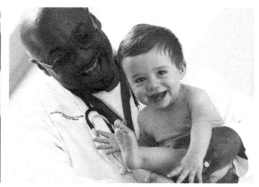

UCLA ranked #1 in LA, #1 in California and #5 nationwide

U.S. News & World Report

The doctors, nurses, staff and volunteers of UCLA are proud to be at the top of *U.S. News & World Report*'s Best Hospitals rankings for 2016 – 2017. And, for the 27th consecutive year we ranked Best in the West. Still, our greatest honor is to bring outstanding care — from the routine to the most complex — to you and your family. Rankings come once a year, but you inspire us every day. And for this, we thank you.

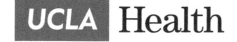 Health | it begins with U

To find a UCLA doctor near you, just call us at
1-800-UCLA-MD1 or visit uclahealth.org

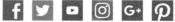

uclahealth.org/getsocial

	COMPLEX CARE BY SPECIALTY
COMPLEX CARE BY SPECIALTY	● Nationally ranked ● High performing
COMMON PROCEDURES & CONDITIONS	● High performing ● Average ● Below average

Metro Rank / Hospital	CANCER	CARDIOLOGY & HEART SURGERY	DIABETES & ENDOCRINOLOGY	EAR, NOSE & THROAT	GASTROENTEROLOGY & GI SURGERY	GERIATRICS	GYNECOLOGY	NEPHROLOGY	NEUROLOGY & NEUROSURGERY	ORTHOPEDICS	PULMONOLOGY	UROLOGY	COLON CANCER SURGERY	LUNG CANCER SURGERY	HEART BYPASS SURGERY	HEART FAILURE	HEART VALVE SURGERY	ABDOMINAL AORTIC ANEURYSM	HIP REPLACEMENT	KNEE REPLACEMENT	COPD
MIAMI-FORT LAUDERDALE																					
1 Cleveland Clinic Florida, Weston	-	-	-	-	●	●	-	-	●	-	-	-	●	●	●	●	●	●	●	●	●
2 Baptist Hospital of Miami	-	-	-	-	-	●	-	●	-	●	-	●	●	●	●	●	●	●	●	●	●
3 Holy Cross Hospital, Fort Lauderdale	-	-	-	-	-	-	-	-	-	-	-	-	●	●	●	●	●	●	●	●	●
4 Mount Sinai Medical Center, Miami Beach	-	-	-	-	●	-	-	-	-	-	-	-	●	●	●	●	●	●	●	●	●
4 South Miami Hospital, Miami	-	-	-	-	-	-	-	-	-	-	-	-	●	●	●	●	●	●	●	●	●
6 Boca Raton Regional Hospital, Boca Raton	-	-	-	-	-	-	-	-	-	-	-	-	●	●	●	●	●	●	●	●	●
6 Homestead Hospital, Homestead	-	-	-	-	-	-	-	-	-	-	●	-	●	-	●	●	-	-	-	●	●
6 West Kendall Baptist Hospital, Miami	-	-	-	-	●	-	-	-	-	-	-	-	●	●	●	●	●	●	●	-	●
MILWAUKEE																					
1 Froedtert Hospital and the Medical College of Wisconsin	●	-	●	●	●	-	-	-	●	-	●	●	●	●	●	●	●	●	●	●	●
2 Aurora St. Luke's Medical Center	●	●	●	-	●	●	-	●	-	●	●	●	●	●	●	●	●	●	●	●	●
3 Aurora Medical Center Grafton	-	-	-	-	-	-	-	-	-	-	-	-	●	●	●	●	●	●	●	●	●
3 Community Memorial Hospital, Menomonee Falls	-	-	-	-	-	-	-	-	-	-	-	-	●	●	●	●	●	-	●	●	●
3 Wheaton Franciscan Healthcare-St. Joseph Campus	-	-	-	-	-	-	-	-	-	-	●	-	●	●	●	●	●	●	●	●	●
MINNEAPOLIS-ST. PAUL																					
1 Abbott Northwestern Hospital, Minneapolis[11]	-	●	●	-	●	●	●	●	●	●	●	-	●	●	●	●	●	●	●	●	●
2 University of Minnesota Medical Center, Minneapolis	●	-	-	-	-	●	-	●	●	●	-	-	●	●	●	●	●	●	●	●	●
3 Mercy Hospital, Coon Rapids	-	-	-	-	●	-	-	-	-	●	●	-	●	●	●	●	●	●	●	●	●
4 Fairview Southdale Hospital, Edina	-	-	-	-	-	-	-	-	-	-	-	-	●	●	●	●	●	●	●	●	●
4 Park Nicollet Methodist Hospital, St. Louis Park	-	-	-	-	-	-	-	-	-	-	●	-	●	●	●	●	●	●	●	●	●
4 United Hospital of St. Paul	-	-	●	-	-	-	-	-	-	-	-	-	●	●	●	●	●	●	●	●	●
7 North Memorial Hospital, Robbinsdale	-	-	-	-	-	-	-	-	-	-	-	-	●	●	●	●	●	●	●	●	●
7 Regions Hospital, St. Paul	-	-	-	-	-	-	-	-	-	-	-	-	●	●	●	●	●	●	●	●	●
NASHVILLE, TENN.																					
1 Vanderbilt University Medical Center	●	●	●	●	●	●	●	●	●	●	●	●	●	●	●	●	●	●	●	●	●
2 St. Thomas Hospital	-	-	-	-	-	-	-	-	-	-	-	-	●	●	●	●	●	●	●	●	●
3 Baptist Hospital	-	-	-	-	-	-	-	-	-	-	-	-	●	●	●	●	●	●	●	●	●
3 Centennial Medical Center	-	-	-	-	-	-	-	-	-	-	-	-	●	●	●	●	●	●	●	●	●

A (-) in a complex care specialty indicates hospital is neither nationally ranked nor high performing. A (-) in a procedure or condition indicates hospital does not offer the indicated care or has too few patients to be rated.
A footnote indicates that another hospital's results were included or that the hospital has a different name in one or more specialties.
[11] Minneapolis Heart Institute at Abbott Northwestern (Cardiology & Heart Surgery).

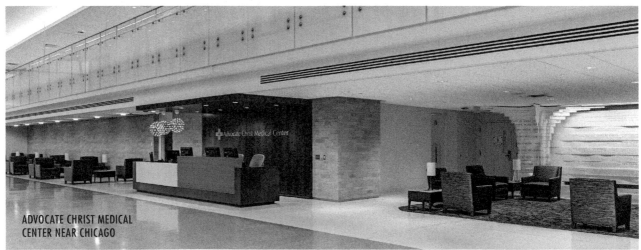

ADVOCATE CHRIST MEDICAL CENTER NEAR CHICAGO

▶ More @ usnews.com/bestmetrohospitals

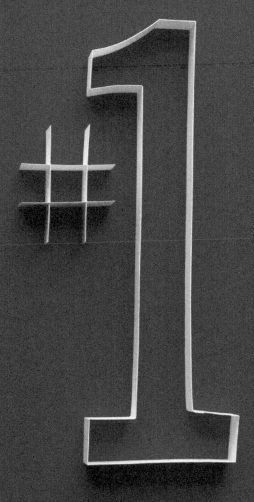
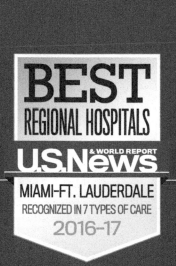
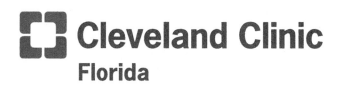

	COMPLEX CARE BY SPECIALTY	COMMON PROCEDURES & CONDITIONS

COMPLEX CARE BY SPECIALTY
- Nationally ranked
- High performing

COMMON PROCEDURES & CONDITIONS
- High performing
- Average
- Below average

Column headers (Complex Care by Specialty): Cancer · Cardiology & Heart Surgery · Diabetes & Endocrinology · Ear, Nose & Throat · Gastroenterology & GI Surgery · Geriatrics · Gynecology · Nephrology · Neurology & Neurosurgery · Orthopedics · Pulmonology · Urology

Column headers (Common Procedures & Conditions): Colon Cancer Surgery · Lung Cancer Surgery · Heart Bypass Surgery · Heart Failure · Heart Valve Surgery · Abdominal Aortic Aneurysm · Hip Replacement · Knee Replacement · COPD

Metro Rank / Hospital	Cancer	Card & Heart Surg	Diabetes & Endo	ENT	Gastro & GI Surg	Geriatrics	Gynecology	Nephrology	Neuro & Neurosurg	Orthopedics	Pulmonology	Urology	Colon Cancer Surg	Lung Cancer Surg	Heart Bypass Surg	Heart Failure	Heart Valve Surg	Abd Aortic Aneurysm	Hip Replacement	Knee Replacement	COPD
NEW ORLEANS																					
1 Ochsner Medical Center	●	–	●	●	●	●	–	●	●	●	●	●	●	●	●	●	●	●	●	●	●
2 East Jefferson General Hospital, Metairie	–	–	–	–	–	–	–	–	–	–	–	–	●	●	●	●	●	●	●	●	●
NEW YORK																					
1 New York-Presby. Univ. Hospital of Columbia and Cornell	●	●	●	●	●	●	●	●	●	●	●	●	●	●	●	●	●	●	●	●	●
2 NYU Langone Medical Center[12]	●	●	●	●	●	●	●	–	●	●	●	●	●	●	●	●	●	●	●	●	●
3 Mount Sinai Hospital	●	●	●	●	●	●	●	●	●	●	●	●	●	●	●	●	●	●	●	●	●
4 Hackensack University Medical Center, Hackensack, N.J.	●	●	–	●	●	●	●	●	●	●	●	●	●	●	●	●	●	●	●	●	●
5 St. Francis Hospital, Roslyn, N.Y.	–	●	–	●	–	–	–	●	–	●	–	●	●	●	●	●	●	●	●	●	●
6 Morristown Medical Center, Morristown, N.J.	–	●	–	●	●	●	●	●	●	●	–	●	●	●	●	●	●	●	●	●	●
7 Montefiore Medical Center, Bronx	●	●	●	–	●	●	●	–	●	–	●	●	●	●	●	●	●	●	●	●	●
8 Winthrop-University Hospital, Mineola, N.Y.	–	–	●	–	●	–	●	●	–	●	–	●	●	●	●	●	●	●	●	●	●
9 Long Island Jewish Medical Center, New Hyde Park, N.Y.	–	–	–	●	●	●	●	●	●	–	●	●	●	●	●	●	●	●	●	●	●
10 Huntington Hospital, Huntington, N.Y.	–	–	●	–	–	–	–	–	–	–	–	–	●	●	–	●	●	–	●	●	●
11 Robert Wood Johnson Univ. Hospital, New Brunswick, N.J.	●	–	–	–	●	–	●	●	●	–	●	●	●	●	●	●	●	●	●	●	●
12 Lenox Hill Hospital	●	●	–	–	●	●	●	–	●	–	●	●	●	●	●	●	●	●	●	●	●
13 Jersey Shore University Medical Center, Neptune, N.J.	–	–	–	–	–	–	●	–	●	–	●	●	●	●	●	●	●	●	●	●	●
14 Valley Hospital, Ridgewood, N.J.	–	–	–	–	–	–	–	–	–	–	●	–	●	●	●	●	●	●	●	●	●
15 White Plains Hospital, White Plains, N.Y.	–	–	–	–	–	–	–	●	●	–	–	–	●	●	–	●	–	●	●	●	●
16 Englewood Hospital and Medical Center, Englewood, N.J.	–	–	–	–	–	–	–	–	–	–	–	–	●	●	●	●	●	●	●	●	●
16 North Shore University Hospital, Manhasset, N.Y.	–	–	–	–	–	●	●	●	–	–	–	–	●	●	●	●	●	●	●	●	●
18 Ocean Medical Center, Brick Township, N.J.	–	–	–	–	–	–	–	–	–	–	–	–	●	●	●	●	●	–	●	●	●
18 St. Joseph's Regional Medical Center, Paterson, N.J.	–	–	●	–	–	–	–	–	–	–	●	–	●	●	●	●	●	●	●	●	●
18 St. Peter's University Hospital, New Brunswick, N.J.	–	–	–	–	–	–	–	–	–	–	–	–	●	●	●	●	●	–	●	●	●
18 University Medical Center of Princeton at Plainsboro, N.J.	–	–	–	–	–	–	–	–	–	–	–	–	●	●	●	●	●	●	●	●	●
22 Beth Israel Medical Center	–	–	–	–	–	–	–	–	–	–	–	–	●	●	●	●	●	●	●	●	●
22 John T. Mather Memorial Hospital, Port Jefferson, N.Y.	–	–	–	–	–	–	–	–	–	–	–	–	●	●	●	●	●	●	●	●	●
22 Northern Westchester Hospital, Mount Kisco, N.Y.	–	–	–	–	–	–	–	–	–	–	–	–	●	–	●	●	–	●	●	●	●
22 Overlook Medical Center, Summit, N.J.	–	–	–	–	–	–	–	●	–	–	–	–	●	●	–	●	–	●	●	●	●
22 St. Luke's-Roosevelt Hospital Center	–	–	–	–	–	–	●	●	–	–	–	–	●	●	●	●	●	●	●	●	●
22 Stony Brook University Hospital, Stony Brook, N.Y.	–	–	–	–	–	–	–	–	–	–	●	–	●	●	●	●	●	●	●	●	●
22 Westchester Medical Center, Valhalla, N.Y.	●	–	–	–	–	–	–	–	–	–	–	–	●	●	●	●	●	●	●	●	●
OKLAHOMA CITY																					
1 Integris Baptist Medical Center	–	–	–	–	–	–	–	–	–	–	–	–	●	●	●	●	●	●	●	●	●
2 Norman Regional Hospital, Norman	–	–	–	–	–	–	–	–	–	–	–	–	●	●	●	●	–	●	●	●	●
ORLANDO, FLA.																					
1 Florida Hospital Orlando	–	–	●	–	●	●	–	●	●	–	–	●	●	●	●	●	●	●	●	●	●
2 Orlando Regional Medical Center	–	–	●	–	–	–	–	–	–	–	–	–	●	●	●	●	●	●	●	●	●
3 Florida Hospital Waterman, Tavares	–	–	–	–	–	–	–	–	–	–	–	–	●	–	●	●	●	●	●	●	●
PHILADELPHIA																					
1 Hospitals of the Univ. of Pennsylvania-Penn Presbyterian	●	●	●	●	●	●	●	●	●	●	●	●	●	●	●	●	●	●	●	●	●
2 Thomas Jefferson University Hospital[13]	●	●	●	●	●	●	●	●	●	●	●	●	●	●	●	●	●	●	●	●	●
3 Christiana Care Christiana Hospital, Newark, Del.	–	–	●	–	●	●	●	●	●	–	●	–	●	●	●	●	●	●	●	●	●
4 Pennsylvania Hospital†	–	–	–	–	●	–	●	–	●	●	–	●	●	●	●	●	●	●	●	●	●
4 Abington Memorial Hospital, Abington	–	–	–	●	–	–	–	–	–	–	–	–	●	●	●	●	●	●	●	●	●
5 Lankenau Medical Center, Wynnewood	–	–	–	–	●	●	●	–	●	●	–	–	●	●	●	●	●	●	●	●	●

A (–) in a complex care specialty indicates hospital is neither nationally ranked nor high performing.
A (–) in a procedure or condition indicates hospital does not offer the indicated care or has too few patients to be rated.
A footnote indicates that another hospital's results were included or that the hospital has a different name in one or more specialties.
[12]Hospital for Joint Diseases, NYU Langone Medical Center (Orthopedics). [13]Rothman Institute at Thomas Jefferson University Hospital (Orthopedics).
†Due to a data processing error, this hospital was initially omitted from these rankings. Rankings for other hospitals have not been changed.

More @ usnews.com/bestmetrohospitals

Home to the
#1 Hospital in New Jersey

Hackensack Meridian
HEALTH

At the heart of our health network is an unwavering commitment
to quality — a passion for excellence unsurpassed.

That's why having three hospitals ranked in the
top 10 in New Jersey by *U.S. News & World Report*, including
HackensackUMC as #1 again
is a vital sign of our network's good health.

Recognition like this gives us a compelling moment to pause and thank
the 28,000 team members and 6,000 physicians for making our care safer,
our outcomes better, and our experience more human each and every day.

**To learn more about how we are humanizing health,
visit HackensackMeridianHealth.org**

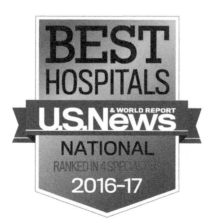

BEST HOSPITALS
U.S.News & WORLD REPORT
NATIONAL
RANKED IN 4 SPECIALTIES
2016-17

Hackensack University Medical Center	**Jersey Shore University Medical Center**	**Ocean Medical Center**
#1 IN NEW JERSEY	#4 IN NEW JERSEY	#8 IN NEW JERSEY
#4 NEW YORK METRO AREA	#13 NEW YORK METRO AREA	#18 NEW YORK METRO AREA
4 NATIONAL RANKINGS		

Plus 37 High Performing Recognitions for Types of Care Throughout Our Integrated Network

HackensackUMC • Jersey Shore University Medical Center • Joseph M. Sanzari Children's Hospital • K. Hovnanian Children's Hospital • Ocean Medical Center
Riverview Medical Center • HackensackUMC Mountainside • HackensackUMC Palisades • Raritan Bay Medical Center in Perth Amboy
Southern Ocean Medical Center • Bayshore Community Hospital • Raritan Bay Medical Center in Old Bridge • HackensackUMC at Pascack Valley

	COMPLEX CARE BY SPECIALTY												COMMON PROCEDURES & CONDITIONS								
Metro Rank / Hospital	CANCER	CARDIOLOGY & HEART SURGERY	DIABETES & ENDOCRINOLOGY	EAR, NOSE & THROAT	GASTROENTEROLOGY & GI SURGERY	GERIATRICS	GYNECOLOGY	NEPHROLOGY	NEUROLOGY & NEUROSURGERY	ORTHOPEDICS	PULMONOLOGY	UROLOGY	COLON CANCER SURGERY	LUNG CANCER SURGERY	HEART BYPASS SURGERY	HEART FAILURE	HEART VALVE SURGERY	ABDOMINAL AORTIC ANEURYSM	HIP REPLACEMENT	KNEE REPLACEMENT	COPD
PHILADELPHIA (CONTINUED)																					
6 Bryn Mawr Hospital, Bryn Mawr	–	–	–	–	–	–	–	●	–	●	–	●	●	●	●	●	●	●	●	●	●
6 Chester County Hospital, West Chester	–	–	–	–	●	–	●	–	–	●	●	●	●	●	●	●	●	●	●	●	●
8 Paoli Hospital, Paoli	–	–	–	–	–	–	–	–	–	●	–	●	●	●	●	–	●	●	●	●	●
9 Riddle Hospital, Media	–	–	–	–	–	–	–	–	–	●	–	●	●	–	●	–	–	–	●	●	●
10 Virtua Voorhees, Voorhees, N.J.	–	–	–	–	–	–	–	–	–	●	–	●	●	●	●	●	●	●	●	●	●
11 St. Mary Medical Center, Langhorne	–	–	–	–	–	–	–	–	–	–	–	●	●	●	●	●	●	●	●	●	●
PHOENIX																					
1 Mayo Clinic	●	●	●	●	●	●	–	●	●	●	●	●	●	●	●	●	●	●	●	●	●
2 Banner University Medical Center Phoenix	–	–	●	–	●	●	●	●	●	●	●	●	●	●	●	●	●	●	●	●	●
3 Banner Estrella Medical Center	–	–	●	–	–	●	–	●	–	●	●	●	●	●	●	●	–	–	●	●	●
4 St. Joseph's Hospital and Medical Center	–	–	–	–	●	–	●	●	●	–	●	●	●	●	●	●	●	●	●	●	●
5 Banner Desert Medical Center, Mesa	–	–	–	–	–	–	●	–	–	–	●	●	●	●	●	●	●	●	●	●	●
6 Banner Boswell Medical Center, Sun City	–	–	–	–	–	–	–	–	–	–	●	●	●	●	●	●	●	●	●	●	●
7 Banner Baywood Medical Center, Mesa	–	–	●	–	–	–	–	–	–	–	●	–	–	–	●	●	–	–	●	●	●
7 HonorHealth Scottsdale Shea Medical Center, Scottsdale	–	–	–	–	–	–	–	–	–	–	●	●	●	●	●	●	●	●	●	●	●
9 HonorHealth Scottsdale Osborn Med. Cen., Scottsdale	–	–	–	–	–	–	–	–	–	–	●	●	●	●	●	●	●	●	●	●	●
9 HonorHealth Scottsdale Thompson Peak Med. Cen., Scottsdale	–	–	–	–	–	–	–	–	–	–	–	●	–	–	●	●	–	–	●	●	●
PITTSBURGH																					
1 UPMC Presbyterian Shadyside	●	●	●	●	●	●	–	●	●	●	●	●	●	●	●	●	●	●	●	●	●
2 West Penn Hospital	●	–	–	–	–	●	–	–	–	–	●	–	–	●	●	●	●	–	●	●	●
3 UPMC St. Margaret	–	–	–	–	●	–	–	–	–	–	–	●	●	●	–	●	●	–	●	●	●
4 St. Clair Hospital	–	–	–	–	–	–	–	–	–	–	–	●	●	●	●	●	●	●	●	●	●
4 UPMC Passavant	–	–	–	–	–	–	–	–	–	–	–	●	●	●	●	●	●	●	●	●	●
6 Excela Westmoreland Hospital, Greensburg	–	–	–	–	–	–	–	–	–	–	–	●	●	●	●	●	●	●	●	●	●
PORTLAND, ORE.																					
1 Oregon Health and Science University Hospital	●	●	●	●	●	●	–	●	●	●	–	●	●	●	●	●	●	●	●	●	●
2 Providence Portland Medical Center	●	–	●	–	●	●	●	–	–	●	–	●	●	●	●	●	●	●	●	●	●
3 Providence St. Vincent Medical Center	–	–	–	–	–	●	–	–	–	–	●	●	●	●	●	●	●	●	●	●	●
4 Kaiser Permanente Sunnyside Medical Center, Clackamas	–	–	–	–	–	–	–	–	●	●	–	●	●	●	●	●	●	●	●	●	●
5 Legacy Good Samaritan Hospital and Health Center	–	–	–	–	–	–	–	–	–	–	–	●	●	●	●	●	●	–	●	●	●
5 Legacy Meridian Park Medical Center, Tualatin	–	–	–	–	–	–	–	–	–	–	–	–	–	–	●	●	–	–	●	●	●
PROVIDENCE, R.I.																					
- Miriam Hospital	–	–	–	–	●	–	–	–	–	–	–	●	●	–	●	●	–	●	●	●	●
RALEIGH-DURHAM, N.C.																					
1 Duke University Hospital, Durham	●	●	●	–	●	●	●	●	●	●	●	●	●	●	●	●	●	●	●	●	●
2 University of North Carolina Hospitals, Chapel Hill	●	–	●	●	●	●	●	●	–	●	●	●	●	●	●	●	●	●	●	●	●
3 UNC Rex Hospital, Raleigh	–	–	–	–	–	–	–	–	–	–	–	●	●	●	●	●	●	●	●	●	●
4 Duke Raleigh Hospital, Raleigh	–	–	–	–	–	–	–	–	–	–	–	●	●	●	●	●	●	●	●	●	●
4 WakeMed Health and Hospitals, Raleigh Campus	–	–	–	–	–	–	–	–	–	–	–	●	●	●	●	●	●	–	●	●	●
6 Duke Regional Hospital, Durham	–	–	–	–	–	–	–	–	–	–	●	●	●	●	●	●	●	–	●	●	●
RICHMOND, VA.																					
1 Virginia Commonwealth University Medical Center	●	–	–	–	●	●	●	●	●	–	●	●	●	●	●	●	●	●	●	●	●
2 Bon Secours Memorial Reg. Med. Center, Mechanicsville	–	–	●	–	–	●	–	–	–	–	●	●	●	●	●	●	●	●	●	●	●
3 Bon Secours St. Mary's Hospital	–	–	–	–	–	–	–	–	–	–	–	●	●	●	●	●	●	●	●	●	●

Legend:

COMPLEX CARE BY SPECIALTY
● Nationally ranked
● High performing

COMMON PROCEDURES & CONDITIONS
● High performing
● Average
● Below average

A (-) in a complex care specialty indicates hospital is neither nationally ranked nor high performing.
A (-) in a procedure or condition indicates hospital does not offer the indicated care or has too few patients to be rated.

▶ **More @ usnews.com/bestmetrohospitals**

Out of 5,000 hospitals, we're honored to be ranked #12 in the nation.

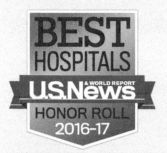

UPMC has once again been named to the *U.S. News & World Report* Honor Roll of America's Best Hospitals with rankings in 15 specialties. We're proud to be one of only 20 hospitals in the country to be named to this prestigious list, and we're still the #1 ranked hospital in Pittsburgh. But the greater honor is to continue to provide the best care to those who rely on us every day. To learn more, visit UPMC.com/HonorRoll.

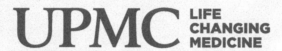

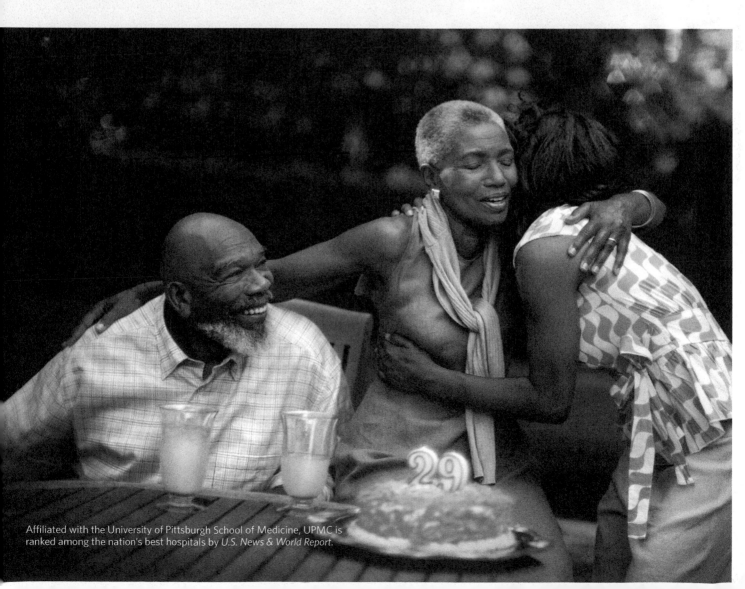

			COMPLEX CARE BY SPECIALTY												COMMON PROCEDURES & CONDITIONS								
Metro Rank	Hospital	CANCER	CARDIOLOGY & HEART SURGERY	DIABETES & ENDOCRINOLOGY	EAR, NOSE & THROAT	GASTROENTEROLOGY & GI SURGERY	GERIATRICS	GYNECOLOGY	NEPHROLOGY	NEUROLOGY & NEUROSURGERY	ORTHOPEDICS	PULMONOLOGY	UROLOGY	COLON CANCER SURGERY	LUNG CANCER SURGERY	HEART BYPASS SURGERY	HEART FAILURE	HEART VALVE SURGERY	ABDOMINAL AORTIC ANEURYSM	HIP REPLACEMENT	KNEE REPLACEMENT	COPD
RIVERSIDE-SAN BERNARDINO, CALIF.																						
1	Eisenhower Medical Center, Rancho Mirage	–	–	–	–	–	–	–	–	–	–	–	–	●	●	●	●	●	●	●	●	●
2	Kaiser Permanente Fontana-Ontario Med. Ctrs., Fontana	–	–	–	–	–	–	–	–	–	–	–	–	●	●	–	●	●	–	–	●	●
2	Loma Linda University Medical Center, Loma Linda	–	–	–	–	–	–	–	–	–	–	●	–	●	●	●	●	●	●	●	●	●
ROCHESTER, N.Y.																						
1	UR Medicine Strong Memorial Hospital	–	●	●	–	–	●	–	●	●	●	●	●	●	●	●	●	●	●	●	–	●
2	Rochester General Hospital	–	–	–	–	●	●	–	–	●	●	–	–	●	●	●	●	●	●	●	●	●
3	Highland Hospital	–	–	–	–	–	–	–	–	–	–	–	–	●	●	–	–	–	–	●	●	●
SACRAMENTO, CALIF.																						
1	University of California, Davis Medical Center	●	●	–	●	●	●	●	●	●	●	●	●	●	●	●	●	●	●	●	●	●
2	Sutter Medical Center	●	–	–	–	–	–	–	–	●	–	–	–	●	●	●	●	●	●	●	●	●
3	Mercy General Hospital	–	–	–	–	–	–	–	–	–	–	–	–	●	●	●	–	●	●	●	●	●
3	Sutter Roseville Medical Center, Roseville	–	–	–	–	–	–	–	–	–	–	–	–	●	●	●	●	–	●	–	●	●
SALT LAKE CITY																						
1	University of Utah Hospitals and Clinics[14]	●	–	–	–	–	●	–	●	●	●	●	●	●	●	●	●	●	●	●	●	●
2	Intermountain Medical Center, Murray	–	–	–	–	–	●	–	–	●	–	●	–	●	●	●	●	●	●	●	●	●
SAN ANTONIO																						
1	University Hospital	●	–	–	–	–	●	●	–	–	●	–	●	●	–	●	●	●	–	●	●	●
2	Baptist Medical Center	–	–	–	–	–	–	–	–	–	–	–	–	●	●	●	●	●	●	●	●	●
SAN DIEGO																						
1	UC San Diego Medical Center-UC San Diego Health	●	●	●	–	●	●	–	●	●	●	●	●	●	●	●	●	●	●	●	●	●
2	Scripps La Jolla Hospitals and Clinics, La Jolla	–	●	●	–	●	●	–	●	●	●	●	●	●	●	●	●	●	●	●	●	●
3	Sharp Memorial Hospital	–	–	–	–	–	–	–	–	–	–	●	●	●	●	●	●	●	●	●	●	●
4	Scripps Mercy Hospital	–	–	●	–	●	–	–	●	–	–	●	●	●	●	●	●	●	●	●	●	●
5	Sharp Grossmont Hospital, La Mesa	–	–	–	–	–	–	–	–	–	–	–	–	●	●	●	●	●	●	●	●	●

A (–) in a complex care specialty indicates hospital is neither nationally ranked nor high performing.
A (–) in a procedure or condition indicates hospital does not offer the indicated care or has too few patients to be rated.

A footnote indicates that another hospital's results were included or that the hospital has a different name in one or more specialties.
[14]Huntsman Cancer Institute at the University of Utah Hospitals and Clinics (Cancer).

Legend:

COMPLEX CARE BY SPECIALTY
● Nationally ranked
● High performing

COMMON PROCEDURES & CONDITIONS
● High performing
● Average
● Below average

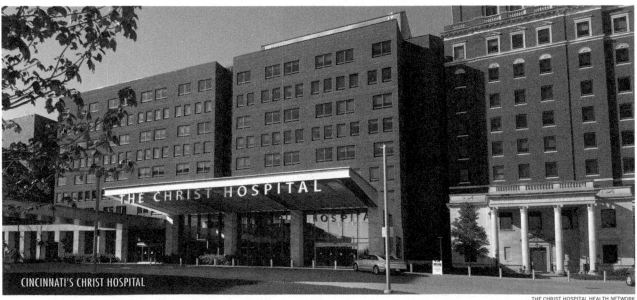

CINCINNATI'S CHRIST HOSPITAL

THE CHRIST HOSPITAL HEALTH NETWORK

▶ More @ usnews.com/bestmetrohospitals

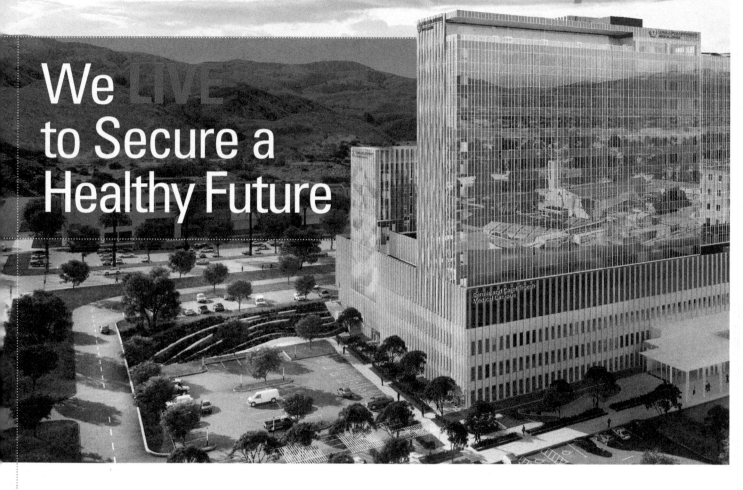

For Our Community

We LIVE to Secure a Healthy Future

From our humble beginnings over a century ago, Loma Linda University Health has developed into a world-class leader in health and education. Today, our determination to deliver unsurpassed service and care is only rivaled by our desire to grow and meet the needs of our communities. That is why we have embarked on an ambitious and transformative campaign that will bring into the region new state-of-the-art hospitals designed to enhance the health and healing process, as well as restore lives and families.

Providing world class care for our community is why we
LIVE TO SECURE A HEALTHY FUTURE.

Find out more about Loma Linda University Health's Vision 2020.
Visit **lluhvision2020.org**

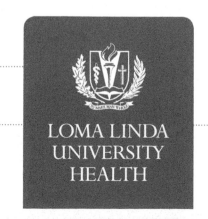

MANY STRENGTHS. ONE MISSION.
A Seventh-day Adventist Organization

LOMA LINDA
UNIVERSITY
HEALTH

COMPLEX CARE BY SPECIALTY
- ● Nationally ranked
- ● High performing

COMMON PROCEDURES & CONDITIONS
- ● High performing
- ● Average
- ● Below average

Metro Rank	Hospital	CANCER	CARDIOLOGY & HEART SURGERY	DIABETES & ENDOCRINOLOGY	EAR, NOSE & THROAT	GASTROENTEROLOGY & GI SURGERY	GERIATRICS	GYNECOLOGY	NEPHROLOGY	NEUROLOGY & NEUROSURGERY	ORTHOPEDICS	PULMONOLOGY	UROLOGY	COLON CANCER SURGERY	LUNG CANCER SURGERY	HEART BYPASS SURGERY	HEART FAILURE	HEART VALVE SURGERY	ABDOMINAL AORTIC ANEURYSM	HIP REPLACEMENT	KNEE REPLACEMENT	COPD
SAN FRANCISCO																						
1	UCSF Medical Center	●	●	●	●	●	●	●	●	●	●	●	●	●	●	●	●	●	●	●	●	●
2	John Muir Medical Center, Walnut Creek	–	–	●	–	●	●	●	–	●	●	●	●	●	●	●	–	●	–	●	●	●
3	Kaiser Permanente San Francisco Medical Center	●	●	●	–	●	●	–	–	–	–	–	–	●	●	●	●	●	●	●	●	●
4	John Muir Medical Center, Concord	–	–	●	–	●	●	●	–	–	●	–	●	●	●	●	●	●	●	●	●	●
5	California Pacific Medical Center	–	–	–	–	●	–	–	–	●	–	–	–	●	●	●	●	●	●	●	●	●
6	Sequoia Hospital, Redwood City	–	–	–	–	–	–	–	–	–	–	–	–	●	●	●	●	●	●	●	●	●
7	Mills-Peninsula Health Services, Burlingame	–	–	–	–	–	–	–	–	–	–	–	–	●	●	●	●	●	●	●	●	●
8	Washington Hospital, Fremont	–	–	–	–	–	–	–	–	–	–	–	–	●	–	●	●	●	–	●	●	●
SAN JOSE, CALIF.																						
1	Stanford Health Care-Stanford Hospital, Stanford	●	●	●	●	●	●	●	●	●	●	●	●	●	●	●	●	●	●	●	●	●
2	El Camino Hospital, Mountain View	–	–	–	–	–	–	–	–	–	–	–	–	●	●	●	●	●	●	●	●	●
3	Kaiser Permanente Santa Clara Medical Center	–	–	–	–	–	–	–	–	–	–	–	–	●	●	●	●	●	–	●	●	●
SEATTLE																						
1	University of Washington Medical Center[15]	●	●	●	●	●	●	●	●	●	●	●	●	●	●	●	●	●	●	●	●	●
2	Swedish Medical Center-First Hill	–	–	–	–	–	–	–	–	●	–	●	–	●	●	●	–	●	–	●	●	●
2	Virginia Mason Medical Center	–	–	–	–	●	–	●	–	–	–	–	–	●	●	●	●	●	●	●	●	●
4	Swedish Medical Center-Cherry Hill	–	–	–	–	–	–	–	–	●	●	●	–	–	–	●	●	●	●	–	–	●
5	Evergreen Health Medical Center, Kirkland	–	–	–	–	●	–	–	●	–	●	–	–	●	●	●	●	●	●	●	●	●
5	Providence Regional Medical Center, Everett	–	–	–	–	–	–	–	–	–	–	–	–	●	●	●	●	●	●	●	●	●
7	Overlake Hospital Medical Center, Bellevue	–	–	–	–	–	–	–	–	–	–	–	–	●	●	●	●	●	●	●	●	●

A (–) in a complex care specialty indicates hospital is neither nationally ranked nor high performing.
A (–) in a procedure or condition indicates hospital does not offer the indicated care or has too few patients to be rated.

A footnote indicates that another hospital's results were included or that the hospital has a different name in one or more specialties.
[15]Seattle Cancer Care Alliance/University of Washington Medical Center (Cancer).

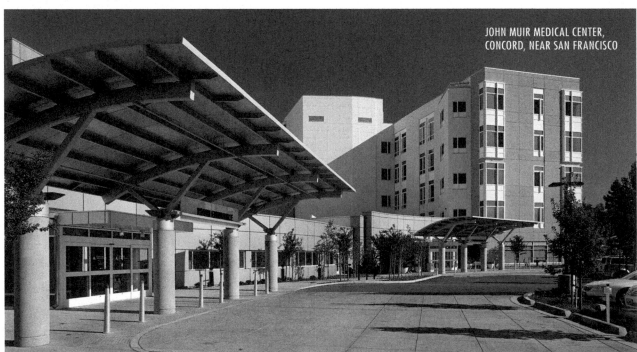

JOHN MUIR MEDICAL CENTER, CONCORD, NEAR SAN FRANCISCO

MICHAEL O'CALLAHAN

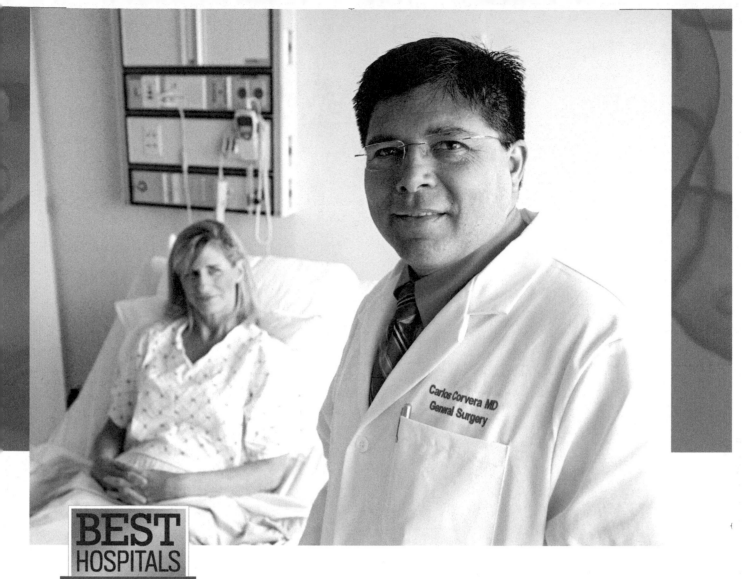

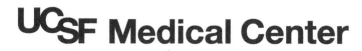

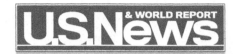
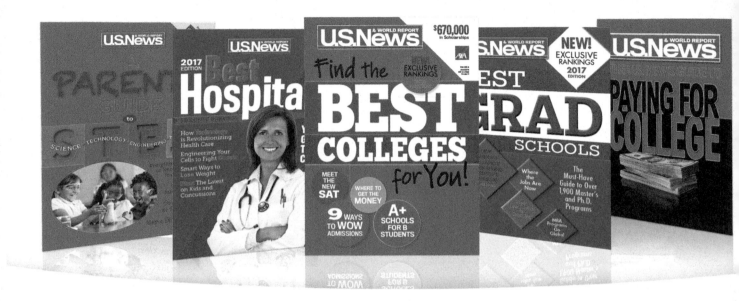
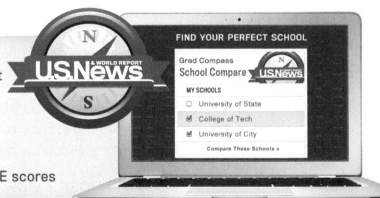

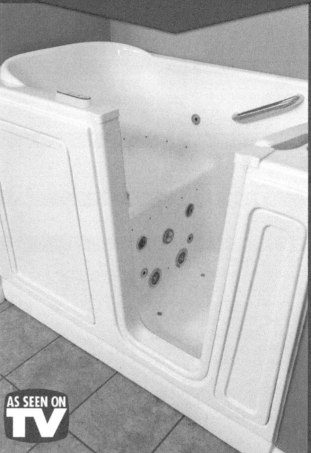

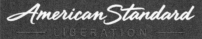

	COMPLEX CARE BY SPECIALTY	COMMON PROCEDURES & CONDITIONS
Nationally ranked ● / High performing ●	High performing ● / Average ● / Below average ●	

COMPLEX CARE BY SPECIALTY — **COMMON PROCEDURES & CONDITIONS**

Metro Rank Hospital	CANCER	CARDIOLOGY & HEART SURGERY	DIABETES & ENDOCRINOLOGY	EAR, NOSE & THROAT	GASTROENTEROLOGY & GI SURGERY	GERIATRICS	GYNECOLOGY	NEPHROLOGY	NEUROLOGY & NEUROSURGERY	ORTHOPEDICS	PULMONOLOGY	UROLOGY	COLON CANCER SURGERY	LUNG CANCER SURGERY	HEART BYPASS SURGERY	HEART FAILURE	HEART VALVE SURGERY	ABDOMINAL AORTIC ANEURYSM	HIP REPLACEMENT	KNEE REPLACEMENT	COPD
ST. LOUIS																					
1 Barnes-Jewish Hospital/Washington University	●	●	●	●	●	●	●	●	●	●	●	●	●	●	●	●	●	●	●	●	●
2 Missouri Baptist Medical Center	–	–	–	–	–	–	–	–	–	–	–	–	●	●	●	●	●	●	●	●	●
3 Mercy Hospital St. Louis	–	–	–	–	–	–	–	–	●	–	–	–	●	●	●	●	●	●	●	●	●
4 St. Luke's Hospital, Chesterfield	–	–	–	–	–	–	–	–	–	–	–	–	●	●	●	●	●	●	●	●	●
TAMPA-ST. PETERSBURG, FLA.																					
1 Tampa General Hospital	–	●	●	–	●	●	●	●	●	●	●	●	●	●	●	●	●	●	●	●	●
2 Morton Plant Hospital, Clearwater	–	●	–	–	–	–	–	–	–	–	–	–	●	●	●	●	●	●	●	●	●
2 St. Joseph's Hospital, Tampa	–	●	–	–	–	–	–	–	–	–	–	–	●	●	●	●	●	●	●	●	●
VIRGINIA BEACH-NORFOLK-NEWPORT NEWS, VA.																					
1 Sentara Norfolk General Hospital[16]	–	●	●	–	–	●	–	●	–	●	●	●	●	●	●	●	●	●	–	–	●
2 Sentara Leigh Hospital, Norfolk	–	–	–	–	–	–	–	●	–	●	–	–	●	●	–	●	–	–	●	●	●
WASHINGTON, D.C.																					
1 MedStar Georgetown University Hospital	–	–	●	–	–	–	–	●	●	–	●	●	●	●	●	–	●	●	●	●	●
2 MedStar Southern Maryland Hospital Center, Clinton	–	–	●	–	●	●	●	●	–	–	–	–	●	–	●	●	●	–	●	●	●
3 MedStar Washington Hospital Center	–	●	–	–	–	●	–	●	●	–	–	–	●	●	●	●	●	●	●	●	●
4 Mary Washington Hospital, Fredericksburg, Va.	–	–	–	–	●	–	–	–	–	–	–	–	●	●	●	●	●	●	●	●	●
5 Virginia Hospital Center, Arlington	–	–	–	–	–	–	–	–	–	–	–	–	●	●	●	●	●	●	●	●	●
6 Inova Fairfax Hospital, Falls Church, Va.	–	–	–	–	–	–	–	–	–	–	–	–	●	●	●	●	●	●	●	●	●
6 Suburban Hospital, Bethesda, Md.	–	–	–	–	–	–	–	–	●	–	–	–	●	●	●	●	●	●	●	●	●
8 Inova Fair Oaks Hospital, Fairfax, Va.	–	–	–	–	–	–	–	–	–	–	–	–	●	–	–	●	–	●	●	●	●

A (-) in a complex care specialty indicates hospital is neither nationally ranked nor high performing.
A (-) in a procedure or condition indicates hospital does not offer the indicated care or has too few patients to be rated.

A footnote indicates that another hospital's results were included or that the hospital has a different name in one or more specialties.
[16] Sentara Norfolk General Hospital-Sentara Heart Hospital (Cardiology & Heart Surgery).

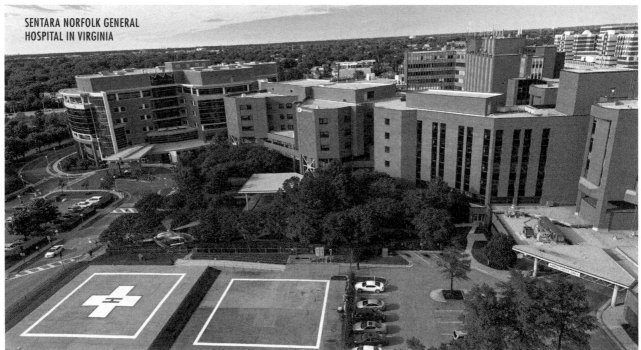

SENTARA NORFOLK GENERAL HOSPITAL IN VIRGINIA

SENTARA HEALTHCARE

▶ **More** @ usnews.com/bestmetrohospitals

CPSIA information can be obtained
at www.ICGtesting.com
Printed in the USA
BVOW05s0717200117

473647BV00003B/1/P